NEURAL PROSTHESES

Neural Prostheses

Replacing Motor Function After Disease or Disability

Edited by

Richard B. Stein
P. Hunter Peckham
Dejan B. Popović

New York   Oxford
OXFORD UNIVERSITY PRESS
1992

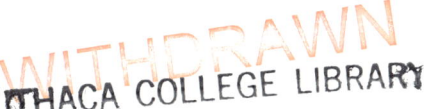

Oxford University Press

Oxford New York Toronto
Delhi Bombay Calcutta Madras Karachi
Petaling Jaya Singapore Hong Kong Tokyo
Nairobi Dar es Salaam Cape Town
Melbourne Auckland

and associated companies in
Berlin Ibadan

Copyright © 1992 by Oxford University Press, Inc.

Published by Oxford University Press, Inc.,
200 Madison Avenue, New York, New York 10016

Oxford is a registered trademark of Oxford University Press

All rights reserved. No part of this publication may be reproduced,
stored in a retrieval system, or transmitted, in any form or by any means,
electronic, mechanical, photocopying, recording, or otherwise,
without the prior permission of Oxford University Press.

Library of Congress Cataloging-in-Publication Data
Neural prostheses : replacing motor function after disease or disability /
edited by Richard B. Stein, P. Hunter Peckham, Dejan B. Popović
p. cm. Includes bibliographical references and index.
ISBN 0-19-507216-2
1. Neural stimulation. I. Stein, Richard B., 1940–
II. Peckham, P. Hunter. III. Popović, Dejan B.
[DNLM: 1. Electric Stimulation. 2. Extremities—physiology.
3. Muscles—physiology. 4. Paralysis—rehabilitation. 5. Prosthesis.
WE 172 N494] , RC350.N48N475 1992 , 616.8'42—dc20
DNLM/DLC for Library of Congress 91-45144

9 8 7 6 5 4 3 2 1

Printed in the United States of America
on acid-free paper

Preface

Returning function to limbs paralyzed as a result of an accident or a disease process is an ancient dream. Only in the last few years, however, have technology and neuroscience advanced to the point that practical systems can be envisaged to realize this dream even partially. Progress in replacing function through electrical stimulation has been more rapid in other biological systems. For example, by means of a simple, repetitive stimulation, cardiac pacemakers have provided life support for large numbers of heart patients in the community for a number of years. Restoration of auditory function has also advanced rapidly by means of cochlear prostheses. Stimulation of sensory pathways with a single channel can provide sensation of sounds in the environment and multichannel stimulators can provide the means for deaf individuals to recognize speech under many conditions.

Replacement of limb function has been slowed by the need to control substantial numbers of different muscles reliably and to provide sensors and sophisticated strategies to adapt to the variety of environmental conditions we experience on a daily basis. However, through the efforts of scientists and engineers around the world, practical solutions are beginning to emerge. This book is an attempt to review and synthesize recent developments in biomedical engineering and neuroscience in a way that will be catalytic for future progress in the field.

Although authors inevitably highlight recent, exciting developments in their laboratories, we have asked them to place these in a context that would be useful for students or others entering this rapidly expanding field. This is not an easy task since neural prostheses draw from the fields of biology, medicine, engineering and computer science that have advanced to different levels. Thus, the reader should not expect a textbook that logically develops the concepts underlying neural prostheses from commonly understood principles. This may be possible in 10 to 20 years when present controversies are resolved. Instead, one finds a series of essays from acknowledged experts in various aspects of the field, presenting their view of this complex area from their own vantage points in as interesting and authoritative a way as present knowledge permits.

Some describe their work with the term prosthesis (an artifical substitute for a missing part), while others prefer the term orthosis (which originally referred to straightening a deformity, but is sometimes used to refer to other external, assistive devices). Similarly, some authors prefer the term functional electrical stimulation (FES) while others use the more restricted term functional neuromuscular stimulation (FNS). In this book they are synonymous. Sorting out the best terminology may have to wait until the major conceptual questions in the field are resolved and practical devices are being produced.

There have been few recent books on neural prostheses for motor systems. Agnew and McCreery (1990) concentrated on the problems associated with the safety and biocompatability of electrodes in the nervous system. To avoid duplication, we have largely omitted these questions from the present volume. Kralj and Bajd (1989) reviewed the selection of patients, their training methods and their experience in applying electrical stimulation with simple systems to produce standing and walking in a number of patients. Rose et al. (1989) described the experience with neuromuscular stimulation in rehabilitation, ranging from basic neurophysiology and pathology to clinical application. Lazorthes and Upton (1985) discussed the use of nerve stimulation primarily for the purpose of controlling pain and movement disorders. Finally, a series of books has emerged from regular meetings held in Yugoslavia over the past 25 years. The most recent (Popović, 1990) provides a good flavor of some current trends in the field, but as with many symposium volumes, it is directed to the specialist and does not provide enough background for the more general reader or the student entering the field.

Although this volume is loosely based on a meeting (Neural Prostheses: Motor Systems III) held in Banff, Canada in August 1991 under the sponsorship of the Engineering Foundation and the World Neuroscience Congress, the chapters were selected, written and edited independently of the meeting in an effort to reach the widest possible readership. It is the first book to focus on control strategies for neural prostheses. Past work, outlined in the Agnew and McCreery and the Kralj and Bajd books, indicates that at least some of the problems relating to stimulating electrodes and to training methods have been solved. However, with the increasing complexity of prostheses that will be feasible in the coming years, more elaborate strategies become essential to control them effectively. The aim of this book is to build in a logical fashion from the past to the present and the future.

In the first chapter, Dr. Terry Hambrecht outlines the historical context for recent developments. Dr. Hambrecht has directed the NIH program in Neural Prostheses for more than 20 years and has had a strong continuing interest in the historical background that has made possible the explosive developments of the last decade. There have been remarkable parallel developments as well in the field of robotics. Certain common problems must be solved in controlling natural movements, in attempting to replace these movements by electrical stimulation of muscles after spinal cord injury and in controlling the movements of the motors or other actuators

Preface

that comprise a robotic system. These are reviewed by Doctors John Hollerbach and David Bennett, who have worked extensively both on biological and robotic systems.

Muscles have tremendous advantages when compared to man-made actuators (Lehninger, 1975). The power-to-weight ratio is enormously greater than available motors. Its use of 0.1 V, 1 ms wide pulses for control is hard to match. The ability, for example, of heart muscle to reliably pump fluids for 70 years or more without servicing and to adapt its output readily to a wide range of demands over varying environmental conditions is truly amazing. Yet, muscles present a number of problems when considered as actuators for replacement of motor function in paralyzed subjects. Their output is highly nonlinear and varies with time (for example, as a result of fatigue) in a way that has defied mathematical description. Dr. George Zahalak provides an overview of attempts to model muscles effectively at levels from the basic molecular events, involving cross-bridges between sliding filaments, to whole muscles described by a few lumped parameters. Dr. William Durfee extends this analysis to identify models that may be most useful in systems for stimulating paralyzed muscles.

Control can be open-loop, by using preset patterns of stimulation, or closed-loop, by feeding back sensory information to modify the pattern of stimulation during a movement. With the difficulty of specifying muscle properties precisely over time, closed loop control has obvious advantages. Nonetheless, because of a lack of adequate sensors, most current systems function essentially without feedback, except for the subject's vision or any proprioception that is preserved. Dr. John Webster reviews the artificial sensors that are available and might be incorporated into stimulation systems, while Dr. Andy Hoffer and Morten Haugland discuss the possibilities for recording from the body's own sensors and using this information to control stimulation systems.

Natural control is exerted by the motor cortex and other brain centers. In the last few years it has been possible to use magnetic fields to excite the cortex and Dr. John Rothwell describes results obtained by stimulation of normal subjects and those with motor disorders. This chapter is somewhat different in orientation since electricity is being used to analyze normal and abnormal connections, rather than to replace missing function.

In attempting to replace hand function, for example in quadriplegics, the most successful and widespread system to date has involved placement of electrodes in a variety of muscles, combined with surgery where required to "simplify" control of hand function. This is discussed by Doctors Hunter Peckham and Mike Keith, an engineer and a surgeon closely involved with these developments.

The replacement of walking in paraplegia involves problems of stability as well as propulsion. Simple conceptual models for these processes have been applied over the years with notable success in a wide range of animals by Dr. McNeill Alexander. Recent promising attempts to develop a specific system that provides stability with bracing and propulsion with electrical stimulation are described by Dr. Moshe Solomonow. A broader overview and a discussion of possible future trends are provided by Dr. Dejan Popović and Doctors Scott Tashman and Felix Zajac.

Walking must take place over a variety of terrains. Dr. Richard Stein reviews what is known about the general control strategies used by the body and how sensory feedback and central pattern generators are utilized to modify control adaptively and rapidly under different conditions. Current prosthetic systems use relatively simple control strategies, but potential ways of providing more sophisticated control are reviewed by Dr. Howard Chizeck. To have a practical impact on the lives of many paralyzed individuals, devices developed in a laboratory need to be produced commercially. In the final chapter Drs. Gerry Loeb and Joe Shulman outline the very real problems of transferring suitable technology to industry.

Organizing and editing a book of this scope requires the help of a number of people. We are indebted to the authors and to the staff of Oxford University Press for their excellent cooperation. We are also grateful for support for the conference, and indirectly for this book, which was provided by the U.S. National Institute on Disability and Rehabilitation Research, the U.S. Department of Veterans Affairs, the Paralyzed Veterans of America, the Alberta Heritage Foundation for Medical Research and the Rick Hansen Man in Motion Legacy Fund.

Edmonton Richard B. Stein
Cleveland P. Hunter Peckham
Belgrade Dejan B. Popović
1992

REFERENCES

Agnew, W.F., and McCreery, D.B. (1990). *Neural prostheses: Fundamental studies.* Englewood Cliffs, NJ: Prentice Hall.
Kralj, A., and Bajd, T. (1989). *Functional electrical stimulation: Standing and walking after spinal cord injury.* Boca Raton, FL: CRC Press.
Lazorthes, Y., and Upton, A.R.M. (1985). *Neurostimulation: An overview.* Mt. Kisco, N.Y.: Futura.
Lehninger, A.L. (1975). *Biochemistry, 2nd ed.* New York: Worth Publishers.
Popović, D.B. (1990). *Advances in external control of human extremities X.* Belgrade: Nauka.
Rose, F.C., Jones, R., and Vrbová, G. (1989). *Neuromuscular stimulation: Basic concepts and clinical applications.* New York: Demos.

Contents

1. A Brief History of Neural Prostheses for Motor Control of Paralyzed Extremities   3
   F. Terry Hambrecht

PART I. MUSCLES AND SENSORS

2. An Overview of Muscle Modeling   17
   George I. Zahalak

3. Model Identification in Neural Prosthesis Systems   58
   William K. Durfee

4. Artificial Sensors Suitable for Closed-Loop Control of FNS   88
   John G. Webster

5. Signals from Tactile Sensors in Glabrous Skin Suitable for Restoring Motor Functions in Paralyzed Humans   99
   J.A. Hoffer and M.K. Haugland

PART II. CONTROL OF UPPER EXTREMITIES

6. Feed-forward versus Feedback Control of Limb Movements   129
   John M. Hollerbach and David J. Bennett

7. What Transcranial Stimulation of the Brain Can Reveal About the Control of Arm Movements in Man   148
    John C. Rothwell

8. Motor Prostheses for Restoration of Upper Extremity Function   162
    P. Hunter Peckham and Michael W. Keith

PART III. CONTROL OF LOWER EXTREMITIES

9. Simple Models of the Mechanics of Walking   191
    R. McNeill Alexander

10. Biomechanics and Physiology of a Practical Functional Neuromuscular Stimulation Powered Walking Orthosis for Paraplegics   202
    Moshe Solomonow

11. Functional Electrical Stimulation for Lower Extremities   233
    Dejan B. Popović

12. Control of Multijoint Lower Limb Motor Tasks with Functional Neuromuscular Stimulation   252
    Scott Tashman and Felix E. Zajac

PART IV. ADAPTIVE CONTROL AND TECHNOLOGY TRANSFER

13. Feedback Control of Normal and Electrically Induced Movements   281
    Richard B. Stein

14. Adaptive and Nonlinear Control Methods for Neural Prostheses   298
    Howard J. Chizeck

15. The Transfer of Technology From the Laboratory to the Real World   329
    Gerald E. Loeb and Joseph H. Schulman

Index   343

Contributors

R. McNeill Alexander, D.Sc., F.R.S.
Department of Pure and Applied Biology
University of Leeds
Leeds, England LS2 9JT

David J. Bennett, Ph.D.
Postdoctoral Fellow
Massachusetts Institute of Technology
Department of Brain and Cognitive Sciences
Cambridge, MA 02139

Howard J. Chizeck, Ph.D.
Systems Engineering
Case Western Reserve University
Cleveland, OH 44106

William K. Durfee, Ph.D.
Department of Mechanical Engineering
Massachusetts Institute of Technology
Cambridge, MA 02139

F. Terry Hambrecht, M.D.
Head, Neural Prosthesis Program
National Institute of Neurological Disorders and Stroke
National Institutes of Health
Bethesda, MD 20892

M. K. Haugland, M.Sc. EE
Department of Medical Informatics and Image Analysis
Institute of Electronic Systems
Aalborg University
Fredrik Bjersvej 7D
DK9220 Aalborg Denmark

J. A. Hoffer, Ph.D.
University of Calgary
Health Sciences Center
Calgary, Alberta T2N 4N1

John M. Hollerbach, Ph.D.
Department of Biomedical Engineering
NSERC/CIAR
McGill University
Montreal, Quebec H3A 2B4

Michael W. Keith, M.D.
Department of Orthopedic Surgery
Case Western Reserve University
Cleveland, OH 44106

Gerald E. Loeb, M.D.
Abramsky Hall
Queen's University
Kingston, Ontario K7L 3N6 Canada

P. Hunter Peckham, Ph.D.
Rehabilitation Engineering
    Department
Metro/Highland View Hospital
3395 Scranton Road
Cleveland, OH 44109

Dejan B. Popović, Ph.D.
Department of Electrical Engineering
University of Belgrade
Belgrade, Yugoslavia and
Division of Neuroscience
University of Alberta
Edmonton AB T6G 2S2 Canada

John C. Rothwell, M.A., Ph.D.
MRC Human Movement and Balance
    Unit
Institute of Neurology
London, England WC1N 3BG
United Kingdom

Joseph H. Schulman, Ph.D.
A.E. Mann Foundation
12744 San Fernando Road
Sylmar, CA 91342

Moshe Solomonow, Ph.D.
Director of Bioengineering
Department of Orthopaedic Surgery
Louisiana State University Medical
    Center
New Orleans, LA 70112

Richard B. Stein, D.Phil.
Director, Division of Neuroscience
University of Alberta
Edmonton, AB T6G 2S2 Canada

Scott Tashman, M.Eng.
Department of Mechanical
    Engineering
Rehabilitation Research and
    Development Center
VA Medical Center
Palo Alto, CA

John G. Webster, Ph.D.
Department of Electrical and
    Computer Engineering
University of Wisconsin-Madison
Madison, WI 53706

George I. Zahalak, D.En.Sc.
Department of Mechanical
    Engineering
Washington University
St. Louis, MO 63130

Felix E. Zajac, Ph.D.
Biomechanical Engineering Program
Department of Mechanical
    Engineering
Stanford University
Stanford, CA 94305

Neural Prostheses

1
A Brief History of Neural Prostheses for Motor Control of Paralyzed Extremities

F. TERRY HAMBRECHT

When did the biological and technological discoveries originate that made possible the utilization of electrical stimulation for functional control of paralyzed extremities? By whom were these discoveries made and how did they depend on their predecessors for the orderly and increasingly rapid advancement of the necessary scientific foundation that occurred? This brief history will attempt to outline some of the most important milestones and identify those investigations that first focused on solving some of the specific problems of neural prostheses for motor control.

EARLY HISTORY

The involuntary contraction of skeletal muscles triggered by external sources of energy was observed in ancient times. For example, touching an electric fish was a well-known cause of muscle contractions. It was also observed that a newly caught torpedo fish when thrown on a pile of "dead" fish seemingly caused the latter to come to life (Kellaway, 1946). Despite these early observations, the use of electricity to control muscle contractions in a functional manner had to await the development of more practical means of generating it.

In the eighteenth century, static electric machines were developed to a high degree of sophistication. These were based on the principle of using friction on insulators such as glass to dislodge electrons and thus develop high voltages due to the resulting charge separation. The first electrical capacitor, known as the Leyden jar, was invented in 1746 to store the charge. A typical glass static electric machine and a discharging electrometer for measuring the potential generated are shown in Figure

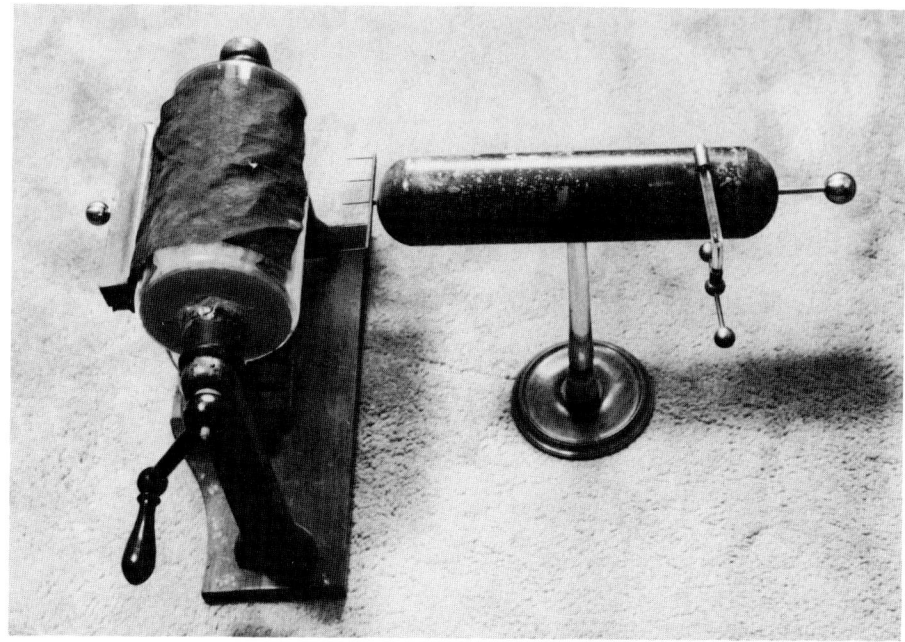

Figure 1-1 Static electric machine and discharging electrometer used in the eighteenth century. (Courtesy The Bakken—A Library and Museum of Electricity in Life, Minneapolis, MN.)

1-1. Benjamin Franklin, among others, experimented with machines like this one to treat paralyzed individuals. He noted that in many cases he could produce involuntary contractions of paralyzed muscles, but he gave up his attempts when he failed to note any long-term benefits (Franklin, 1757). However, other investigators reported "cures." It is likely that these cures were a combination of cases of hysterical paralysis, a disorder that was not as well recognized then as it would be in the next century, and of recovery following regeneration of injured lower motor neurons. It does not appear that any of these early investigators considered the possibility of a neural prosthesis to produce functional movements in paralyzed individuals based on externally applied electricity.

By the end of the eighteenth century the basic principles of electricity were understood, and it was known that electricity was the physical phenomenon by which a static electric machine caused muscle contractions. It was not proven, however, that muscles and nerves normally utilized electricity to function or that they generated their own electricity. Luigi Galvani suggested the latter possibility in his theory of animal electricity in 1791 (Galvani, 1791). He performed an extensive number of animal experiments in which he used metallic bridges to connect different parts of nerve-muscle preparations and studied the conditions under which muscle contraction occurred. From these experiments he concluded that the animal generated its own electricity and that the metallic bridge completed the circuit, allowing the electricity to flow.

Galvani's conclusion was challenged by Alessandro Volta, the inventor of the battery known as the voltaic pile (Volta, 1800). Volta claimed that the metallic bridges used by Galvani had actually generated the electricity by utilizing dissimilar metals just as in his voltaic pile. This probably occurred in some of the experiments, especially when both zinc and copper wires were used, but Galvani was able to counter Volta by showing that if the metallic conductors were eliminated and the end of a cut nerve was looped back to touch its attached muscle, a contraction would occur. Galvani called this driving force "animal electricity."

Neither static electricity machines nor voltaic piles produce sustained muscle contractions, but instead cause brief contractions at the moment of circuit closure or contact with the device. To produce functional motor prostheses, a means was needed to induce sustained muscle contractions.

At the beginning of the nineteenth century, scientists were well aware of the phenomena of electricity and magnetism, but their relationship was not understood. This was changed by a combination of empirical observations and a set of consolidating mathematical equations. Hans Christian Oersted described the effect of current flowing through a wire on a magnetized needle in 1820. This provided a connection between electricity and magnetism. Similarly, Michael Faraday, in 1821, showed that a magnet could exert a force on current-carrying wires. He also discovered magnetic induction, which is the induced flow of current in one circuit that is close to another current-carrying circuit. John Clerk Maxwell collected and unified these observations and other previously known relationships into four basic equations of electromagnetic theory which bear his name. These empirical findings and equations are the basis of transformers, motors, and generators, and made possible the design of electrical stimulators capable of producing sustained muscle contractions.

The first practical device for producing sustained muscle contractions was the magnetoelectric generator. One of the more elaborate varieties that was used in the 1850s for stimulating nerves and muscles is shown in Figure 1–2. It consists of a coil, which is coupled by pulleys to a hand crank, and an adjacent horseshoe magnet separated by an air gap from the coil. As the coil was rotated in the magnetic field, an alternating sinusoidal current was generated at the frequency of rotation of the coil. This alternating current produced repetitive muscle contractions. Magnetoelectric stimulators had the disadvantage of requiring an external source of rotational energy. The control of the output level was accomplished by positioning a soft metal magnetic shunt across the ends of the horeshoe magnet. This was difficult to control and resulted in poor output reproducibility. Some of the more sophisticated magnetoelectric generators had elaborate gears and linkages connecting the moveable shunt with a "calibrated" mechanical output indicator in the cover of the device. Despite the drawbacks, it is interesting to note that Albert Hyman in 1930 used a modified magnetoelectric generator in his pioneering work on heart stimulation to reverse cardiac standstill. He named his stimulator "the artificial pacemaker" (Hyman, 1930).

A more practical neuromuscular stimulator was the induction coil stimulator, or the faradaic stimulator, as it was popularly known. It consisted of a mechanical interrupter in series with a battery and the primary of a transformer. The output from the secondary of the transformer is a series of pulses at the frequency of the interrupter. A ninteenth-century model which used a wet battery is shown in Figure 1–3. The faradaic stimulator was the first device that could produce carefully controlled and sustained muscle contractions. It was self-contained with its own power source, was portable, and its output frequency could be adjusted to easily exceed

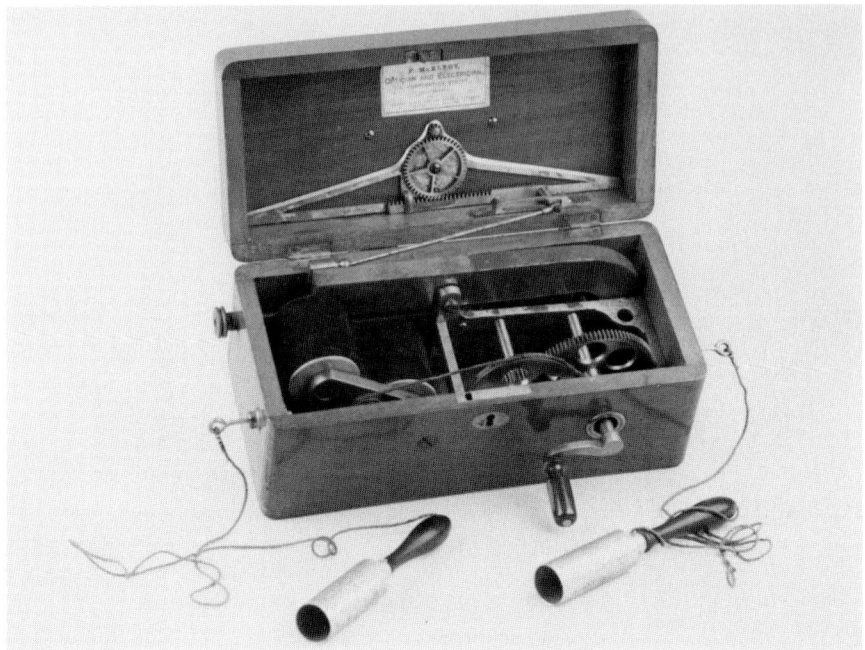

Figure 1-2 Magnetoelectric generator of the type popular from about 1840-1860. (Author's collection.)

100 Hz. The output level was often controlled by varying a rheostat in the primary circuit. A device of this type was used to great advantage by Guillaume Benjamin Armand Duchenne to study the anatomy and functional movements of specific muscles by using moistened electrodes on the skin surface over the muscles (Duchenne, 1867). A typical focal stimulating electrode designed for placement over a muscle motor point, and sponge electrode for diffuse stimulation or for use as a return electrode are shown in Figure 1-4.

THE PRESENT CENTURY

The early twentieth century brought the discovery of the diode tube by Fleming in 1904 and De Forest's invention of the triode in 1906. These new devices made possible totally electronic oscillators, stimulators, amplifiers, and cathode ray oscilloscopes for neurophysiological studies. An understanding of action potentials in nerve and muscle, conduction velocities, membrane biophysics, myoneural junction transmission, and the biophysics of muscle contraction soon followed.

Electronic stimulators using vacuum tubes replaced the earlier electromechanical stimulators, resulting in improved reliability and stimulus control. Although portable devices were made with vacuum tubes, they were hardly wearable because of the bulk and weight of the batteries they required.

A major breakthrough occurred in 1947 when Bardeen, Brattain, and Shockley invented the transistor at the Bell Telephone Laboratoties (Bardeen and Brattain,

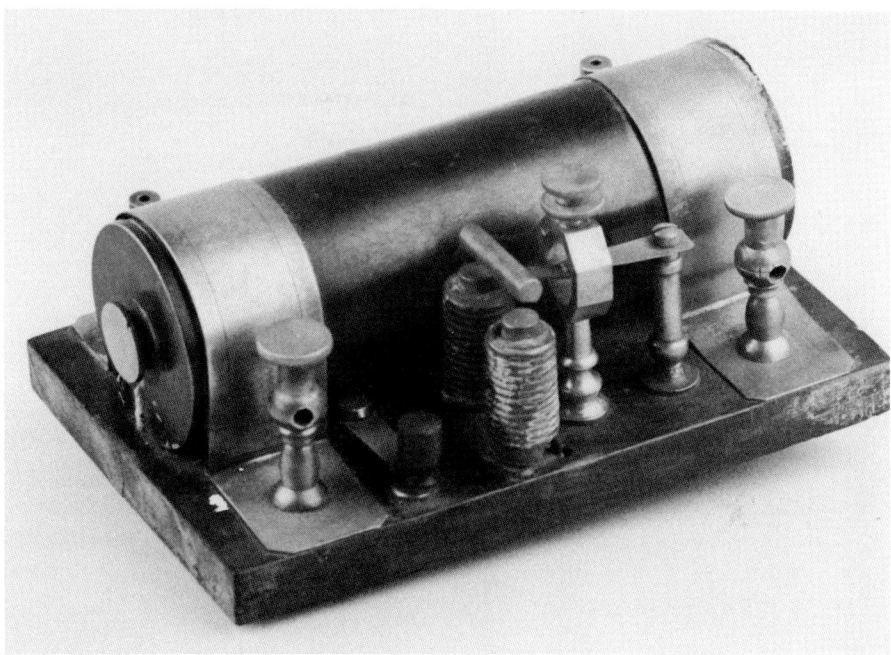

Figure 1-3 Faradaic or induction coil stimulator as used from the mid to late nineteenth century. (Author's collection.)

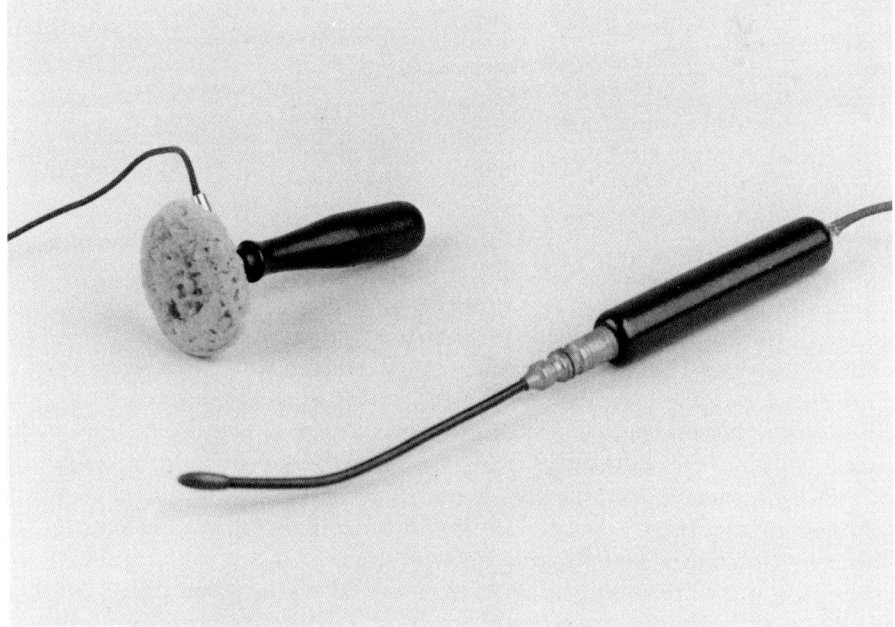

Figure 1-4 Focal stimulation electrode and sponge-type diffuse stimulating electrode from the late nineteenth and early 20th century, respectively. (Author's collection.)

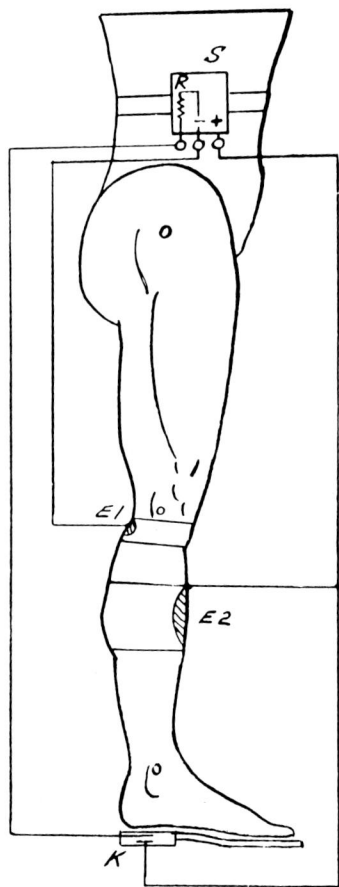

Figure 1–5 Diagram of FNS system used by Liberson and his colleagues to overcome footdrop in stroke patients by stimulating the peroneal nerve. (Adapted with permission from Liberson et al., 1961.)

1948; Shockley, 1948). This device could operate as an amplifier or as an oscillator at a fraction of the power consumption of previous devices. The age of true electronic portability had arrived. Later, Kilby and Noyce developed techniques to simultaneously manufacture multiple transistors together with other electronic components such as resistors, capacitors, and diodes into monolithic integrated circuits. This permitted sophisticated electronic circuits to be incorporated into very small packages. Following their early application in radios, transistors and integrated circuits were soon incorporated into battery-powered stimulators for activating muscles.

Liberson and his co-workers are generally credited as the first investigators to utilize electrical stimulation to restore functional control of a paralyzed limb muscle on a continuing basis (Liberson et al., 1961). They treated footdrop in hemiplegic patients by placing conductive rubber electrodes on the skin over the peroneal nerve. Activation of this nerve by a transistorized stimulator resulted in contraction of the tibialis anterior muscle and elevation of the foot. A switch was placed in the sole of the shoe, causing current to flow through the nerve during periods when the foot was lifted off the ground, as shown in Figure 1–5. Over 100 patients were treated with this technique, and it was claimed that all of them obtained some degree of gait improvement (Liberson, 1972). However, patient acceptance was limited by factors such as skin irritation caused by the electrodes, the need for precise electrode placement each time the system was to be used, breakage of electrode wires, and limited benefits as compared to the hassle of applying and maintaining the equipment.

Liberson called his technique "functional electrotherapy." For some reason this term did not gain widespread acceptance, but instead, "functional electrical stimulation" (FES), introduced by Moe and Post, did (Moe and Post, 1962). Functional electrical stimulation is generally used to mean the neural prosthetic technique that utilizes stimulation of neural tissue for the purpose of restoring function. Because this can include a broad range of neural systems, the term functional neuromuscular stimulation is often used to indicate the subcategory of FES that restricts stimulation to the neuromuscular system.

Long and Masciarelli, intrigued by the novel application of FES to the lower extremity reported by Liberson and his colleagues, developed an FES-assisted splint for control of the hand in high quadriplegic patients (Long and Masciarelli, 1963). Incorporated in the hand splint was an electrode which applied electrical stimulation over the motor point of the extensor digitorum. The splint braced the thumb and wrist in a fixed position. The middle and index fingers were held together in a hinged splint and brought into opposition by a spring. By controlling the amplitude of stimulation to the extensor digitorum muscle, the patient could overcome the spring force and separate the fingers from the thumb. Proportional control of the stimulation channel was made possible by a potentiometer in series with the output of the stimulator. The potentiometer was mounted beneath the bearings of a balanced forearm orthosis of the opposite arm, permitting voluntary control of the system. The splint was used by a patient with C4-5 quadriplegia for over 16 months, permitting activities such as grasping and releasing tiles in mosaic construction, holding typing sticks and page turners, performing grasp-and-release activities during board games, and some feeding with adapted eating equipment. Although the patient's tolerance of the device was reported as excellent, the system did not see widespread clinical acceptance.

Peckham and his colleagues, working with C5 quadriplegic patients, provided two types of functional hand grasp (palmar prehension and release as well as lateral prehension and release) using electrical stimulation with percutaneous electrodes implanted chronically in the forearm muscles (Peckham et al., 1980a). The same investigators also reported augmenting tenodesis grip in C6 quadriplegic patients using similar techniques (Peckham et al., 1980b).

In spinal-cord-injured paraplegic patients, restoration of the functional abilities to stand from a sitting position and to walk with a minimum of bracing has been the goal of several research groups. In 1960 Kantrowitz reported a paraplegic patient with surface electrodes over the quadriceps and gluteal muscles who was able to rise from a sitting to a standing position without braces and who was able to maintain the standing position for a few minutes when stimulated (Kantrowitz, 1960). Cooper and his co-workers implanted electrodes bilaterally on the femoral and sciatic nerves in a T11-12 paraplegic individual. They claimed the patient was able to ambulate up to 40 feet when using a walker for stability (Cooper et al., 1973). Using implanted stimulators with electrodes on branches of the femoral nerves bilaterally, Brindley and co-workers were able to demonstrate standing from a sitting position and limited biped gait assisted by elbow crutches, but without braces or a walker, in a paraplegic individual. In this case, femoral nerve stimulation was essentially providing knee splinting which the patient controlled with a switch (Brindley et al., 1978). These early studies were soon followed by more sophisticated multichannel systems (Kralj et al., 1983; Marsolais and Kobetic, 1983).

The above-cited early attempts to restore limited upper and lower limb functions were valuable prototypes for elucidating the problems that needed to be solved before truly practical neural prostheses could be developed for control of paralyzed extremities. Some of the more significant problems were lead and electrode breakage, electrode positioning and stabilization, inadequate stimulus specificity, insufficient muscle force, muscle fatigue, involuntary muscle spasms, hyperactive muscle contractions, reliable sources of control signals, and limited functional gains for the patients.

Most serious FNS investigators soon became convinced that the future of FNS required the abandonment of skin-surface-stimulating electrodes except for short-term laboratory investigations. The alternative was implanted electrodes. Practical considerations dictated that these either be inserted into or on the surface of the paralyzed muscles near the motor points or on the surface of the nerves innervating the muscles. Ideally, an electrode was needed which could be easily implanted without a major surgical operation, could be tested at various implantation sites before a final location was selected, and would be resistant to breakage during movements. One type of chronic implanted electrode which meets some of these requirements and has been the basis for more advanced electrodes is the Caldwell coiled-wire percutaneous electrode (Caldwell, 1970). These electrodes were wound on a mandrel and were terminated at the implanted end by straightening a portion of the wire and bending it back to act as a hook. The Caldwell electrode was originally developed for both long-term recording of electromyographic (EMG) activity as part of a myoelectric control system for orthoses and prostheses, and for electrically stimulating paralyzed muscles. The original electrode could be inserted into a muscle through a 23-gauge hyperdermic needle. In the process of insertion and initial testing, when the desired electrode tip location was found, the hypodermic needle was withdrawn while the hook caused the electrode to remain in place. These early electrodes were insulated with either polyurethane or nylon and were filled with medical-grade silicone rubber, except for the active tip. They utilized either dispersion-strengthened platinum-10% iridium, Karma (a nickel-chrome alloy), or 304 stainless steel. None of these metals was ideal with respect to both mechanical properties and freedom from corrosion during electrical stimulation, resulting in the eventual change to 316 LVM stainless steel. Although these electrodes have been extensively modified over the past 20 years and are now more reliable, they still are susceptible to breakage during long-term implantation and require excessive attention in cleaning the percutaneous site and making connections with leads outside of the body.

Other early FNS electrodes include epimysial electrodes and various types of peripheral nerve electrodes (Glenn et al., 1977; Grandjean and Mortimer, 1986; Thoma et al., 1981; Jeglic et al., 1967). Although each type had advantages over the others in specific applications, each required compromises between reliability, stimulus specificity, and ease of implementation.

A better understanding of how nerve fibers are excited by externally applied electric fields has resulted in new and improved electrode designs. In a now classical paper, McNeal analyzed a mathematical model of myelinated nerve which described the time course of events following stimulus application up to the initiation of the action potential (McNeal, 1976). This model and extensions of it have been valuable tools for rapidly determining the effects of changes in electrode geometries and surrounding insulators.

The causes of muscle fatigue and weakness were analyzed and methods of preventing them were studied (Peckham, 1972). Peckham and others found that if the lower motor neurons were intact, weakness associated with disuse atrophy could be overcome and muscle strength restored to functional levels with electrically induced exercise (Peckham et al., 1976). Another problem is related to the fact that electrical stimulation excites the largest motor neurons at the lowest stimulus thresholds, and these tend to innervate the more easily fatigued muscle fibers, which is just the opposite of normal physiological activation. Attempts were made by several groups to convert fatigue-sensitive muscle fibers to fatigue-resistant types by patterned electrical stimulation. Mortimer, using the model of the cat tibialis anterior muscle, demonstrated that converted muscle fibers with increased capacity for aerobic metabolism and slowed twitch contraction times could improve the ability of stimulated muscle to sustain repeated contraction (Mortimer, 1981). Methods of reducing fatigue have been introduced which utilize sequential stimulation of multiple electrodes activating different motor units in the same muscle. This permits lowering the actual stimulus frequency of individual motor units while maintaining a relatively constant muscle contraction. Multiple electrodes on the surface of nerves and multiple electrodes implanted within a single functional muscle have been investigated (Starbuch et al., 1966; Peckham et al., 1970).

Methods of alleviating involuntary spasms and hyperactive muscle contractions have been evaluated. It was demonstrated that electrical stimulation of cutaneous nerves such as the sural nerve could cause periods of reflex inhibition of excessive motor activity (Morris et al., 1968). However, a practical method of producing such inhibition in a controlled manner over a long period of time has not been developed.

The study of simple and reliable sources of voluntary control signals and their information content was undertaken (Vodovnik and Rebersek, 1971). Position control, pressure control, and myoelectric control derived from the shoulder area were compared and found to be potentially valuable sources. In terms of information content, including the number of distinguishable levels of output, position control was found to produce the highest signal-to-noise levels and myoelectric control gave the lowest. One of the earliest practical position transducers was a two-axis shoulder-position transducer, which in modified form is still popular for control of FNS systems (Bayer et al., 1972).

The term functional neuromuscular stimulation was coined as a subcategory of FES at the first international workshop devoted exclusively to FNS, which was held at the National Institutes of Health, April 27–28, 1972. This meeting brought together most of the leading investigators in the field. They participated in intense discussions of the problem areas previously cited (FNS Workshop, 1972). The workshop had been preceded by three international symposiums on external control of human extremities held in Yugoslavia (Yugoslav Committee for Electronics and Automation, 1964–1970). These symposiums, which are still held every 3 years, include FNS sessions and serve as a valuable forum for sharing recent research results.

As the component density of integrated circuits increased and their reliability improved, it became possible to place the principal components of a digital computer in a single, monolithic chip and to think about "smart" multichannel, implantable systems, with and without lead wires. These have been envisioned to couple sensors of force and position into closed-loop, adapting, feedback-control systems, and to incorporate features such as refreshable memories containing current information about each muscle's contraction properties in response to stimulation. But this takes us from history into present and future research.

REFERENCES

Bardeen, J., and Brattain, W.H. (1948). Three-electrode circuit element utilizing semiconductor materials. *U.S. Patent No. 2,524,035.*

Bayer, D.M., Lord, R.H., Swanker, J.W., and Mortimer J.T. (1972). A two-axis shoulder position transducer for control of orthotic prosthetic devices. *IEEE Trans. Ind. Electron. Cont. Instr.*, **19**(2), 61–64.

Brindley, G.S., Polkey, C.E., and Ruston, D.N. (1978). Electrical splinting of the knee in paraplegia. *Paraplegia*, **16**, 434–441.

Caldwell, C.W. (1970). A high strength platinum percutaneous electrode for chronic use. *Report No. EDC 4-70-30.*, Cleveland OH: Engineering Design Center, Case Western Reserve University.

Cooper, E.B., Bunch, W.H., and Campa, J.H. (1973). Effects of chronic human neuromuscular stimulation. *Surg. Forum*, **24**, 477–479.

Duchenne, G.B.A. (1867). Physiologie des mouvements demontree a l'aide l'experimentation electrique et de l'observation clinique, et applicable a l'etude des paralysies et des deformations. Paris.

Franklin, B. (1757). On the effects of electricity in paralytic cases. *Phil. Trans.*, **50**, 481–483.

Galvani, L. (1791). De viribus electricitatis in motu musculari, commentarius. *De Bononiensi Scientiarum et Artium Instituto atque Academia*, **7**, 363–418.

Glenn, W.W.L., Holcomb, W.G., Hogan, J.F., Kaneyuki, T., and Kim, J. (1977). Long-term stimulation of the phrenic nerve for diaphragm pacing. In: F.T. Hambrecht and J.B. Reswick, eds., *Functional Electrical Stimulation: Applications in Neural Prostheses*, pp. 97–122. New York: Marcel Dekker.

Grandjean, P.A., and Mortimer, J.T. (1986). Recruitment properties of monopolar and bipolar epimysial electrodes. *Ann. Biomed. Eng.*, **14**, 53–66.

Hyman, A.S. (1930). Resuscitation of the stopped heart by intracardiac therapy. *Arch. Intern. Med.*, **46**, 553–568.

Jeglic, A., Vavken, E., Strbenk, M., and Benedik, M. (1967). Electrical stimulation of skeletal muscle by directly powered implanted rf receivers. In M.M. Gavrilovic and A.B. Wilson, eds., *External Control of Human Extremities*, pp. 42–53. Belgrade, Yugoslavia: Yugoslav Committee for Electronics and Automation.

Kantrowitz, A. (1960). In: *Electronic Physiologic Aids: A Report of the Maimonides Hospital*, pp. 4–5. Brooklyn, NY.

Kellaway, P. (1946). The part played by electric fish in the early history of bioelectricity and electrotherapy. *Bull. Hist. Med.*, **20**, 112–137.

Kralj, A., Bajd, T., Turk, R., Krajnik, J., and Benko, H. (1983). Gait restoration in paraplegic patients: A feasibility demonstration using multichannel surface electrode FES. *J. Rehabil. Res. Dev.*, **20**, 3–20.

LeBlanc, M.A., ed. (1972). Functional neuromuscular stimulation: Report of a workshop. Washington, DC: National Academy of Sciences.

Liberson, W.T., Holmquest, H.J., Scot D., and Dow, M. (1961). Functional electrotherapy: Stimulation of the peroneal nerve synchronized with the swing phase of the gait of hemiplegic patients. *Arch. Phys. Med. Rehabil.*, **42**, 101–105.

Liberson, W.T. (1972). Functional neuromuscular stimulation: Historical background and personal experience. In: M.A. LeBlanc, ed., *Functional Neuromuscular Stimulation: Report of a Workshop. April 27–28, 1972*, pp. 147–156. Washington, DC: National Academy of Sciences.

Long, C., and Masciarelli, V. (1963). An electrophysiological splint for the hand. *Arch. Phys. Med. Rehabil.*, **44**, 449–503.

Marsolais, E.B., and Kobetic, R. (1983). Functional walking in paralyzed patients by means of electrical stimulation. *Clin. Orthop.*, **175**, 30–36.

McNeal, D.R. (1976). Analysis of a model for excitation of myelinated nerve. *IEEE Trans. Biomed. Eng.*, **23**, 329–337.

Moe, J.H., and Post. H.W. (1962). Functional electrical stimulation for ambulation in hemiplegia. *Lancet*, **82**, 285–288.

Morris, J.M., Pollack, S.F., and Hinchliffe, H.A. (1968). Elicitation of periods of inhibition in human muscle by stimulation of cutaneous nerves. *Technical Report 59*, Berkeley, CA: Biomechanics Laboratory, University of California.

Mortimer, J.T. (1981). Motor prostheses. In: J.M. Brookhart, V.B. Mountcastle, V.B. Brooks, and S.R. Geiger, eds., *Handbook of Physiology. Section 1: The Nervous System, Vol II: Motor Control*, pp. 155–187. Bethesda, MD: American Physiological Society.

Peckham, P.H., Van Der Meulen, J.P., and Reswick, J.B. (1970). Electrical activation of skeletal muscle by sequential stimulation. In: N. Wolfson and A. Sances Jr., eds., *The Nervous System and Electrical Currents*, pp. 45–50.

Peckham, P.H. (1972). Electrical excitation of skeletal muscle: Alterations in force, fatigue and metabolic properties. *Report No. EDC 4-72-32. Eng. Design. Ctr.*, Cleveland, OH: Case Western Reserve University.

Peckham, P.H., Mortimer, J.T., and Marsolais, E.B. (1976). Alteration in the force and fatigability of skeletal muscle in quadriplegic humans following exercise induced by chronic electrical stimulation. *Clin. Orthop.*, **114**, 326–334.

Peckham, P.H., Mortimer, J.T., and Marsolais, E.B. (1980a). Controlled prehension and release in the C5 quadriplegic elicited by functional electrical stimulation of the paralyzed forearm musculature. *Ann. Biomed. Eng.*, **8**, 369–388.

Peckham, P.H., Marsolais, E.B., and Mortimer, J.T. (1980b). Restoration of key grip and release in the C6 tetraplegic patient through functional electrical stimulation. *J. Hand Surg.*, **5**, 462–469.

Shockley, W.B. (1948). Circuit element utilizing semiconductor material. *U.S. Patent No. 2,569,348*.

Starbuck, D.L., Mortimer, J.T., Shealy, C.N., and Reswick, J.B. (1966). An implanted electrode system for nerve stimulation. *Proceedings of the 19th Annual Conference on Medicine and Biology*, p. 38. San Francisco, CA.

Thoma, H., Frey, M., Holle, J., Losert, U., Rosen Kranz, D., and Stohr, H. (1981). Experiments on the electrode nerve connection. *Proceedings of the 7th International Symposium on External Control of Human Extremities*, pp. 121–135. Belgrade, Yugoslavia: Yugoslav Committee for Electronics and Automation.

Vodovnik, L., and Rebersek, S. (1971). Information content of myocontrol signals for orthotic and prosthetic systems. Final Report. *Development of Orthotic and Prosthetic Systems Using Functional Electrical Stimulation and Myoelectric Control*, pp. 96–106. Washington, DC: Project 19-P-58391-F-01, Social and Rehabilitation Service, HEW.

Volta, A. (1800). Letter to Sir Joseph Banks, March 20, 1800. On electricity excited by the mere contact of conducting substances of different kinds. *Phil. Trans. Roy. Soc.*, **90**, 403–431.

Yugoslav Committee for Electronics and Automation. (1964–1991). Advances in external control of human extremities. *Proceedings of International Symposium I-X on External Control of Human Extremities.* Belgrade, Yugoslavia.

I
Muscles and Sensors

2
An Overview of Muscle Modeling

GEORGE I. ZAHALAK

A broad, though not exhaustive, survey is presented of various models that have been proposed as mathematical representations of isolated skeletal muscle. The main purposes of muscle models (*comprehension* and *prediction*), and their desirable characteristics (*credibility* and *tractability*) are considered briefly. For purposes of discussion the models are grouped into three main classes depending on the level of structure they address primarily: (1) microscopic (cross-bridge, sarcomere) models; (2) fiber models; and (3) macroscopic (whole muscle) models. Group (1) is subdivided further into "conventional" (Huxley-type) and "unconventional" cross-bridge models; group (3) is subdivided into Hill-type models, viscoelastic models, and systems (blackbox) models. The two main currents in present muscle modeling are Huxley-type microscopic models and Hill-type macroscopic models: the former offer superior credibility while the latter are much more tractable. If the intractability of the crossbridge models could be reduced they could be pressed into service in macroscopic biomechanics; it may be possible to achieve this desirable goal via the distribution-moment (DM) model, or some other approach which accomplishes the same purpose. Future muscle models may have to focus more on the effects of sarcomere inhomogeneity within fibers and differences in fiber architecture among muscles.

PURPOSE AND SCOPE

A major purpose of neural prostheses, the subject of this book, is to restore normal musculoskeletal function to the maximum extent possible. The analysis and design of such prostheses must therefore take into account the potentialities and limitations—in short, the operating characteristics—of the actuators of the motor control system: the skeletal muscles. Although muscle has been the object of intense interest and study for hundreds of years, and despite the enormous progress which has been made in understanding its structure and function during the past few decades, the formulation of a completely satisfactory quantitative representation of contraction dynamics has been elusive. A great variety of muscle models has evolved over the years, differing in intended application, mathematical complexity, level of structure considered, and fidelity to the biological facts. The goal of this chapter is to provide a brief survey of the several currents evident in contemporary muscle modeling, and thus contribute (along with other chapters on sensors, electrodes, and parameter identification) to a basis for discussion of neural prostheses.

The literature on muscle is vast, even when restricted to its modeling. This overview does not aim to be exhaustive, but rather to present a representative sample from the broad spectrum of muscle models which have been proposed. I will only consider models for muscle as an isolated entity. Thus the interactions of muscles within a group, or interactions between different groups of muscles, will not be considered, although these are certainly essential aspects of overall neuromuscular function. Also removed from the purview of this chapter are models which combine the actuator functions of muscle with the associated neural circuitry into integrated descriptions of feedback control systems—for example, those regulating the reflex stiffness of a limb (Astaryan and Fel'dman, 1965; Houk and Rymer, 1983; Hogan 1985a). Some of these important topics will be addressed in other chapters of this volume. Finally, I will not provide a separate discussion of models for muscle under artificial external stimulation, designed specifically for applications of particular interest in neural prostheses. Such models, and the experimental determination of their parameters, are discussed by Durfee in Chapter 3.

WHY MODEL?

Before embarking on an examination of the various extant muscle models, it seems worthwhile to consider briefly why we bother to model muscle at all, and what the desirable characteristics of a model are. In the present context, an appropriate working definition is that a model is a reduced or truncated representation of reality; for engineering purposes the representation is usually mathematical. The model must be reduced in the sense of lacking *some* of the properties of the object or process it represents, for otherwise it would be isomorphic with and equivalent to that object or process. In return for giving up some, possibly much, of the detail of the reality, a model is usually compensatingly simpler to understand and manipulate. A good model is one which is as simple as possible while simultaneously retaining the essential characteristics of the thing it represents. "Essential" is, of course, a relative term connected with the purpose of the model; what is essential to a biophysicist may not be so to a control engineer, and vice versa.

What purposes does modeling serve? Probably the two most important are that a model can promote an understanding of its object and, further, it can predict the behavior of that object. Here "understanding" may be taken to signify the description of a complicated phenomenon in terms of a limited number of simpler concepts, and this is what a good model will provide in stripping away all but the bare essentials, which may have been obscured by the inevitable complexity of physical reality. A good model will also enable one to infer how a system will behave in circumstances which may be far removed from the necessarily limited range of experimental experience. By their very nature models cannot predict *all* aspects of system behavior, but a good model will predict those which are most important. These two functions of *comprehension* and *prediction* are not necessarily linked. A model that promotes a correct appreciation of a system's behavior in terms of more elementary concepts will usually enable the prediction of that behavior. But of course there is always a danger that the prediction may be incorrect in a specific case because an attribute of the system which is important in that particular case has been omitted from the model. Conversely, there are purely formal predictive models, often arrived at via statistical considerations, which add little if anything to an understanding of the system whose behavior they predict. Although such formal models have considerable power and generality within the realm of linear systems, muscle is grossly nonlinear and the application of a purely predictive model to circumstances other than those under which it was derived is always suspect.

These two primary functions of models, comprehension and prediction, appeal primarily to different constituencies. The scientist, in particular the biophysicist or physiologist, is concerned with understanding how muscle works, whereas the engineer wishes to predict its behavior as an element of a larger control system. Obviously these two goals are not mutually exclusive. Indeed the best models would do both things well: they would permit the calculation of behavior under varied experimental conditions and also provide insight about what physical mechanisms are responsible when the predictions are correct, and also when they are not. The functions of comprehension and prediction are related by the following: *the degree to which one can place confidence in the predictions of a model beyond the immediate range of experimental experience is proportional to one's confidence that the model includes all important relevant physical mechanisms.*

It should be borne in mind that mathematical models need not always be numerically very accurate in order to be useful. They may indicate important qualitative relations between variables. For example, model predictions that "muscle stiffness decreases with increasing shortening velocity at constant stimulation," or "the rate of change of elastic energy in a tendon is usually small compared to the rate of energy released by phosphocreatine hydrolysis in calcium pumping" may be valuable conclusions even if the absolute values of the predicted stiffness or elastic energy are somewhat in error. Also, quite apart from its numerical accuracy, a model may be useful for rendering dimensionless and scaling the responses of systems of different sizes and properties (Zajac, 1989); or it may suggest appropriate *forms* of simpler, more tractable models which may be useful in applications. Another example in this vein is that relatively crude and inaccurate models of system elements may nevertheless provide important insights about the interaction of those elements within the system. An extreme example of this is the analysis by Hogan (1985a,b) of the significance of multiarticular muscles and cocontraction, which is based on a representation of muscles as simple springs.

What, then, are the desirable qualities of a model? It seems, in the main, there are two: *credibility* and *tractability*. Credibility refers to the fact that the predictions of a model should be believable statements about the nature of the system the model represents. This has both qualitative and quantitative aspects. The model should certainly predict at least qualitatively the phenomena of interest and, further, should correctly identify the salient physical mechanisms responsible for these phenomena. Further, credibility requires that the model predictions be quantitatively accurate within some tolerance, although mere orders of magnitude may be acceptable in some cases. These aspects—qualitative and quantitative—reinforce each other: if a model is known to include the important physics, then its numerical predictions are regarded with more confidence. Conversely, a model which predicts accurately a sufficiently wide range of phenomena provides presumptive evidence that it includes the most important physics.

Tractability, on the other hand, refers to the ease with which a model can be manipulated mathematically and interpreted. A credible model may not be useful if it is so complex mathematically that it is very difficult to extract any conclusion from it. This is not simply a matter of whether or not the equations of the model can be solved; given burgeoning computer power, the degree of complexity of models whose behavior can be calculated is constantly increasing. It is possible, however, to view a model as simultaneously computable and intractable. Although numerical results can be obtained, they may be in such complicated form and so far removed from measurable variables of interest that intuitive grasp of their significance may be lost. Further, for possible real-time applications in neural prosthetics, models must not be so computationally burdensome that responses cannot be calculated rapidly, and even in applications to controller design and simulation it is highly desirable to use reasonably simple models which give a short turnaround time.

As Wilkie (1954) remarked about facts and theories, credibility and tractability are to some extent "natural enemies." The more of the known physical mechanisms which operate in a given system that are included in its model, presumably the more believable the model will become, but it will also probably become less tractable. Conversely, deleting features of the system from the model will make it more tractable but less credible. The art of modeling consists of knowing what to put in and what to leave out. It must be emphasized, however, that simply increasing the complexity of a model, and thus decreasing its tractability, will not necessarily improve credibility. As an example, consider the differential equation governing the classic A.V. Hill muscle model [see equation (16)].

$$\dot{L} = C(P)\dot{P} - F(P; P_0) \tag{1}$$

where L is the muscle length, P is the force, P_0 is the isometric force, C is the series elastic compliance, and F is the shortening velocity of the contractile element as a function of muscle force. Under the simplest assumptions C can be taken to be constant and F to be given by Hill's equation $[F = b(P_0 - P)/(a + P)]$; thus the muscle is characterized by the four parameters C, a, b, and P_0. It has been shown, however, that even if C and F are taken to be arbitrary functions, which amounts to characterizing the muscle by an infinity of parameters, equation (1) is incapable of predicting the phenomenon of "yielding" on stretch (Zahalak, 1981). Thus decreasing tractability simply by increasing the number of parameters in this model will not improve the credibility of its qualitative predictions in this experiment. The structure of the model is incorrect and must be replaced, either in an ad hoc manner (Winters, 1990) or with a different set of physical postulates (Zahalak, 1981).

TYPES OF MUSCLE MODELS

There exists a plethora of different muscle models; indeed it seems sometimes that each investigator has his own particular model. In an attempt to impose some order on this diversity, I offer the classification scheme illustrated in Figure 2-1. The scheme is certainly not unique and the categories are not mutually exclusive, but this ordering does provide a framework for exposition. Muscle models are divided initially into three classes on the basis of the level of structure that they address primarily. These three classes are: (1) cross-bridge/sarcomere, or microscopic, models; (2) fiber models; and (3) whole-muscle, or macroscopic, models. The distinctions between these classes are not absolute; thus a cross-bridge model can be used to represent a whole muscle which is assumed to be a homogeneous assembly of identical sarcomeres. Conversely, A.V. Hill-type models which were developed originally for whole muscles have been used to represent the dynamics of individual sarcomeres within a fiber (Hatze, 1981; Morgan et al., 1982). The microscopic and macroscopic classes are subdivided further. The first contains two subcategories: (1) cross-bridge models of the type first introduced by A.F. Huxley (1957) and elaborated by T.L. Hill (1977) and many others (these will be referred to as "conventional" cross-bridge models); and (2) a diverse group of cross-bridge models based on postulates significantly different from those of Huxley (these are labeled "unconventional" microscopic models). The macroscopic whole-muscle models have been divided into three subcategories for purposes of discussion: (1) viscoelastic models, which consider muscle to be a viscoelastic material; (2) Hill-type models which are variations on the prototype model proposed by A.V. Hill in his classic 1938 paper (Hill, 1938); and (3) systems models which regard muscles as "black boxes," the contents of which are to be determined by formal parameter identification procedures. Again, these categories can overlap. Systems models are so general that they could subsume viscoelastic and Hill-type models, and Hill-type models can be considered formally as a special class of viscoelastic models. Nevertheless, order will be maintained by assigning to any specific model a primary affiliation with one of the classes.

One more category of muscle models appears in Figure 2-1: the distribution-moment (DM) models (Zahalak, 1981, 1990; Zahalak and Ma, 1990). These are models for sarcomeres or whole muscles which are extracted via a formal mathematical approximation from Huxley-type cross-bridge models. As such they are not assigned to one of the primary categories, but rather from a bridge between the microscopic and macroscopic domains.

The various types of muscle models which have been identified in this section will be discussed more extensively in the following sections.

CONVENTIONAL (HUXLEY-TYPE) MICROSCOPIC MODELS

These are models patterned after the prototype introduced by A.F. Huxley in his seminal 1957 paper. Thirty years later they appear to be the models of choice among the great majority of active muscle biophysicists, although the specific details of the models have changed considerably since Huxley's original version, which he has recently referred to as a "skeleton model" (Huxley, 1988); indeed, these models

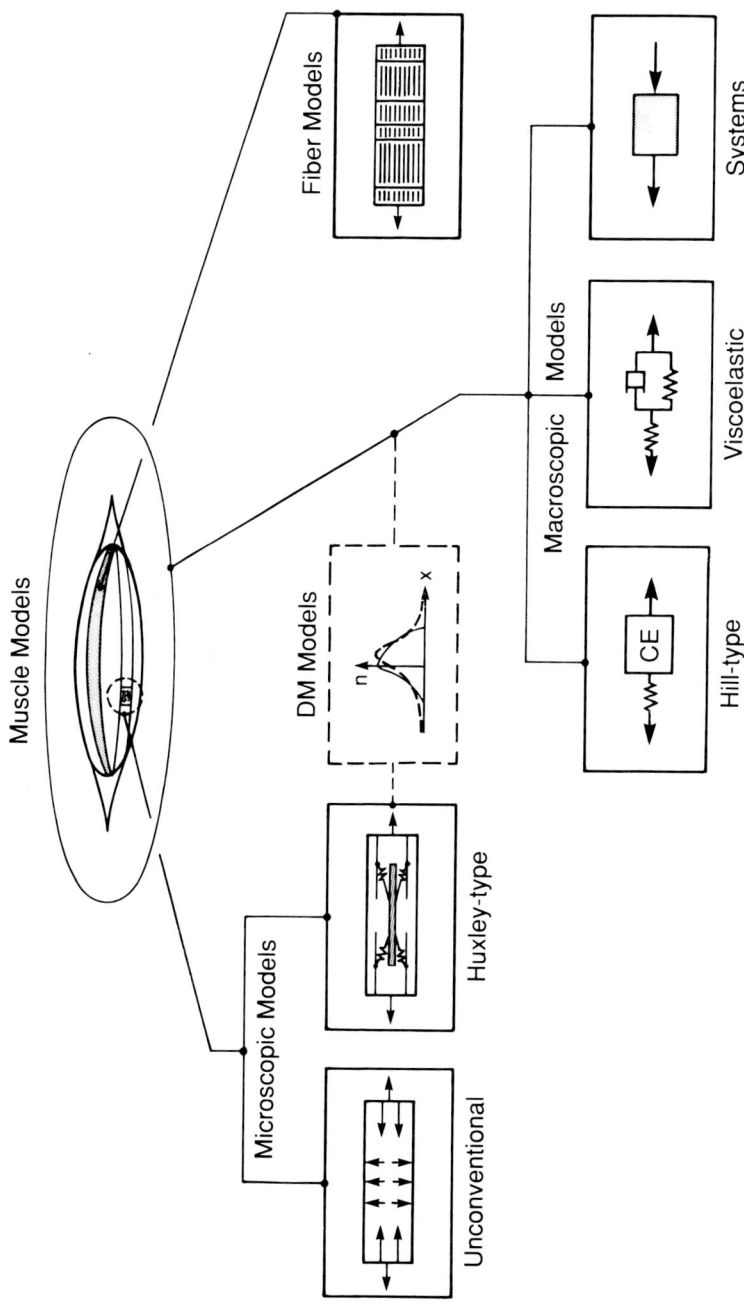

Figure 2–1 Classification of muscle models.

AN OVERVIEW OF MUSCLE MODELING

continue to evolve. Nevertheless, the basic schema underlying Huxley's theory has withstood the test of time (Huxley, 1980, 1988) and provides a concise mathematical description of the way that muscle is believed to work. Huxley's original model is well known and is illustrated in Figure 2–2A. Cross-bridges are assumed to be linked to the myosin filament backbone by an elastic connection and to be in continuous random thermal motion about a neutral equilibrium position; the cross-bridges act independently, uninfluenced by the motions of neighboring cross-bridges. It is assumed that each cross-bridge may be in one of two states—either attached to a specific binding site on a thin actin filament, or detached from actin. When attached, the cross-bridge exerts a force of interaction between the actin and myosin filaments because its elastic linkage is deformed. The basic variable of the theory is the *bond distribution function*, $n(x,t)$, which gives the fraction of cross-bridges at time t that are linked to actin with bond length (i.e., displacement from the equilibrium position) x. Assuming first-order kinetics for the actin-myosin reaction, Huxley (1957) showed that n satisfied his celebrated rate equation

$$\left(\frac{\partial n}{\partial t}\right)_x - v(t)\left(\frac{\partial n}{\partial x}\right)_t = f - (f + g)n \qquad (2)$$

where $v(t)$ is the relative myofilament sliding velocity (shortening positive), f is the bonding rate constant, and g is the unbonding rate constant. Actually, the rate "constants" were assumed to be functions of the bond length, x, and indeed this is what makes the theory work. Figure 2–2B shows the variations of f and g originally assumed by Huxley, and Figure 2–2C shows the time evolution of n, computed from equation (2) and these rate functions, when a block of contractile tissue is rapidly shortened at constant speed, starting from an isometric state.

Once the bond-distribution function has been determined, macroscopic quantities of interest such as force, stiffness, and chemical energy liberation can be easily computed as appropriate integrals involving n if a whole muscle, or at least a muscle fiber, is assumed to be a *collection of identical sarcomeres*; this has been invariably assumed in all applications of cross-bridge theories to experiments [but has been questioned in the fiber theory of Morgan (1990a,b)]. If, as is usually assumed, the stiffness of a cross-bridge is constant, then it can be shown for the Huxley two-state model that the muscle stiffness, K, the muscle force, P, and the elastic energy stored in the cross-bridges, U_c, are proportional to the first three *moments* of n (Zahalak and Ma, 1990). That is

$$K \sim Q_0 \quad P \sim Q_1 \quad U_c \sim Q_2 \qquad (3)$$

where the moments are defined as

$$Q_\lambda = \int \xi^\lambda n(\xi,t)d\xi \,, \quad \lambda = 0, 1, 2 \ldots \qquad (4)$$

and the integration extends over all values of ξ. The normalized bond-length ξ is defined as x/h where h is a scaling parameter which measures the range of bond-lengths over which there is significant probability of bonding. Huxley was able to secure excellent fits of this model to two major experimental results which had been obtained by A.V. Hill: the force-velocity relation and the rate of heat production (both for maximally stimulated shortening muscle).

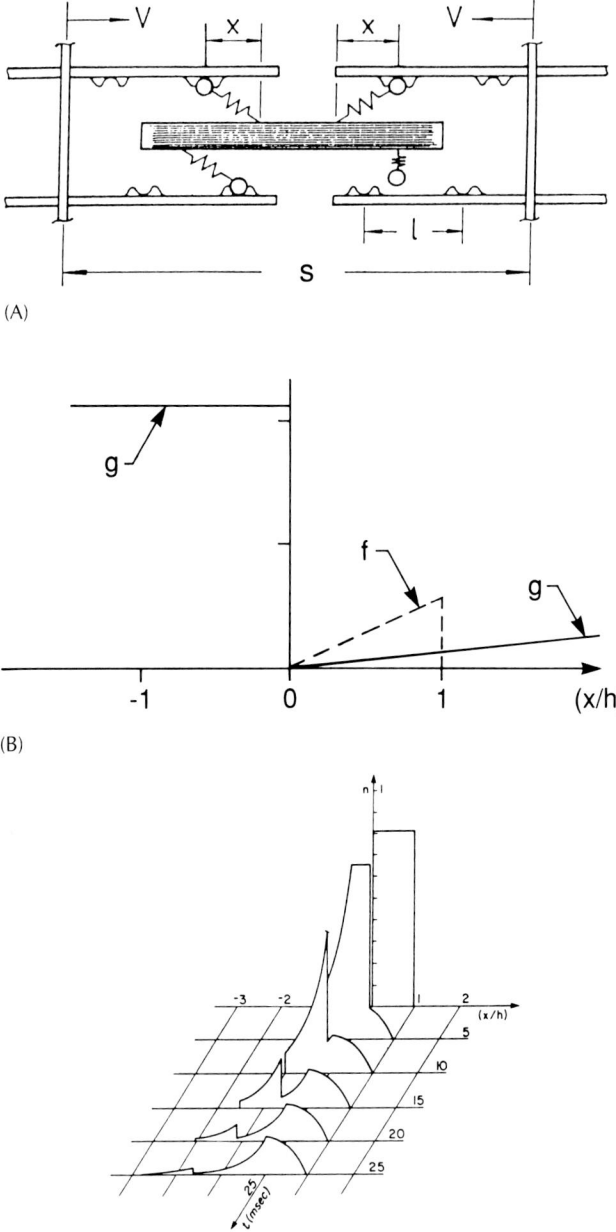

Figure 2-2 The A.F. Huxley 1957 cross-bridge model. (A) Cartoon illustrating bonding of cross-bridges, linked elastically to the thick myosin filaments, to the thin actin filaments. (B) Variation of the rate functions f and g with bond length x (h is a scaling parameter measuring the range of bond lengths over which there exists a significant probability of bonding). (C) Evolution of the bond-distribution function $n(x, t)$ when the Huxley model is shortened at maximum (unloaded) speed. (From Zahalak, 1981, with permission.)

With this model Huxley founded a thriving industry. Many subsequent investigators have elaborated the model and applied it to the interpretation of a growing repertoire of mechanical, biochemical, energetic, and structural experiments. The theoretical framework of the Huxley theory was formalized by T.L. Hill and his associates (Hill et al., 1975; Hill, 1977), who also introduced the thermodynamic requirement of *self-consistency* into the model. Thus Hill considers a cross-bridge which may exist in an arbitrary number, N, of biochemical states, some attached and some detached. If p_i represents the probability that a cross-bridge is in state i (or, equivalently, the fraction of cross-bridges in that state), then the state probabilities satisfy the coupled system of rate equations

$$\left(\frac{\partial p_i}{\partial t}\right)_x - v(t)\left(\frac{\partial p_i}{\partial x}\right)_t = \sum_{\substack{j=1 \\ j\neq i}}^{N} f_{ji}(x)p_j - p_i \sum_{\substack{j=1 \\ j\neq i}}^{N} f_{ij}(x) \qquad i = 1, 2, \ldots N-1 \quad (5)$$

with the constraint

$$\sum_{i=1}^{N} p_i = 1 \qquad (6)$$

as the p_i are by definition probabilities of mutually exclusive events. The self-consistency condition asserts that not all the rate functions $f_{ij}(x)$ are independent because they must satisfy $N(N-1)/2$ equations of the from

$$f_{ij}/f_{ji} = e^{-(A_j - A_i)/K_B T} \qquad (7)$$

where K_B is Boltzmann's constant, T is the absolute temperature, and A_i is the free energy of state i (which includes the strain energy of the elastic link if this state is an attached one). Equations (5) must be solved subject to appropriate auxiliary conditions to yield the $p_i(x, t)$ which in turn will yield the macroscopic variables of interest as weighted integrals of these functions. Thus, for example, the force is given by

$$P(t) = \text{const.} \int \left(\sum_i p_i(x,t) P_i(x)\right) dx \qquad (8)$$

where $P_i(x)$ is the force developed by the elastic link when the cross-bridge is in state i. If these force functions admit of series representations (in particular, if the link is linearly elastic)

$$P_i(x) = \sum_j A_{ij} x^j \qquad (9)$$

then clearly the force is a linear combination of the moments, with

$$P(t) = \sum_i \sum_j B_{ij} Q_{ij}(t) \qquad (10)$$

where

$$Q_{ij}(t) = \int \xi^j P_i(\xi, t) d\xi \qquad (11)$$

Hill emphasized that in order for any such cross-bridge model to produce net

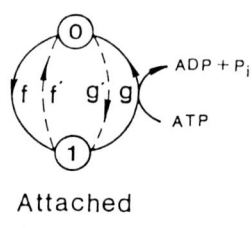

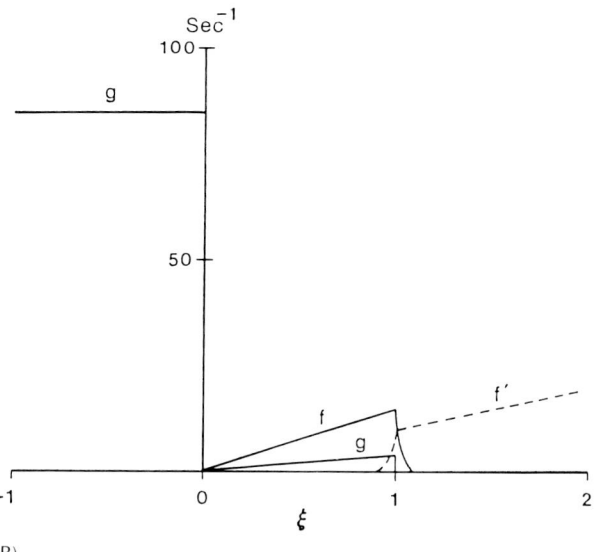

Figure 2–3 (A) The Huxley-Hill model showing two distinct reaction paths between the attached and detached states. (B) Typical variation of the rate functions with normalized bond length $\xi = x/h$. The "exponential tails" at $\xi = 1$ are a consequence of the detailed balance relations, equation (7). The bonding rate g', determined from g by the detailed balance relations, is too small to be visible on the scale of this figure. (From Zahalak and Ma, 1990, with permission.)

work in a steady-state contraction there must exist at least one *cycle* containing both detached and attached states, where a cycle is a closed sequence of reactions beginning and ending at some particular state (Hill, 1977). In the special case of a two-state model (Hill et al., 1975), the existence of a cycle implies that there are two distinct reaction paths between the attached and detached states; this could result if either or both of the states contained substates that were transient intermediates or were in a fast equilibrium with each other (Hill, 1977). This is illustrated in Figure 2–3A, where f and f' denote the forward and reverse rate functions in one path, and g and g' in the other. Then if $n = p_1$, equations (5) reduce to

$$\left(\frac{\partial n}{\partial t}\right)_x - v(t)\left(\frac{\partial n}{\partial x}\right)_t = [f(x) + g'(x)][1 - n(x, t)] - [f'(x) + g(x)]n(x, t) \quad (12)$$

which is identical in form to the Huxley original two-state model, but with f and g

replaced respectively by $f + g'$ and $f' + g$. Further, it is believed that one molecule of adenosine triphosphate (ATP) is hydrolyzed to adenosine diphosphate (ADP) in each cycle of cross-bridge attachment and detachment (Woledge et al., 1985; Squire, 1986), and this may be accounted for by coupling the hydrolysis to one of the reaction steps. In Figure 2-3A the ATP binding and hydrolysis is shown coupled to the unbonding step in the g-path, and this is consistent with the role of ATP as a "relaxing factor" in rigor muscle. With this assumption one may calculate (Hill et al., 1975; Ma and Zahalak, 1987, 1991) the rate of ATP hydrolysis in cross-bridge cycling, $\dot{E}$, as

$$\dot{E}(t) = \text{const.} \int_{-\infty}^{\infty} \{g(x)n(x, t) - g'(x)[1 - n(x, t)]\} \, dx \qquad (13)$$

It is a great virtue of the Huxley-type cross-bridge models that they maintain a close coupling between the mechanics and the biochemical energetics, as is the case in real muscle.

A central theme of recent research into the biophysics of muscular contraction has been the correlation of biochemical states identified by in vitro experiments on actin-myosin solutions with the presumed distinct mechanical states of the in vivo cross-bridge cycle (Eisenberg and Greene, 1980; Eisenberg, 1986). As solution experiments have revealed more biochemical states, the number of states assigned to a cross-bridge cycle has grown. Also, additional states have been postulated to account for mechanical behaviors revealed by experiments carried out with high precision on fast time scales, such as the T_1-T_2 phenomenon discovered by Huxley and Simmons (1971). Table 2-1, reproduced from a recent paper by D.A. Smith (1990), summarizes the performance of eight Huxley-type cross-bridge models vis-à-vis several desirable criteria and experimental behaviors. These models range in complexity from 2 to 18(!) states. In spite of this, none of the models satisfy *all* the chosen performance criteria. This illustrates the point made earlier that a model can never be *completely* realistic. The reader is referred to Smith's paper for a more extensive discussion of multistate cross-bridge models.

In addition to a proliferation of states hypothesized for an individual cross-bridge, there have been efforts to generalize the Huxley model in other ways. The original assumptions that a cross-bridge interacts with only one actin-binding site at any time instant has been removed in some studies, and a cross bridge is permitted to bind to several alternative binding sites (Wood and Mann, 1981; Schoenberg, 1985). There have been other analyses that recognize the existence of two separate globular heads (the S_1 fragments) in each cross-bridge, and postulate the possibility that the two heads may compete with each other for actin binding sites (Tozeren and Schoenberg, 1986; Tozeren, 1987). Further, while almost all cross-bridge models specify linearly elastic cross-bridges it is also possible to consider nonlinear force-deformation relations (Harry et al., 1990). It is fair to say, I believe, that none of these enhancements produces radical changes in model behavior or confers on the model a substantially improved capability of predicting the entire spectrum of known muscle behavior.

Most analyses of cross-bridge models have been geared toward interpreting simple isometric and isotonic experiments at maximal activation. Only a few attempts (some, very ad hoc) have been made to incorporate time-varying activation into cross-bridge models (Julian, 1969; Klauss, 1973; Wood, 1976). Variable activation is, of course,

Table 2-1 Comparative properties and predictions available from published models of the in vivo contraction cycle.[a]

	H	JSS	N+M	EHC	WM	P	PC	S
Biochemical basis:								
No. of states	2	3	3	4	5	18	5	5
Are they biochemical?	No	Yes(?)	No	Yes	Yes	Yes	Yes	Yes
Rate fns. from chemical kinetics?	No	No	No	No	Yes(?)	Yes(?)	No	Yes
Predictions								
Steady-state:								
T_0 large, k small*	No	No	No(?)	No	Yes	Yes	No	Yes
ν_0 (≥ 2 μm sec^{-1})	No	Yes	Yes	Yes	Yes	Yes	Yes	Yes
Double hyperbolic $T(\nu)$†	No	No	No	No	No	No	No	Yes
T_{max}/T_0 (1·3–2·5)	—	—	Yes	—	—	—	—	Yes
ATP-ase fn. $R(\nu)$	Yes	No	Yes	Yes	—	Yes	—	Yes(?)
Max. in $R(\nu)$	No	No	No	No	—	No	—	No
Efficiency‡	Yes	No	—	Yes	Yes	No	—	—
Length steps:								
$T_1(\Delta l)$, $T_2(\Delta l)$	—	Yes	Yes(?)	Yes	Yes	Yes	—	Yes
Rapid rate $r(\Delta l)$	—	—	—	Yes	—	No	—	Yes(?)
Existence of phase 3	—	Yes	No	No	Yes	Yes	—	Yes
Existence of phase 4	—	Yes	Yes	Yes	Yes	Yes	—	Yes
"Stop and stretch"	—	—	—	—	—	—	—	Yes
AC stiffness:								
$\kappa(\omega)$ (isometric)	—	—	Yes	—	—	—	—	Yes
With a high-freq. tail?	—	—	No	—	—	—	—	Yes
Loop frequencies $r_1 - r_3$	—	—	Yes	—	—	—	—	Yes
$\kappa_\infty(\nu)$ (at $\omega = \infty$)	—	Yes	Yes	—	Yes	Yes	—	Yes
Tension steps	—	Yes	Yes	—	Yes	—	—	Yes
AC stiffness in relaxed state	—	—	—	—	—	—	—	Yes
Partial activation:								
T_0	—	—	—	—	—	—	—	Yes
ν_0	—	—	—	—	—	—	—	No
$T(\nu)$ drops in extension	—	—	—	—	—	—	—	Yes
Nyquist loop amplitudes	—	—	—	—	—	—	—	Yes
second loop frequencies	—	—	—	—	—	—	—	Yes
Phosphate dependence:								
T_0	—	—	—	—	—	—	Yes	Yes
R_0 (ATP-ase rate)	—	—	—	—	—	—	Yes	Yes
ν_0	—	—	—	—	—	—	Yes	Yes
Nyquist loop amplitudes	—	—	—	—	—	—	—	Yes(?)
ATP dependence:								
T_0	—	—	—	—	Yes	—	No	No
R_0	—	—	—	—	Yes	—	Yes	—
ν_0	—	—	—	—	—	Yes	Yes	—
ADP dependence:								
T_0	—	—	—	—	—	—	Yes	No
R_0	—	—	—	—	—	—	Yes	—
ν_0	—	—	—	—	—	—	Yes	—
Same parameter values?	Yes	No	No	Yes	Yes	Yes	Yes	Yes

Source: Adapted from Smith (1980), with permission (see text for details).

[a] The authors of the models are as follows: H, Huxley (1957); JSS, Julian, Sollins, and Sollins (1974); N + M, Nishiyama et al. (1977); Murase et al. (1986); ECH, Eisenberg, Hill, and Chen (1980); WM, Wood and Mann (1981); P, Propp (1986); PC, Pate and Cooke (1989); S, Smith (1990). A null entry under "predictions" means not considered by the author(s).

a central concern in modeling muscle for motor-control studies and functional electrical stimulation, and much remains to be done on this topic within the context of cross-bridge theory. (See later section dealing with the DM model for further remarks on introducing activation into cross-bridge theories).

UNCONVENTIONAL MICROSCOPIC MODELS

Although the models described in the last section are widely accepted by active muscle researchers, they do not account completely for all known aspects of muscle behavior, and this gives rise to occasional calls for a fundamental revision of conventional hypotheses (Pollack, 1983). Indeed, over the years there have appeared and continue to appear models at the cross-bridge/sarcomere level which proceed from assumptions quite different from those of Huxley's school. The fact that they differ from the conventional viewpoint appears to be the only thing that models in this class of "unconventional" microscopic models have in common. A sample of such models will be described in this section.

Bornhorst and Minardi (1970), building on earlier work by Caplan (1966), modeled individual cross-bridges as linear energy converters employing the formalism of near-equilibrium irreversible thermodynamics. Thus they assumed that for the i-th typical cross-bridge in steady-state shortening

$$V_i = L_{11}^i(-P_i) + L_{12}^i A_i \tag{14}$$

$$v_i = L_{21}^i(-P_i) + L_{22}^i A_i \tag{15}$$

where P_i is the cross-bridge force, V_i is the cross-bridge velocity relative to the actin filaments, v_i is the flux of the energy-yielding chemical species driving the contraction reaction, and A_i is the affinity of that reaction. The L_{mn}^i are phenomenological transport coefficients, which were assumed to be constant and satisfy the Onsager reciprocal relations $L_{12}^i = L_{21}^i$. On this basis the authors of the model were able to calculate: (1) how the number of bonded cross-bridges must vary with velocity to reproduce Hill's force-velocity relation; and (2) the relation between the energy liberation rate (total chemical flux), v, and the force or velocity, in terms of three measurable (not "adjustable") parameters. The energy predictions in shortening agreed well with measurements. Indeed, this correlation between mechanics and biochemistry appears to be the main objective and achievement of the model, which is otherwise quite limited in being restricted to steady-state shortening and heavily dependent on fitting (rather than predicting) force-velocity and tension-length characteristics.

Iwazumi (1978) has proposed an unconventional microscopic model in which there is no direct bonding between myosin and actin. Instead, ATP hydrolysis is assumed to generate separated charges on the cross-bridges which produce electric fields in which the thin filaments are suspended. A thin actin filament surrounded by a cage of thick myosin filaments is supposed to behave something like a coaxial cylindrical capacitor. In this system energy decreases as the tip of the internal rod moves farther into the interior of the surrounding cylinder, and this electrostatic mechanism is assumed in Iwazumi's theory to be the source of contractile force. The published accounts of this theory present interesting qualitative arguments that it explains many muscle phenomena, but do not provide a mathematical formulation and detailed numerical comparisons with experimental data, so the theory is not particularly useful to those wishing to predict the behavior of muscle as a control system element. Further, although it was originally proposed 20 years ago, this model has not gained acceptance within the muscle biophysics community.

Another unconventional theory of contraction which denies direct bonding between actin and myosin is the "hydrodynamic" theory of Tirosh et al. (1978). This appears to be a modern version of hydraulic-pneumatic theories of muscle contraction whose origins have been traced back to the third century B.C. (McMahon, 1984). The basic idea in this model is that ATP hydrolysis by the myosin ATP-ase creates a directed stream of protons within the sarcomere. This stream, in turn, produces pressure gradients and flow of the sarcoplasm inward from the Z-disks toward the M-line. As the sarcomere is incompressible, the inward axial flow at the ends is balanced by an outward radial flow around the center, resulting in a shortening of the sarcomere if it is unconstrained, or force development if it is constrained. As with the Iwazumi model, a detailed mathematical formulation and analysis of this muscle model does not appear to be available in the published reports, which are confined largely to qualitative arguments. There seems to be no support for this mechanism of muscle contraction among experimentalists.

As a final example of an unconventional cross-bridge theory I will cite the work of Hatze (1990). This model is somewhat closer to the mainstream cross-bridge models of Huxley et al. than theories of Iwazumi and Tirosh. The main features which distinguish Hatze's work from Huxley-type models are: (1) an attempt to describe in detail the mechanism of force generation by a cross-bridge in terms of charge transfer induced by ATP hydrolysis; and (2) the assumption that the cross-bridges are rigidly attached to the myosin backbone, and that the "series" elasticity resides in the Z-disks and M-lines, and not the cross-bridges. Hatze originally proposed a similar charge-transfer mechanism in 1973 (Hatze, 1973). The published references provide a complete description of the mathematical formulation and detailed calculations which indicate that the model predictions of steady-state force-velocity relations and energy rates in shortening, as well as the maintained extra tension on stretch, are plausible. This does not necessarily prove the validity of the theory as, for example, all conventional cross-bridge models also produce plausible force-velocity relations in shortening. Further, as discussed later in the section on fiber models, there are growing indications that the phenomenon of sustained extra tension in stretch is a consequence of sarcomere inhomogeneity, and is not determined by cross-bridge properties as in the Hatze model. No direct confirmation of the charge transfer hypothesis is available from experimentalists because current techniques do not measure this level of detail. The model's assumption of a passive exponential series elasticity outside the cross-bridges has been considered previously several times in the muscle biophysics literature (Podolsky and Nolan, 1973; Julian and Sollins, 1975; Ford et al., 1981) and rejected as incompatible with experimental measurements.

Other unconventional theories of contraction have appeared, but the four examples cited will suffice to illustrate this class. While they may offer some fresh and provocative views of how muscle hypothetically *could* work, these models share the problem that they are not considered as serious alternatives to Huxley-type models by most active muscle biophysicists. And indeed, the proponents of these models have not established that they explain as wide a range of experimental facts as conventional theory, or that they explain them better.

MACROSCOPIC MODELS

Viscoelastic

These models view muscle as a viscoelastic material. The process of electrical stimulation somehow transforms this material from a compliant, fluent state to a stiff, viscous state. Models of this type were among the first attempts at quantitative characterization of muscle mechanics, and were popular in the 1920s and 1930s. In their classic early experiments, Gasser and Hill (1924) went so far as to actually build a physical viscoelastic muscle model consisting of an elastic tube filled with a viscous fluid, and claimed that this system mimicked many of the mechanical behaviors they measured in tetanized frog sartorius muscle (Gasser and Hill, 1924). Shortly thereafter, Levin and Wyman (1927) published their ergometer studies and proposed a three-element model of muscle consisting of an "undamped elastic element" in series with a "damped elastic element" equivalent to a parallel combination of a spring and dashpot (Figure 2–4A). Prior to 1938, experiments on muscle mechanics were usually interpreted in terms of viscoelastic behavior (see Hill, 1938, for a bibliography).

In 1938, A.V. Hill emphatically rejected his previous acceptance of the viscoelastic theory of muscle (Hill, 1938), based on his measurements of heat production during contraction. He found, for example, that the heat is produced by muscle during slow stretches at a lower rate than in the isometric state, whereas a viscoelastic model would predict increased viscous energy dissipation. In place of the then-current viscoelastic models, Hill proposed the famous alternative model which bears his name and which will be discussed in the next section. The fact, however, that muscle researchers accepted viscoelastic models for many years confirms that muscle does exhibit viscoelastic-like behavior. Indeed, muscle is truly to some extent a viscoelastic material, with internal structures and fluids providing some stiffness and viscosity, but these viscoelastic properties do not appear to be of primary importance for the mechanical behavior of muscle. Relaxation phenomena, like the transient changes in muscle force after a sudden shortening or lengthening, were formerly attributed to muscle "viscoelasticity," but are now regarded as manifestations of chemical reactions between actin and myosin.

In spite of Hill's recantation and modern cross-bridge theory, viscoelastic models continued to appear in the scientific literature. Buchthal and his associates published extensive studies of the viscoelastic properties of muscle in the 1940s, with no mention of A.V. Hill's 1938 critique (Buchthal, 1942). Bioengineers, in particular, are familiar with viscoelastic behavior and appear comfortable with models of this type (Apter, 1970; Williams and Edwin, 1971). Biorheologists are also prone to use viscoelastic models to describe the results of experiments on the flow properties of passive or active muscle (Ohnishi, 1963; Little, 1969; Truong, 1972). Most of these models are

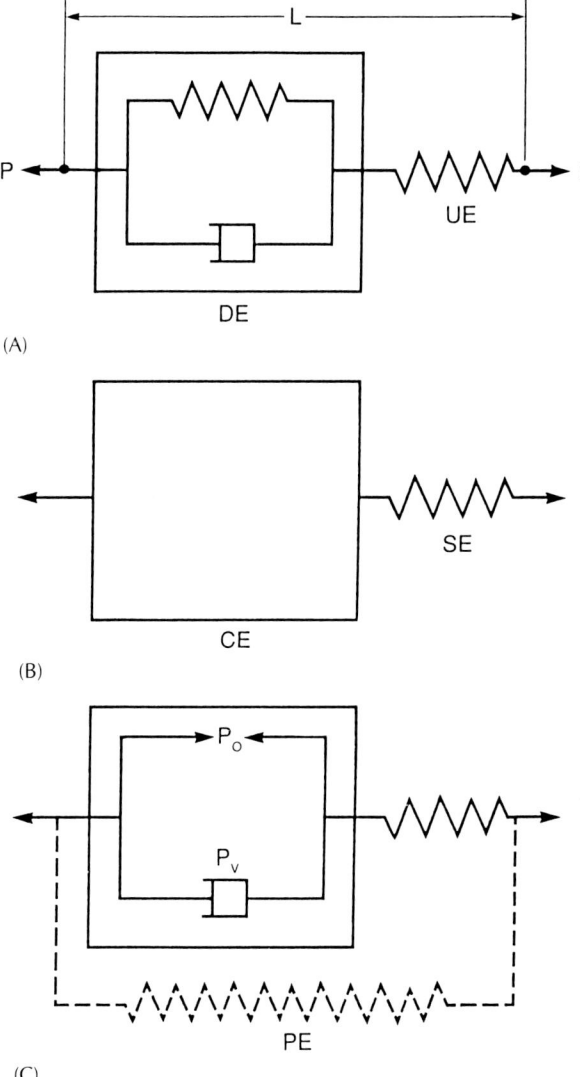

Figure 2–4 Macroscopic muscle models. (A) The Levin-Wyman 1927 viscoelastic model consisting of an undamped elastic element (UE) and a damped elastic element (DE). (B) The A.V. Hill 1938 model consisting of a series elastic element (SE) and a contractile element (CE). (C) Internal structure of the CE of the Hill model showing the active state force P_0 and the quasi-viscous internal resisting force $P_V = BV$. Shown in dashes is the parallel elastic element (PE) which may be added to model the passive elastic properties of unstimulated muscle. (From Zahalak, 1990, with permission.)

confined to constant-activation conditions, and are based on experiments restricted to those conditions. Therefore, while they may have some utility for estimating the impedance of muscle subjected to constant stimulation (in studies, for example, like those of Hogan 1985a,b), they are inadequate for predicting muscle behavior under time-varying activation and loading.

Hill-Type

These are the models derived from the famous original introduced by A.V. Hill in his classic study of heat production in muscle (Hill, 1938). They are by far the most popular models among engineers and scientists studying the dynamics and control of movement. The basic Hill model is illustrated in Figure 2–4B and consists of two elements connected in series: *a series elastic element* (SE), which models the mechanical response of muscle to rapid length changes, and a *contractile element* (CE), which represents the active force-generating capacity derived from chemical free energy stores. A third element, the *parallel elastic element* (PE), is often added to account for the resistance of passive muscle to stretch, but in many skeletal muscles this element generates significant forces only at long muscle lengths and can often be ignored. The length of the SE is assumed to be a (usually nonlinear) function of the force it supports, which in the absence of a PE is the muscle force. The velocity of the CE is assumed to be uniquely determined by the force it supports, which is the same as the SE force. Thus the CE cannot change length abruptly in response to any finite force increment (in this it resembles the Levin-Wyman "damped elastic element"), and this is the basis of the standard *isotonic quick-release test* for determining the dependences of both the SE length and the CE velocity on the force (Zahalak, 1990). Ignoring the PE, the behavior of the prototypical Hill model is described mathematically by the single nonlinear ordinary differential equation.

$$\dot{L} = C(P)\dot{P} - F(P; P_0) \tag{16}$$

where the superposed dots denote time differentiation, L is the muscle length, P the force, $C(P)$ the compliance of the SE, and $F(P; P_0)$ the shortening velocity of the CE as a function of P. The parameter P_0 is a measure of activation of the contractile tissue and is defined as the force exerted by the CE when it is neither shortening nor lengthening, that is $F(P_0; P_0) = 0$. Clearly, under isometric steady-state conditions, the muscle force P is equal to P_0; thus P_0 is called the *isometric force*. But more generally P_0 is assumed to depend on time and the history of stimulation; in this role it is called the *active state*.

The procedures for measuring $C(P)$ and $F(P; P_0)$ in quick-release experiments are well known (Aidley, 1971; McMahon, 1984). The SE behaves operationally as a "hard" spring with a compliance that decreases with increasing force. The CE can be characterized by Hill's famous hyperbolic force-velocity relation; based partially on thermodynamic arguments, Hill deduced the following specific form from his 1938 experiments

$$F(P; P_0) = b \frac{P_0 - P}{a + P} \tag{17}$$

where a and b are constants characteristic of a given muscle. Although Hill's later experiments (Hill, 1964) invalidated the original thermodynamic arguments, equation (17) remains a good empirical approximation to the steady-state force-velocity behavior of many muscles under isotonic shortening conditions and is used extensively.

Formally, the Hill model and its progeny may be considered as a special class of complex viscoelastic models. This is evident from an algebraic manipulation. Thus we can write for the CE

$$P = F^{-1}(V; P_0) = P_0 - B(V, P_0)V \qquad (18)$$

where

$$B = V^{-1}[P_0 - F^{-1}(V; P_0)] \qquad (19)$$

In the preceding equations F^{-1} is the inverse of the function F at constant P_0. Equation (18) states that the force generated by the CE can be regarded as the sum of the active state force P_0, and a velocity-dependent force BV; the "viscosity" of the damper $B(V, P_0)$ depends nonlinearly on both velocity and active state. This internal decomposition of the CE is illustrated in Figure 2–4C. Thus the Hill model is basically a *viscoelastic analogy*, containing an internal force generator.

As with Huxley's 1957 cross-bridge model, Hill's 1938 whole-muscle model provoked an enormous experimental and theoretical effort designed to clarify it and extend its range of applicability. This development is reviewed elsewhere (Aidley, 1971; Carlson and Wilkie, 1974; McMahon, 1984; Winters, 1990; Zahalak, 1990) and I will omit a repetition here. Thus, although Hill's model was originally formulated to describe *shortening* muscle at *maximal* stimulation over a *small range of muscle lengths* near the mean length of the muscle in the body, successive investigators have introduced modifications to account for (1) response in *lengthening* as well as shortening, (2) *submaximal time-varying* stimulation, and (3) *large variations in muscle length*. Although many researchers have contributed to the development of the Hill model, particularly Wilkie and his associates (Abbott and Wilkie, 1953; Ritchie and Wilkie, 1958; Jewell and Wilkie, 1958), for purposes of this overview I will survey briefly three modern engineering versions of the model—those of Hatze, Winters, and Zajac—which amply illustrate the nature of the enhancements. It is widely perceived that these latter forms are the most likely to be useful for FNS applications in the near future.

In several papers which are summarized in Hatze (1981), Hatze introduced what he called a *myocybernetic control model of skeletal muscle* which he characterized as "complete in the sense that it adequately describes all possible contractive states normally occurring in living muscle" (Hatze, 1977). The model is complicated and it is not possible to describe it here in any detail. The very complexity of the Hatze model tends to obscure the fact that it is *au fond* a Hill-type model, albeit with some interesting special features. The model is developed starting with the *assumption* that each sarcomere behaves like an individual Hill-type element, with its own PE, SE, and CE. A series of phenomenological assumptions, claimed to be substantiated by experiment, are invoked to relate electrical pulse stimulation and sarcoplasmic free calcium to troponin sites with bound calcium. Known structural relations between sarcomeres, fibers, and connective tissue in whole muscle are introduced, and after some laborious averaging calculations, the equations of the Hatze model are derived in state-variable format as

$$\dot{\mathbf{x}} = F(\mathbf{x}; \mathbf{u}) \qquad (20)$$

where $\mathbf{x} = (n, r, \psi, \gamma, \xi)$ is the vector of state variables and $\mathbf{u} = (v, z)$ is the vector of control variables (Hatze, 1981). The state variables n and r measure the sizes of two subpopulations of motor units: those which are currently stimulated, and those which are currently unstimulated but still in a contractile state, respectively. The state variables ψ and γ represent "pseudo-calcium concentrations" related to the activation of the n and r groups of motor units. Finally, ξ represents the normalized length of the lumped muscle's CE. The two control variables v and z reflect two accepted mechanisms by which muscle force is graded: v is the mean firing frequency of the active motor units, and z is the rate of motor unit recruitment. Hatze has published the results of several simulations employing this model, both for isolated muscle and whole-body motion (Hatze, 1981).

The most interesting contribution of the Hatze model is the introduction of the two separate control variables, v and z, representing rate coding and recruitment; in this it is unique among contemporary theoretical muscle models. Unfortunately, no practical techniques are available at present to experimentally separate these two contributions to activation for muscle functioning normally in vivo [although such a separation is now possible for artificially stimulated muscles in experimental animals (Fang and Mortimer, 1987; Zhou et al., 1987)]. The complexity of this model is formidable [a single muscle requires the specification of 28 parameters (Hatze, 1981)]. Although several experimental phenomena have been simulated, the model hardly predicts *all* known behaviors of muscle. Further, in spite of its genesis the model offers little insight about muscle behavior at the microscopic level in relation to whole-muscle behavior, as sarcomeres are assumed to be Hill elements *ab initio* and intersarcomere dynamics are not accounted for as in Morgan's theory (see later section on fiber models).

The generalized Hill model of Winters (Winters, 1990) is a simple and straightforward enhancement of the original, which makes no claim to be based within the microstructure. Winters has assembled and combined ideas proposed by several workers since 1938 into a model that aims to account for muscle behavior under arbitrary activation and loading and, most important, is in a form which is relatively easy to use. The model is specifically intended to describe the actions of antagonistic muscles about a joint, and all synergists are lumped into two opposed "equivalent muscles." For each equivalent muscle, force-length-velocity relations are translated into moment–joint-angle–angular-velocity relations. Each equivalent muscle is characterized by the basic Hill structure shown in Figure 2–4B; the central element in this structure is the CE, which in the Winters model is described by the following equations

$$M = M_0 - B\dot{\theta} \quad \text{and} \quad M_0 = AM_{0m}f(\theta) \qquad (21)$$

where M is the muscle moment exerted about the joint, M_0 is the isometric, or *active state* moment with a maximum possible value of M_{0m}, θ is the joint angle corresponding to the current "CE length" (which is in general not equal to the actual joint angle because of the presence of a compliant SE element), A is a normalized

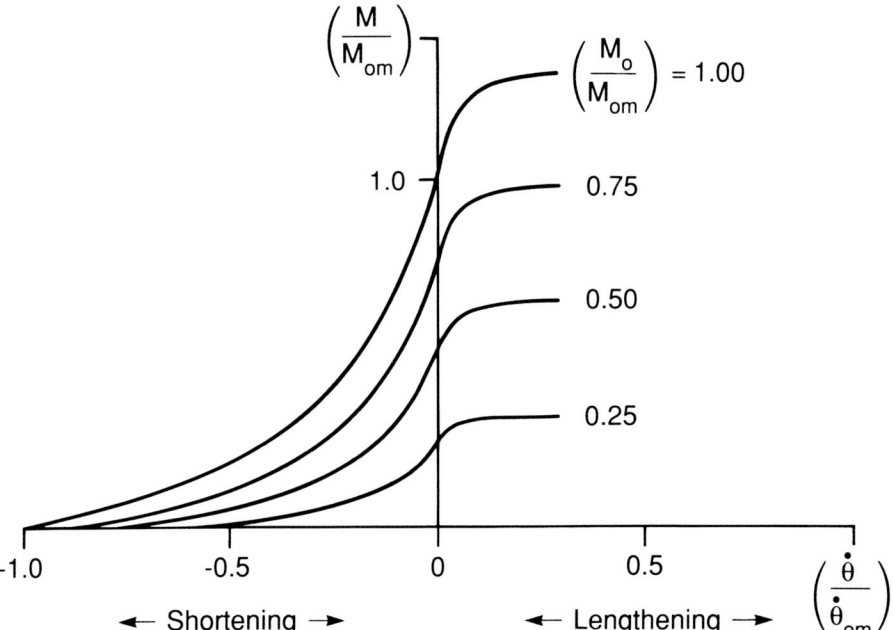

Figure 2–5 Typical force-velocity relations at several levels of activation for Winters's Hill-type model.

activation variable ($A = 0$ for relaxed muscle and $A = 1$ for tetanized muscle), $f(\theta)$ is the normalized tetanic length-tension relation, and B is a variable damping coefficient. For *shortening* muscle

$$B = M_0(1 + \alpha)/(\dot{\theta} + \alpha\dot{\theta}_0), \quad \dot{\theta}_0 < \dot{\theta} < 0 \tag{22}$$

whereas for *lengthening* muscle

$$B = M_0(1 - \beta)/(\dot{\theta} + \gamma\dot{\theta}_0), \quad \dot{\theta} > 0 \tag{23}$$

where α, β, and γ are constants. The unloaded shortening velocity $\dot{\theta}_0$ is assumed to depend on the active state and muscle length according to the equation

$$\dot{\theta}_0 = -[\dot{\theta}_{0m} - \{\mu(1 - M_0/M_{0m})\}]f(\theta) \tag{24}$$

Typical force velocity curves corresponding to these assumptions are illustrated in Figure 2–5.

The model is completed by specifying exponential force-elongation relations for both the SE and PE. Finally the "activation" variable, A, is related to an "excitation" variable, E, by piecewise linear dynamics of the form

$$\dot{A} + \tau^{-1}A = \rho\tau^{-1}E \tag{25}$$

where ρ is a constant and the time constant τ has a larger value for *deactivation* (A decreasing) than for activation (A increasing). The excitation variable E can be identified with an EMG, and this assumption connects the model with experimental reality. (In Winter's model, E is itself the output of a first-order neural controller

AN OVERVIEW OF MUSCLE MODELING

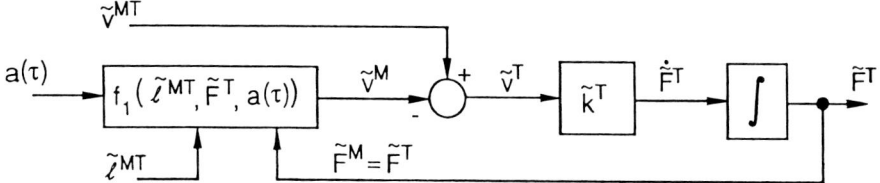

Figure 2-6 Block diagram of Zajac's generic musculotendon actuator, a Hill-type model. (From Zajac, 1989, with permission.)

which presumably receives inputs from higher brain centers, but this detail is irrelevant to the muscle model per se.)

An extensive discussion of this model is available in Winters (1990). Its greatest virtues are its relative simplicity and the provision by its author of design protocols to estimate the numerous parameters needed for simulating specific muscle groups, from available anatomical data (Winters, 1985). With this model, Winters and his associates have been able to match simulations reasonably well to experimental measurements on several musculoskeletal subsystems, including forearm flexion, ankle flexion, head rotation, and eye movements. Recently, Winters (1990) has shown that by making certain ad hoc assumptions about the dependence of activation on the history of contraction, it is even possible to simulate the phenomenon of yielding in stretch—something which conventional Hill-type models cannot do. This is achieved by adding to the "active state" of the Hill model yet another conceptual construct called "attachment."

In an excellent recent review article, Zajac has proposed an appealing new version of the Hill model designed primarily for use in studies of mechanical interactions in multiple muscle systems (Zajac, 1989). The model, illustrated in the block diagram of Figure 2-6, describes the dynamics of what Zajac calls the "dimensionless musculotendon actuator." He has presented arguments to support the concept that the model of Figure 2-6 is *generic*—that is, it represents the dynamics of *any* muscle. The variables are all dimensionless: $\tilde{v}^{MT}$ and $\tilde{v}^{M}$ are, respectively, the muscle and contractile element velocities normalized by the maximum speed of unloaded shortening, v_m; $\tilde{F}^{M} = \tilde{F}^{T}$ represent the common tendon and contractile element force normalized by the maximum isometric force F_0^M; $\tilde{\ell}^{MT}$ is the muscle length normalized by ℓ_0^M, the length at which the maximum isometric force is produced; τ is time normalized by ℓ_0^M/v_m. The function f_1 is a Hill force-velocity relation which expresses the dimensionless CE velocity as a function of dimensionless muscle force, length, and an activation variable $a(\tau)$ which can be regarded as a dimensionless active state. The parameter $\tilde{k}^T$ is the dimensionless stiffness of the tendon (series elastic element), which is approximated as a constant (see Zajac's, 1989 for supporting arguments). This stiffness is shown to be approximately inversely proportional to a single dimensionless tendon parameter $\tilde{\ell}_s^T = \ell_s^T/\ell_0^M$, the ratio of the tendon *slack length* to the optimal muscle length, and this parameter also enters the function f_1. The equation governing the dynamics of the dimensionless musculotendon actuator is

$$\frac{d\tilde{F}^T}{d\tau} = \tilde{k}^T \left\{ \tilde{v}^{MT} - f_1[\tilde{\ell}^{MT}, \tilde{F}^T, a(\tau); \tilde{\ell}_s^T] \right\} \tag{26}$$

According to this theory the *dimensionless* dynamic response of *any* muscle for a given activation and length history is *completely determined by a single tendon parameter*, ℓ_s^T. (This assumes that the pennation angle is small; otherwise this angle enters as an additional parameter). The physical response can be recovered from the dimensionless response if three generally available scaling parameters are known: maximum force (F_0^M), maximum shortening velocity (V_m), and optimal length (ℓ_0^M). This scaling is an extremely attractive feature of Zajac's version of the Hill model, as it permits the calculation of the mechanical behavior of many different muscles on the basis of four simple characteristic quantities. The benefit of such simplicity would seem to be worth the cost of some loss of fidelity in the representation of the complexities of muscle mechanics.

In closing this section, it is appropriate to note that in spite of their wide acceptance and pervasive influence, Hill-type models suffer from several deficiencies, some which have been reviewed in Zahalak (1990). The two major problems are:

1. These models are basically viscoelastic analogies with only the most tenuous connections to the current physiological views of how muscle actually works.
2. The fundamental assumption underlying these models (that at constant length, activation, and force, the muscle velocity is uniquely determined) is not true in general.

These shortcomings affect, respectively, the models' potential for comprehension and prediction. With respect to point (1), it is difficult to relate in any precise quantitative sense the "series elasticity" to the stiffness of cross-bridges and connective tissues, or the "active state" to actually measured action potentials or calcium concentrations. Indeed, "series elasticity" and "active state" are conceptual constructs which depend on the Hill model for their definition, and cannot be measured apart from it. With respect to point (2), Jewell and Wilkie showed 30 years ago that the Hill model could not predict accurately the rise of force in an isometric tetanus (Jewell and Wilkie, 1958). Further, it has long been known that if a constant force in excess of isometric is imposed suddenly on a tetanized muscle, the stretch velocity will not remain constant but rather will exhibit a transient variation (Katz, 1939). More recent studies specifically addressing the issue (Joyce and Rack, 1969; Joyce et al., 1969; van Ingen Schenau et al., 1988) have not found a unique relation between force and velocity, particularly in lengthening and at submaximal activation. The conclusion to be drawn from these considerations is that while the basic Hill model may be a useful approximation in many circumstances, one should resist the temptation to assume that, as far as mechanical behavior is concerned, this model *is* muscle.

Systems

I have called "systems" models those which are derived from experiments via the formal identification techniques of systems engineering, and which rely minimally on a basis in muscle physiology and biophysics. These are "black-box" models whose major purpose is the prediction of muscle behavior under appropriately restricted conditions. The simplest such models are *linear* single-input single-output time-invariant models which are characterized by integral representations of the form

$$y(t) = \int_{-\infty}^{t} G(t - \tau)\dot{x}(\tau)d\tau \tag{27}$$

where x is the input $\dot{x}$ is its time derivative, and y is the output; the system function $G(t)$ (called the step response, weighting function, or kernel) characterizes the intrinsic dynamics of the system. (In control theory it is more common to express system response in terms of the derivative of G, which is called the "impulse response" function). The object of system identification is to determine $G(t)$ through appropriate experiments; once this is accomplished, then the response $y(t)$ can be computed from any input $x(t)$. If $G(t)$ satisfies certain restrictions, then equation (27) can be converted to an equivalent linear differential equation relating x and y.

Linear systems models have been applied to muscle with the (input/output) pairs (EMG/force) or (stimulation rate/force) in isometric experiments, and (displacement/force) in small amplitude perturbation experiments at constant mean length and activation. Several investigators have concluded that isometric muscle exhibits a second-order relation between the activation, A, (as measured by mean stimulation frequency or appropriately processed EMG) and the muscle force, P, which in Laplace transform notation takes the form

$$\frac{P(s)}{A(s)} = sG(s) = \frac{\alpha}{s^2 + \beta s + \gamma} \tag{28}$$

where α, β and γ are constants. This form of transfer function has been found in naturally activated human muscles (Coggshall and Bekey, 1970; Gottlieb and Agarwal, 1971; Soechting and Roberts, 1975), in artificially stimulated human muscle (Crochetiere et al., 1967; Aaron and Stein, 1976; Bawa and Stein, 1976), and in isolated muscle preparations (Mannard and Stein, 1973; Bawa et al., 1976; Robles and Soechting, 1979). To account for the observed phase response at higher frequencies (above 5 Hz) it was found necessary to multiply the right side of equation (28) by the factor $e^{-s\tau}$, thus introducing an *activation time delay*, τ, with a value of the order of $0.01s$ (Crochetiere et al., 1967; Mannard and Stein, 1973; Bawa et al., 1976; Baratta and Solomonow, 1990).

If the length is not held constant, then muscle can be regarded as a two-input one-output system, with the force depending on both the activation and the length. Some studies of such multiple-input systems have been reported (Zahalak and Heyman, 1979; Robles and Soechting, 1979; Cannon and Zahalak, 1982). For example, based on forced and voluntary oscillation tests of the human flexors and extensors, Cannon and Zahalak (1982) proposed the model of Figure 2–7 to describe the relations between the *perturbations* (about a state of isometric contraction) of the muscle force (δP), the muscle length (δx), and the activation measured by the EMG (δE). Under isometric conditions ($\delta x = 0$) this model reduces to the second-order model described in the last paragraph.

Such linear dynamic models are expected to be applicable to sufficiently small excursions in muscle length and activation about a steady-state (usually isometric) operating point. In general, the values of the model parameters depend on the

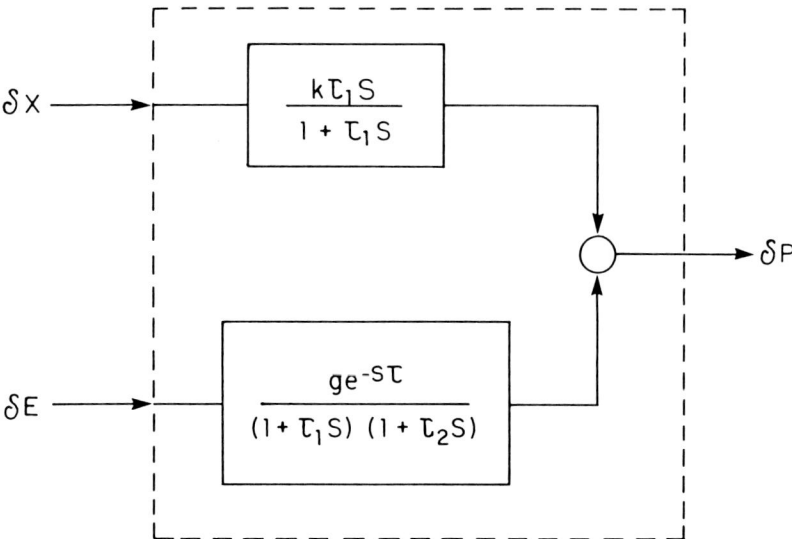

Figure 2–7 Block diagram of linear two-input (muscle length, δx, and activation, δE) one-output (muscle force, δP) model relating the *perturbations* of these variables about a steady operating point. (From Cannon and Zahalak, 1982, with permission.)

operating point. For example, it can be shown that the model of Figure 2–7 can be derived from the Hill model of muscle if it is assumed that perturbations are sufficiently small and a first-order (possibly nonlinear) process transforms the excitation signal (EMG or stimulation rate) into the active state (Zahalak and Heyman, 1979; see also Stein and Wong, 1974). Given these constraints, it is not surprising that the predictive power of linear models is limited. They certainly cannot be expected to work well for large variations of muscle length and/or activation, and even when restricted to small perturbations in these variables the models may not be entirely consistent between different types of movements—for example, oscillations versus steps (Ma and Zahalak, 1985). Their greatest virtue is their simplicity, and they can be useful in providing some qualitative insights [see, for example, Zajac's analysis of musculotendon actuator function (Zajac, 1989)]. And, of course, there are circumstances in which the length and activation variations are genuinely small; the prime example of this is *tremor*. In this case the linear models may even have some quantitative validity (Stein and Oguztoreli, 1976; Zahalak, 1983).

Beyond whatever narrow range of validity the linear models may possess, one must turn to nonlinear descriptions of muscle—a much more difficult proposition. Formally, nonlinear functionals can be expanded in functional series (Volterra, 1930). For a single-input single-output time-invariant system such an expansion has the form

$$y(t) = \int_{-\infty}^{t} G(t - \tau)\dot{x}(\tau)d\tau + \int_{-\infty}^{t}\int_{-\infty}^{t} H(t - \tau, t - \eta)\dot{x}(\tau)\dot{x}(\eta)d\tau d\eta + \ldots \quad (29)$$

where the first term on the right represents the linear approximation. While experimental techniques exist to determine the higher-order kernal functions, $H(\tau, \eta)$, $I(\tau, \eta, \xi)$, ... in biological systems (Marmarelis and Naka, 1974; Krausz, 1975; Marmarelis and Marmarelis, 1978), this approach is very laborious and functional series expansions have seen little application to muscle. The difficulties of developing nonlinear models for muscle can be reduced if certain a priori assumptions can be made about the model structure. Thus, for example, one could assume, under circumstances restricted to a single input, that muscle dynamics are adequately described by a linear dynamic system, but either preceded by a static nonlinearity (Hammerstein cascade) or followed by one (Wiener cascade). This approach has been discussed by Hunter and Korenberg (1986), and applied by Durfee and MacLean (1989) to isometric muscle. Another example of this type of nonlinear modeling has been the "fading memory" muscle models of Bergel and Hunter (1979), and Fung (1981). These are special Hammerstein and Wiener cascade models where the nonlinearity is associated with the Hill force-velocity relation.

A rather extreme example of formal black-box modeling of muscle has been the application of autoregressive moving average (ARMA) algorithms to define the relation between EMG and force in cat leg muscles (Sherif et al., 1983), and between foot moment and knee rotation in human leg muscles (Mote and Kuo, 1989). These procedures construct formal linear models to predict the history of muscle force (knee rotation) from the measured history of EMG (foot moment), using standard statistical criteria to determine the optimal order of the model. No account whatever is taken of muscle physiology in these models, and they can only be expected to be valid for the restricted conditions of activation and motion under which they were derived.

Most recent muscle models developed specifically for FNS applications appear to be of the "systems" type, relying minimally on muscle biology, and maximally on direct experimentation and parameter identification. Solomonow and his associates, for example, have developed an experimental system which permits separate control of stimulation frequency and recruitment level (Zhou et al., 1987). They have applied this system to isolated cat muscles and identified relations between EMG and force under isometric conditions, as a function of fiber recruitment strategy (Solomonow et al., 1987). Further experiments by this group, involving length and velocity variations, will presumably result in a muscle model valid under more general conditions. As mentioned previously, Durfee and MacLean (1989) have modeled isometric cat muscle as a Hammerstein cascade, and have investigated several methods for identifying the parameters of the isometric recruitment curve (IRC), which is the characteristic of the static nonlinearity. Crago et al. (1990) have proposed a discrete-time nonlinear multiplicative model which takes into account the level of stimulation, muscle length, and force-velocity characteristics. They have tested the model and identified its parameters in experiments involving random variations of stimulation and hind limb position in cats (Shue, 1990). The muscle forces predicted by this model compared well with the randomly varying measured forces, particularly if parameter adaptation was permitted, but the model did not predict isometric and isotonic behaviors well. The reader is referred to Chapter 3 by Durfee for further information on systems models and related parameter-identification methods.

FIBER MODELS

This final category of muscle models focuses on the fiber level. In contrast to all other models, which treat fibers as chains of uniform sarcomeres, this theory asserts that important aspects of the macroscopic behavior of muscle can be explained only by taking account of the nonuniformity of a fiber–that is, recognizing that series sarcomeres in a chain may differ in length, activation level, or other properties. Although the physical fact of sarcomere nonuniformity has been known for some time (Huxley and Peachey, 1961), and indeed was an important motivation for A.F. Huxley's introduction of the "spot-follower" apparatus into muscle research (Huxley, 1988), the elucidation of the quantitative implications of this fact for muscle mechanics is due largely to the work of David Morgan (Morgan et al., 1982; 1990a,b).

In its latest version (Morgan, 1990a,b) Morgan's theory of intersarcomere dynamics is based on three fundamental assumptions about the mechanical behavior of individual sarcomeres at constant activation. These assumptions are:

1. Active isometric tension varies with sarcomere length as revealed in the classic experiments of Gordon et al. (1966). That is, isometric tension increases with sarcomere length at short lengths (ascending limb), remains constant at intermediate lengths (plateau), and decreases at long lengths (descending limb).
2. At any length a sarcomere is characterized by an A.V. Hill-type force-velocity relation which in stretch either asymptotes to a constant force as the stretch velocity increases, or else peaks at a maximum force after which the force decreases with increasing stretch velocity. The maximum force attained by a sarcomere in stretch is referred to as its "yield tension."
3. At long lengths the sarcomere can develop large passive elastic forces.

Morgan assumes that not all the series sarcomeres in a muscle fiber are identical, but rather that there exists a statistical variation in sarcomere properties, including yield tension. This leads to the possibility of internal instability within the fiber. For example, suppose a gradually increasing tension is applied to an actively contracting fiber. When that tension exceeds the isometric force of the weakest sarcomere (i.e., that with the lowest isometric force), that sarcomere will start to stretch in accordance with its force-velocity relation. Assuming further that this weakest sarcomere also has the lowest yield tension, it will lengthen rapidly as that yield tension is approached. If the sarcomere is on the ascending limb of its length-tension curve, then it may for a time resist the increasing applied force by lengthening, but if the force continues to rise, eventually it must lengthen onto first the plateau and then the descending limb. Due to the assumptions about the character of the force-velocity curve the sarcomere cannot generate additional resisting force by simply increasing its stretch velocity, so it will lengthen rapidly and catastrophically until the assumed passive "parallel" elasticity is able to provide a resisting force equal to the current applied load. In short, the sarcomere "pops" from a shorter to a longer length. As the muscle force continues to increase, the preceding scenario is repeated for the sarcomere with the next lowest yield tension, and then the next, and so on.

Morgan has summarized his concept of sarcomere instability very succinctly.

> This, then, is the central mechanism being proposed here; that forced lengthening of a muscle on the plateau or the descending limb of the length tension curve must take place essentially by "popping" of sarcomeres, ideally one at a time, in order from the weakest toward the strongest. The term "popping" is used to describe the uncontrolled, virtually instantaneous lengthening of a sarcomere from a length commensurate with its passive length to a length where passive structures primarily support the tension. If the strength

variations are randomly distributed along most of the fiber, active lengthening will involve extreme lengthening of a few randomly distributed sarcomeres. It is proposed that this is an inescapable consequence of a descending limb of the length tension relation and a tension that does not continue to increase with increasing stretch velocity. [Morgan, 1990a]

A quantitative form has been given to this theory by assuming that a muscle fiber is a chain of 100–500 sarcomeres, each of which is described by a Hill-type model. Computation of model responses have simulated several muscle phenomena which were difficult to understand previously. For example, the model has been able to predict the "permanent" extra tension (Morgan, 1990a,b) observed during stretch of tetanized frog muscle fibers (Julian and Morgan, 1979). This is illustrated in Figure 2–8. Model computations have also predicted (1) a continuously rising force in stretch at constant velocity on the plateau of the length-tension curve (Morgan, 1990a,b), and (2) force "creep" in fixed-end tetani at long sarcomere lengths (Morgan et al., 1982), both of which have been measured experimentally. Morgan has argued persuasively that this theory of "popping sarcomeres" describes a very general mechanism underlying all muscular contraction and explains a wide spectrum of experimental observations.

This theory, however, is still in a relatively early stage of development and not yet incorporated into models capable of predicting muscle behavior under arbitrary activation and loading histories. It makes the mathematical description of muscle much more difficult, in that either partial differential equations or high-order systems of coupled nonlinear ordinary differential equations must be employed, in contrast to a single ordinary differential equation for the Hill model. Initial conditions on such a model may be difficult to set as the initial distribution of nonuniformities may be unknown. In the context of whole-muscle modeling, it should be borne in mind that the effects of sarcomere nonuniformity appear to be most pronounced at long muscle lengths which may be prevented in vivo by skeletal constraints. Further, some of these effects, while they may be of great intrinsic interests, are not very large (see, for example, the experimental records of permanent extra tension shown in Figure 2–8A). It is important to develop the inhomogenous fiber model further to determine when sarcomere nonuniformities should be accounted for, the simplest way to do this, and the quantitative consequences of ignoring the nonuniformities relative to other inaccuracies that may be inherent in the model.

THE DISTRIBUTION-MOMENT (DM) MODEL

Although not considered a separate model in its own right, the distribution-moment (DM) model is an attempt to simplify Huxley-type cross-bridge models so that they may be useful in studies of global musculoskeletal dynamics. The theory, which has been explained in a series of publications (Zahalak, 1981, 1986; Zahalak and Ma, 1990; Ma and Zahalak, 1987, 1991), is based on an a priori approximation of the *forms* of the bond-distribution functions of the cross-bridge models, and it emphasizes the central importance of the *moments* of these functions. Although the DM approach is applicable in principle to multistate cross-bridge models, it has been worked out in detail only for two-state models governed by equations (2) or (12). Under the DM approximation these partial differential equations governing the time evolution

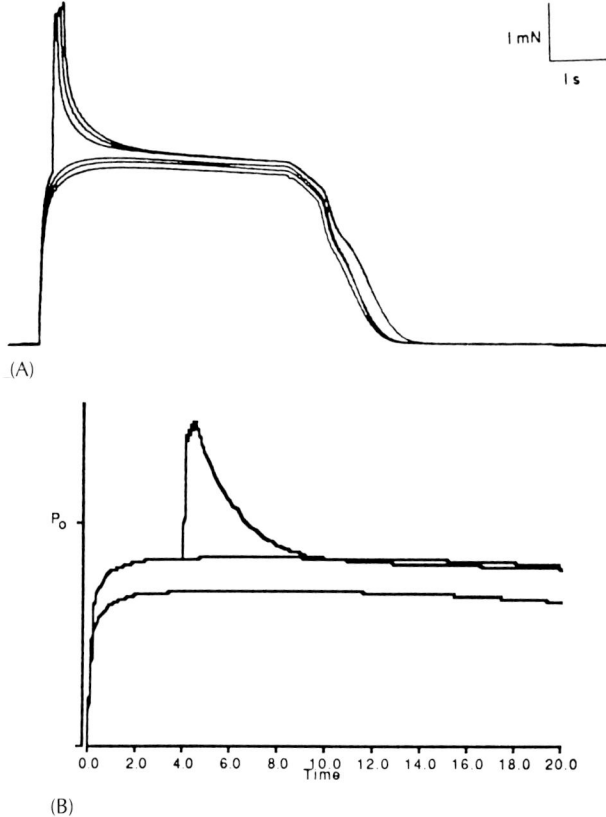

Figure 2–8 (A) Experimental records of force during tetanic stimulation of frog muscle fibers. Three stretches of progressively increasing magnitude were applied either before stimulation (three lower curves) or during stimulation (three upper curves). Note the "permanent extra tension" resulting from stretch during stimulation, which is independent of stretch amplitude. (From Julian and Morgan, 1979, with permission.) (B) Simulation of the experiment in (A) with Morgan's fiber model. Two isometric force traces are shown, with the lower isometric force corresponding to the longer length. The peaked curve represents the model response to a stretch from the shorter to the longer length during stimulation. Note that upon completion of the stretch the force remains above that which would be predicted from the length-tension relation of the longer length. (C) Sarcomere length distributions at the beginning of stretch (top panel) and at two subsequent times during stretch (middle and lower panels). Note the progressively increasing dispersion of sarcomere lengths. Note further the two distinct subpopulations of sarcomeres during stretch: a larger population with lengths near their initial lengths, and a smaller population of "popped" sarcomeres with lengths near 3.7 μm. (From Morgan, 1990, with permission.)

of the bond distribution are converted into ordinary differential equations governing the approximate evolution of the moments $Q_0(t)$, $Q_1(t)$, and $Q_2(t)$ which, as explained in the section on Huxley-type models, earlier, are proportional to stiffness, force, and elastic energy, respectively.

The relation of calcium-activation dynamics to Huxley-type cross-bridge contraction dynamics has also been studied (Zahalak and Ma, 1990) under two different assumptions: *tight coupling* in which calcium can unbond from troponin only if the associated myosin is not bonded to actin, and *loose coupling* in which calcium can unbond from troponin regardless of the state of bonding between actin and myosin.

AN OVERVIEW OF MUSCLE MODELING

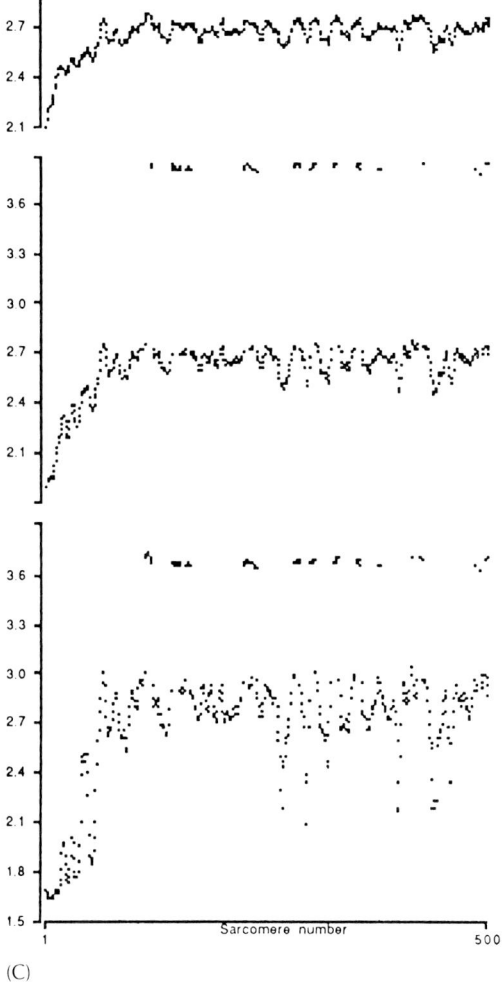

Figure 2-8 (Continued).

The tight-coupling version appears to permit a better representation of experimental reality, so only this version will be discussed here. If some plausible assumptions are made in conjunction with tight coupling, it can be shown that the rate equation for the Huxley-Hill two-state model, equation (12), becomes

$$\frac{\partial n}{\partial t} - v(t)\frac{\partial n}{\partial x} = r(f + g')(\alpha - n) - (f' + g)n \qquad (30)$$

where r is called the *activation factor* and is a pure function of sarcoplasmic free calcium concentration [Ca] according to

$$r([Ca]) = k_1^2[Ca]^2/(k_1^2[Ca]^2 + k_1 k_{-1}[Ca] + k_{-1}^2) \qquad (31)$$

where k_1 and k_{-1} are rate constants; α is a function of contractile tissue length (sometimes called the "overlap function") which represents the fraction of total cross-bridges that can interact with actin. Thus, with tightly-coupled calcium dynamics, the bonding rate of the Huxley-Hill model, $(f + g')$, changes to $r([C_a])(f + g')$ while the unbonding rate, $(g + f')$, remains unchanged.

In the specific applications of the DM approximation that have been developed so far, the bond-distribution function, n, is assumed to have the form of an unnormalized Gaussian probability-density function, which is completely determined by its first three moments. If this approximation is applied to equation (30), and it is assumed further that an elastic tendon is in series with a block of Huxley-type contractile tissue, there results a fifth-order state-variable model of muscle, of the form (Zahalak and Ma, 1990)

$$\dot{C} = \rho(1 - c/c^*)\chi(t) - \tau_0^{-1}[c/(c + k_m)] \quad (32)$$

$$\dot{Q}_\lambda = r\alpha\beta_\lambda - r\phi_{1\lambda}(Q_0, Q_1, Q_2) - \phi_{2\lambda}(Q_0, Q_1, Q_2) - \lambda u(t) Q_{\lambda-1} \quad \lambda = 0, 1, 2 \quad (33)$$

$$\dot{\Lambda} = \kappa(Q_1)\dot{Q}_1 - \gamma u(t) \quad (34)$$

with

$$C = c + 2bQ_0 + r(2 + \mu/c)(1 - bQ_0) \quad (35)$$

and

$$r(c) = c^2(c^2 + \mu c + \mu^2) \quad (36)$$

All variables in the above equations have been normalized except time (see Zahalak and Ma, 1990). The five state variables describing a muscle in this model are: Λ (muscle length), c (sarcoplasmic free calcium concentration), Q_0 (zero-th moment, stiffness), Q_1 (first moment, force), and Q_2 (second moment, elastic energy). The reader is referred to the cited references for an explanation of the functions and parameters appearing in equations (32) through (36); in particular $\chi(t)$ represents a train of stimulus pulses, and it is in this manner that electrical stimulation enters the model. As the model assumes that the stimulation is synchronous, at this stage of development it applies strictly to muscle fibers, motor units, or artificially stimulated whole muscle. If appropriate constraints are applied (e.g., isometric or isotonic), equations (32) through (34) can easily be integrated to simulate the muscle's behavior under those constraints, and this behavior is a good approximation to that exhibited by the Huxley-Hill model [equation (12) plus a series elastic tendon]. Some examples of the performance of the DM activation contraction model are shown in Figures 2–9 through 2–12.

A very attractive feature of biophysical cross-bridge models of the Huxley type is that much of the energetics is implicit in them along with the mechanics, and need not be appended ad hoc as in the Hill model; this virtue is retained in the DM approximation. Based on the DM model of equations (32) through (34), a compatible energetics model has been derived (Ma and Zahalak, 1991). This model is embodied in two equations which give, respectively, the chemical energy release rate, $\dot{E}$, and the heat production rate, $\dot{H}$, in terms of the DM state variables. The dimensionless forms of these equations are

AN OVERVIEW OF MUSCLE MODELING

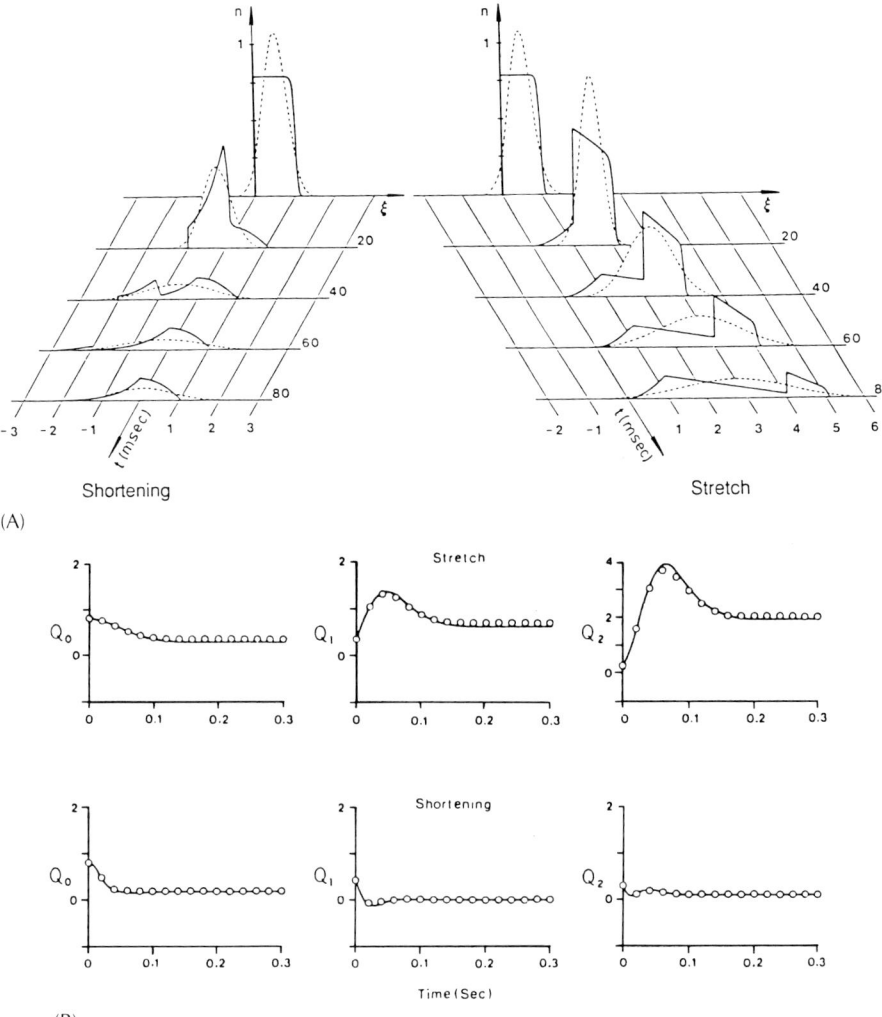

Figure 2–9 Comparison of the DM model [equations (32)–(34)] to the Huxley-Hill model (equation 12) with the rate functions shown in Figure 2–3B. (A) The solid curves are solutions for $n(\xi, t)$ obtained from equation (12) when the muscle is maximally stimulated ($r = 1$) and then either shortened or stretched at the maximum speed of unloaded shortening. The dashed curves are Gaussian approximations with the first three moments, Q_0, Q_1, and Q_2, computed with the DM equations (32)–(34). (B) The first three moments of n as a function of time: open circles are exact values computed with equation (12) and continuous curves are DM approximations computed with equations (32)–(33). [Equation (34) has been omitted due to the absence of a passive series elasticity.] Note that although the Gaussian curves are not accurate pointwise approximations to n, their first three moments are excellent approximations to those of n.

$$\left(\frac{\dot{E}}{P_0 \dot{L}_m}\right) = (Q_1^{(0)} \dot{\Lambda}_m)^{-1} \left[\hat{\nu}_0 \tau_0^{-1} \frac{c}{c + k_m} + \hat{\nu}_1 \Psi(Q_0, Q_1, Q_2, c, \Lambda) \right. \tag{37}$$

$$\left. + \hat{\nu}_2 \zeta(c) \left\{ \tau_0^{-1} \frac{c}{c + k_m} - \rho \left(1 - \frac{c}{c^*}\right) \chi(t) \right\} \right]$$

(continued)

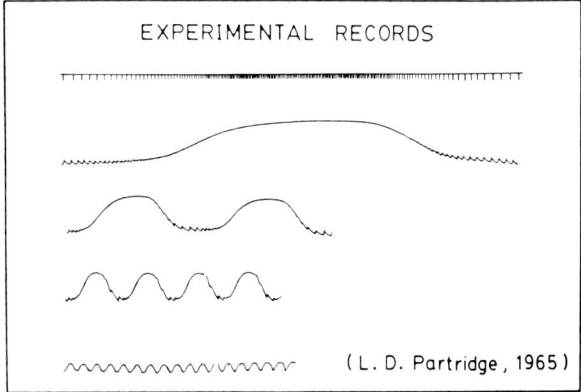

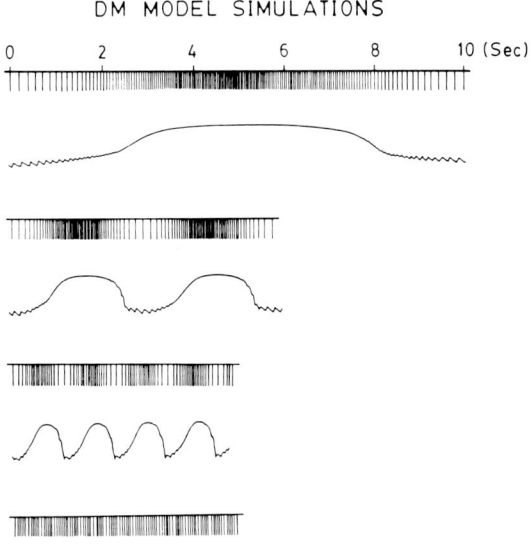

Figure 2–10 DM model simulation of the force generated by an isometric muscle which is subjected to sinusoidally modulated trains of stimulating pulses. The main figure shows pulse trains at four different modulation frequencies together with the resulting force traces. The box shows corresponding experimental data of Partridge. (From Zahalak and Ma, 1990, with permission.)

$$+ \hat{v}_3 \left\{ \rho \left(1 - \frac{c}{c^*}\right) \chi(t) - \tau_0^{-1} \frac{c}{c + k_m} - \dot{c} \right\}$$

$$+ \hat{v}_4 \dot{Q}_0 - \frac{1}{2} \lambda \dot{Q}_2 \Bigg]$$

and

$$\left(\frac{\dot{H}}{P_0 \dot{L}_m}\right) = \left(\frac{\dot{E}}{P_0 \dot{L}_m}\right) + (Q_1^{(0)} \hat{\Lambda}_m)^{-1} (Q_1 \hat{\Lambda} - \kappa Q_1 \dot{Q}_1) \tag{38}$$

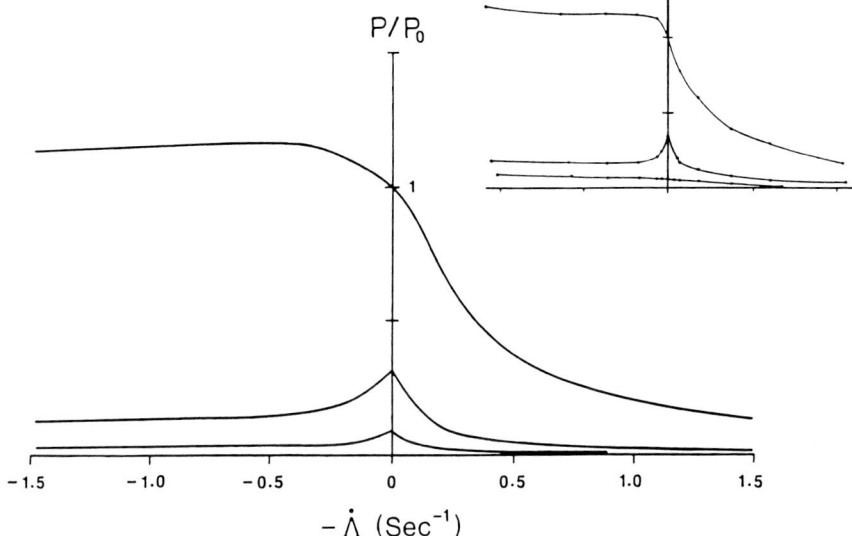

Figure 2-11 Steady-state force-velocity relations for a DM model subjected to constant velocity stretch or shortening, at three activation levels (r = 1.0, 0.2, 0.05). The inset shows corresponding experimental data (of Joyce et al., 1969) for cat soleus at 37°C. (From Zahalak, 1990, with permission.)

Again, the reader must be referred to the cited paper for details, but note that the factors considered in deriving equations (37) and (38) include:

1. Phosphocreatine hydrolysis associated with cross-bridge cycling.
2. Phosphocreatine hydrolysis associated with sarcoplasmic-reticulum pumping of calcium.
3. Passive calcium flux across the sarcoplasmic-reticulum membrane.
4. Calcium-troponin bonding.
5. Cross-bridge bonding at zero strain.
6. Cross-bridge strain energy.
7. Tendon strain energy.
8. External work.

As an illustrative example, Figure 2-12 shows the heat production and variations in sarcoplasmic free calcium occurring during a single twitch of an isometric muscle.

The virtues of the DM approach to muscle modeling have been argued elsewhere (Zahalak, 1981, 1986). Basically, it provides a representation of muscle approaching the analytical and computational simplicity of Hill-type models while retaining much of the presumed physiological veracity and insight of Huxley-type models. The moments form a bridge between microscopic and macroscopic perspectives of contraction as they simultaneously possess microscopic significance (as moments of bond distribution functions) and macroscopic significance (as stiffness, force, and elastic energy). There is no need in this model to "extract" the muscle elasticity associated with the cross-bridges and place it "in series" with the contractile tissue, and there is no need to introduce a nebulous "active state" to couple excitation to contraction. Energetics flow naturally from the model, and do not need to be appended ad hoc.

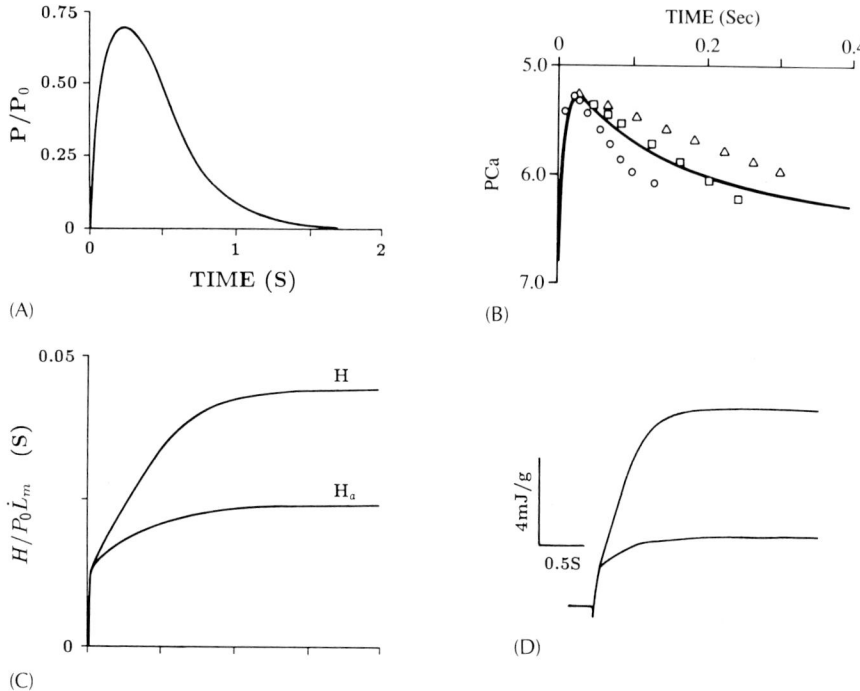

Figure 2–12 Force, calcium release, and heat production during a DM simulation of an isometric twitch in frog sartorius to 0°C. (A) Normalized force. (B) Sarcoplasmic free calcium (as pCa): the solid curve is the DM model prediction and the discrete symbols represent the results of three experiments reported in the literature. (From Zahalak and Ma, 1990, with permission.)

(C) Total heat, H, and activation heat, H_a, as a function of time; the activation heat is the sum of all contributions not associated with cross-bridge cycling. (D) Experimental measurements by Rall (1982) of the total and activation heats in a twitch of frog semitendinosus at 0°C. The activation heat was measured by stretching the muscle until myofilament overlap was eliminated [(A), (C), and (D)]. (From Ma and Zahalak, 1991, with permission.)

On the other hand, the DM model is more complicated than Hill-type models (with the possible exception of Hatze's model), and its parameters enter in a complex nonlinear fashion and are difficult to identify. Indeed, a complete set of mechanical parameters has been identified for only three muscles, which are very well represented in the experimental literature (Ma and Zahalak, 1991). It remains to be seen to what extent this model will prove useful in macroscopic muscle mechanics, but it seems that if the results of biophysical muscle research are ever to be incorporated into studies of global musculoskeletal dynamics, it will be via a DM approximation or something much like it.

CLOSURE

Obviously, there exists a large variety of muscle models. Equally obvious is the fact that no single existing model predicts *all* the known experimental behaviors of muscle, including mechanics and energetics, in shortening and stretch, under time-varying activation, for large variations in length, and subject to arbitrary external loading. Given the known complexities of muscle, it is doubtful that any tractable model will achieve this goal of complete fidelity. Imperfect models will be used and it is therefore important to understand the nature of those imperfections and to estimate, quantitatively if possible, their consequences. On the other hand, models need not be perfect to be useful; a model may predict a wide range of phenomena with acceptable (if modest) accuracy, or it may predict a restricted range of phenomena with high accuracy. There is usually a tradeoff in tuning a model for these two possibilities.

Caution must be observed, especially with phenomenological models like the Hill type which are based entirely on direct experimental measurements, that differences between specific muscles are taken into account. A huge amount of experimental effort has gone into studying the dynamics of tetanized frog sartorius, and the results obtained are often tacitly accepted as characteristic of muscle in general. But this is not necessarily so. For example, tetanized frog sartorius shows a relatively weak tendency to yield on stretch, whereas submaximally activated cat soleus shows a very strong tendency to yield, even at low stretch velocities. Or again, experiments on frog muscles have identified a component of isometric heat production known as the "labile heat," but it would be incorrect to formulate a model for *human* muscle which generates labile heat, as this heat does not appear to be produced by terrestrial animal muscles and indeed may be associated with the presence of the protein parvalbumin found primarily in the muscles of aquatic and amphibious animals (Woledge et al., 1985). Such differences, combined with the well-known differences in the properties of fast and slow fibers (Burke, 1983), and with differences in the arrangement of fibers within muscles (Richmond et al., 1985), make the prospect of a single, *accurate*, generic model to cover all muscles seem somewhat remote.

Although considerable theoretical research has been done on the purely electrical characteristics of muscle excitation, particularly the prediction of the characteristics of the electromyogram from measured or assumed characteristics of individual fiber or motor unit potentials (Agarwal and Gottlieb, 1982), there seems to have been little modeling work to relate these electrical phenomena to muscle's *mechanical* behavior. This is a gap which should be filled. As surface and intramuscular EMG's are used ubiquitously as indicators of muscular activation, it would be very useful to have some models to elucidate expected quantitative relations between the electromyogram and muscle mechanics. Conversely, it would also be useful to have detailed theoretical models relating the geometry of artificial stimulation systems and the characteristics of the stimulation signals to the target muscle's mechanical response. Both of these types of studies would presumably require a combination of volume-conductor theory (Plonsey, 1969; Altman, 1986) with one of the available models for fiber mechanics and energetics.

Each of the models reviewed in this chapter has its partisans, but it seems clear that the two main currents in muscle modeling are Hill-type macroscopic models and Huxley-type microscopic cross-bridge models. Each aims at a general mathematical representation of muscle valid under most, if not all, conditions, and each has deep roots in experimental muscle biology. With regard to the two main purposes of a muscle model, *comprehension* and *prediction*, the cross-bridge models certainly provide a deeper understanding of the function of individual, isolated muscles than the Hill-type models. Both types of models predict some, but not all, experimentally observed muscle phenomena, with the cross-bridge models, particularly in their multistate versions, predicting a wider range. While the Hill-type models may not offer much insight into the nature of contraction in single muscle, they may indeed aid in the understanding of certain aspects of the *interactions* between muscles and body segments in multiple muscle systems.

With regard to the two main desirable characteristics of a muscle model, *credibility* and *tractability*, the cross-bridge models must be regarded as more credible beyond the range of the usual laboratory experiments, as they embody fundamental mechanisms which most biologists believe underlie the process of contraction. The Hill-type models are basically *viscoelastic analogies*, and although they can be fit accurately to limited sets of data, they must be considered suspect when experimental conditions deviate sharply from the standard isometric and isotonic conditions. As noted at the conclusion of the section above, regarding Hill-type macroscopic models, the fundamental assumption of the Hill model is not substantiated by experiment. On the other hand, Hill-type models are *much* more tractable, analytically and computationally, than cross-bridge models, and for this reason variants of the former are likely to be the models of choice in macroscopic biomechanics into the foreseeable future.

But one should not forget the connection between comprehension and credibility. Models that offer a fundamental understanding of contraction dynamics are more than just intellectually satisfying—they carry a presumption of credibility beyond the range of immediate experimental experience. For this reason alone it would be highly desirable to harness the Huxley-type models and the supporting biological knowledge for service in macroscopic biomechanics, if the tractability barrier can be surmounted. For this purpose, the DM approximation or similar approaches which accomplish the same purpose, may serve.

Finally, in view of the subject of this book, it is appropriate to inquire how much relevance the Hill- and Huxley-type models have to the design of neural prostheses. Little application of these physiologically-based models to functional electrical stimulation (FES) control systems is evident so far. Specialists in this field prefer to postulate and identify input-output models directly for their particular applications. This is understandable, as the physiologically-based models tend to be complicated, and have limited accuracy, but it is also somewhat unfortunate because a great deal of information about muscle behavior is embodied in these models. Muscle, in fact, *is* very complicated and wishing things were otherwise will not make them so. Thus simple input-output models can at best represent accurately only a limited range of muscle behavior. Under favorable circumstances this range may be sufficient for a particular neural prosthetic application. [Alternately, proposals have been advanced for "braked" prostheses which try to avoid the problem of actuator complexity altogether (Durfee, 1991)]. Introduction of physiologically-based models into neural prosthesis design is presumably desirable, but may not be feasible at this time because of their level of complexity and high computational costs. This situation may change as computation becomes faster and cheaper. At the very least, the available physiologically-based models can be used to evaluate simplified control model structures and gauge over what operating ranges they are likely to be consistent with the biological facts.

ACKNOWLEDGMENT

This work was supported by the U.S. National Science Foundation under Grant No. BCS-8918641.

REFERENCES

Aaron, S.L., and Stein, R.B. (1976). Comparison of an EMG-controlled prosthesis and the normal human biceps brachii muscle. *Am. J. Phys. Med.*, **55** (1), 1–14.
Abbott, B.C., and Wilkie, D.R. (1953). The relation between the velocity of shortening and the tension-length curve of skeletal muscle. *J. Physiol.*, **120**, 214–223.
Agarwal, G.C., and Gottlieb, G.L. (1982). Mathematical modelling and simulation of the postural control loop: Part I. *CRC Crit. Rev. Biomed. Eng.*, **8**, 93–134.
Aidley, D.J. (1971). In: *The Physiology of Excitable Cells*. London: Cambridge University Press.
Altman, K.W., and Plonsey, R. (1986). A two-part model for determining the electromagnetic and physiologic behavior of cuff electrode nerve stimulators. *IEEE Trans. Biomed. Eng.*, **33** (3), 285–293.
Apter, J.T., and Graessley, W.W. (1970). A physical model for muscular behavior. *Biophys. J.*, **10**, 539–555.
Asatryan, D.G., and Fel'dman, A.G. (1965). Functional tuning of the nervous system with control of movement or maintenance of posture. I. Mechanographic analysis of the work of the joint on execution of a postural task. *Biophys. USSR*, **10**, 925–935.
Baratta, R., and Solomonow, M. (1990). The dynamic response model of nine different skeletal muscles. *IEEE Trans. Biomed. Eng.*, **37** (3), 243–251.
Bawa, P., and Stein, R.B. (1976). Frequency response of the human soleus muscle. *J. Neurophysiol.*, **39** (4), 788–793.
Bawa, P., Mannard, A., and Stein, R.B. (1976). Effects of elastic loads on the contractions of cat muscles. *Biol. Cybern.*, **22**, 129–137.
Bergel, D.H., and Hunter, P.J. (1979). The mechanics of the heart. In: N.H.C. Hwang, D.R. Gross, and D.J. Patel, eds., *Quantitative Cardiovascular Studies*, pp. 151–213. Baltimore: University Park Press.
Bornhorst, W.J., and Minardi, J.E. (1970). A phenomenological theory of muscular contraction. I. Rate equations at a given length based on irreversible thermodynamics. *Biophys. J.*, **10**, 137–154.
Buchthal, F.E. (1942). The mechanical properties of single striated muscle fibre at rest and during contraction and their structural interpretation. *Danske Videnskabernes Selskab Biologiske Meddeleser*, **17**, 1–138.
Burke, R.E. (1983). Motor units: Anatomy, physiology, and functional organization. In: V.B. Brooks, ed., *Handbook of Physiology—the Nervous System*, II, sect. 1, pp. 345–422. Bethesda, MD: American Physiological Society.
Cannon, S.C., and Zahalak, G.I. (1982). The mechanical behavior of active human skeletal muscle in small oscillations. *J. Biomech.*, **15** (2), 111–121.
Caplan, D.R. (1966). A characteristic of self-regulated energy converters: The Hill force-velocity relation for muscle. *J. Theor. Biol.*, **11**, 63–86.
Carlson, F.D., and Wilkie, D.R. (1974). In: *Muscle Physiology*, Engelwood Cliffs, N.J: Prentice Hall.
Coggshall, J.C., and Bekey, G.A. (1970). EMG-force dynamics in human skeletal muscle. *Med. Biol. Eng.*, **8**, 265–270.

Crago, P.E., Lemay, M.A., and Liu, L. (1990). External control of limb movements involving environmental interactions. In: J.M. Winters and S.L-Y. Woo, eds., *Multiple Muscle Systems; Biomechanics and Movement Organization*, pp. 343–359. New York: Springer-Verlag.

Crochetiere, W.J., Vodovnik, L., and Reswick, J.B. (1967). Electrical stimulation of skeletal muscle—a study of muscle as an actuator. *Med. Biol. Eng.*, **5**, 111–125.

Durfee, W.K., and MacLean, K.E. (1989). Methods for estimating isometric recruitment curves of electrically stimulated muscle. *IEEE Trans. Biomed. Eng.*, **36** (7), 654–667.

Durfee, W.K., and Hausdorff, J.M. (1991). Regulating knee joint position by combining electrical stimulation with a controllable friction brake. *Ann. Biomed. Eng.*, in press.

Eisenberg, E., and Greene, L.E. (1980). The relation of muscle biochemistry to muscle physiology. *Ann. Rev. Physiol.*, **42**, 293–309.

Eisenberg, E. (1986). How ATP hydrolysis drives muscle contraction. *Lec. Math. Life Sci.*, **16**, 19–55.

Fang, Z.P., and Mortimer, J.T. (1987). A method for attaining natural recruitment order in artifically activated muscles. *Proc. 9th IEEE/EMBS Conf.*, 657–658.

Ford, L.E., Huxley, A.F., and Simmons, R.M. (1981). The relation between stiffness and filament overlap in stimulated frog muscle fibers. *J. Physiol.*, **311**, 219–249.

Fung, Y.C. (1981). In: *Biomechanics: Mechanical Properties of Living Tissues*, pp. 324–326. New York: Springer-Verlag.

Gasser, H.S., and Hill, A.V. (1924). The dynamics of muscular contraction, *Proc. R. Soc., Lond. [Biol.]*, **96**, 398–437.

Gordon, A.M., Huxley, A.F., and Julian, F.J. (1966). The variation in isometric tension with sarcomere length in vertebrate muscle fibers. *J. Physiol.*, **184**, 170–192.

Gottlieb, G.L., and Agarwal, G.C. (1971). Dynamic relation between isometric muscle tension and the electromyogram in man. *J. Appl. Physiol.*, **30** (3), 345–351.

Harry, J.D., Ward, A.W., Heglund, N.C., Morgan, D.L., and McMahon, T.A. (1990). Cross-bridge cycling theories cannot explain high-speed lengthening behavior in frog muscle. *Biophys. J.*, **57**, 201–208.

Hatze, H. (1973). A theory of contraction and a mathematical model of striated muscle. *J. Theor. Biol.*, **40**, 219–246.

Hatze, H. (1977). A myocybernetic control model of skeletal muscle. *Biol. Cybern.*, **25**, 103–119.

Hatze, H. (1981). In: *Myocybernetic Control Models of Skeletal Muscle*. Pretoria: University of South Africa Press.

Hatze, H. (1990). The charge-transfer model of myofilamentary interaction: Prediction of force enhancement and related myodynamic phenomena. In: J.M. Winters and S.L-Y. Woo, eds., *Multiple Muscle Systems: Biomechanics and Movement Organization*, pp. 24–45. New York: Springer-Verlag.

Hill, T.L., Eisenberg, E., Chen, Y., and Podolsky, R.J. (1975). Some self-consistent two-state sliding filament models of muscle contraction. *Biophys. J.*, **15**, 335–372.

Hill, T.L. (1977). In: *Free Energy Transduction in Biology*. New York: Academic Press.

Hill, A.V. (1938). The heat of shortening and the dynamic constants of muscle. *Proc. R. Soc., Lond. [Biol.]*, **126**, 136–195.

Hill, A.V. (1964). The effect of load on the heat of shortening of muscle. *Proc. R. Soc., Lond. [Biol.]*, **159**, 297–318.

Hogan, N. (1985a). The mechanics of multi-joint posture and movement control. *Biol. Cybern.*, **52**, 315–331.

Hogan, N. (1985b). Impedance control: An approach to manipulation. Part II—Implementation. *J. Dyn. Sys. Meas. Cont.* **107**, 8–16.

Houk, J.C., and Rymer, W.Z. (1983). Neural control of muscle length and tension. In: V.B.

Brooks, ed., *Handbook of Physiology—The Nervous System*, II, pp. 257–323. Bethesda, MD: American Physiological Society.

Hunter, I., and Korenberg, M. (1986). Identification of nonlinear biological systems: Wiener and Hammerstein cascade models. *Biol. Cybern.*, **55**, 135–144.

Huxley, A.F., and Peachey, L.D. (1961). The maximum length for contraction in vertebrate striated muscle. *J. Physiol.*, **156**, 150–165.

Huxley, A.F. (1957). Muscle structure and theories of contraction. *Prog. Biophys. Biophys. Chem.*, **7**, 257–318.

Huxley, A.F., and Simmons R.M. (1971). Proposed mechanism of force generation in striated muscle. *Nature*, **233**, 533–538.

Huxley, A.F. (1980). In: *Reflections on Muscle*. Princeton, NJ: Princeton University Press.

Huxley, A.F. (1988). Muscular contraction. *Ann. Rev. Physiol.*, **50**, 1–16.

Iwazumi, T. (1978). A new field theory of muscle contraction. In: H. Sugi and G.H. Pollack, eds., *Cross-Bridge Mechanisms in Muscle Contraction*, pp. 611–632. Baltimore: University Park Press.

Jewell, B.R., and Wilkie, D.R. (1958). An analysis of the mechanical components in frog's striated muscle. *J. Physiol.*, **143**, 515–540.

Joyce, G.C., and Rack, P.M.H. (1969). Isotonic lengthening and shortening movements of cat soleus muscle. *J. Physiol.*, **204**, 475–491.

Joyce, G.C., Rack, P.M.H., and Westbury, D.R. (1969). The mechanical properties of cat soleus muscle during controlled lengthening and shortening movements. *J. Physiol.*, **204**, 461–467.

Julian, F.J. (1969). Activation in a skeletal muscle contraction model with modification for insect fibrillar muscle. *Biophys. J.*, **9**, 547–570.

Julian, F.J., and Sollins, M.R. (1975). Variation of muscle stiffness with force at increasing speeds of shortening. *Biophys. J.*, **66**, 287–302.

Julian, F.J., and Morgan, D.L. (1979). The effect of tension on non-uniform distribution of length changes applied to frog muscle fibers. *J. Physiol.*, **293**, 379–392.

Katz, B. (1939). The relation between force and speed in muscular contraction. *J. Physiol.*, **96**, 45–64.

Klauss, P.M. (1973). A model of skeletal muscle contraction. *Tech. Rep. No. 6302-12*. Stanford, CA: Information Systems Laboratory, Stanford University.

Krausz, H.I. (1975). Identification of nonlinear systems using random impulse train inputs. *Biol. Cybern.*, **19**, 217–230.

Levin, A., and Wyman, J. (1927). The viscous elastic properties of muscle. *Proc. R. Soc., Lond. [Biol.]*, **101**, 218–243.

Little, R.C. (1969). Dynamics of stress relaxation in skeletal muscle. *Am. J. Physiol.*, **217** (6), 1665–1671.

Ma, S., and Zahalak, G.I. (1985). The mechanical response of the active human triceps brachii muscle to very rapid stretch and shortening. *J. Biomech.*, **18** (8), 585–598.

Ma, S., and Zahalak, G.I. (1987). A simple self-consistent distribution-moment model for muscle: Chemical energy and heat rates. *Math. Biosci.*, **84**, 211–230.

Ma, S., and Zahalak, G.I. (1991). A distribution-moment model of energetics in skeletal muscle. *J. Biomech.*, **24**, 21–35.

Mannard, A., and Stein, R.B. (1973). Determination of the frequency response of isometric soleus muscle in the cat using random nerve stimulation. *J. Physiol.*, **229**, 275–296.

Marmarelis, P.Z., and Naka, K.I. (1974). Identification of multi-input biological systems. *IEEE Trans. Biomed. Eng.*, **21**, 88–101.

Marmarelis, P.Z., and Marmarelis, V.Z. (1978). In: *Analysis of Physiological Systems: The White Noise Approach*. New York: Plenum Press.

McMahon, T.A. (1984). In: *Muscles, Reflexes, and Locomotion*. Princeton, NJ: Princeton University Press.

Morgan, D.L., Mochon, S., and Julian, F.J. (1982). A quantitative model of intersarcomere dynamics during fixed-end contractions of single frog muscle fibers. *Biophys. J.*, **39**, 189–196.

Morgan, D.L. (1990a). New insights into the behavior of muscle during active lengthening. *Biophys. J.*, **57**, 209–221.

Morgan, D.L. (1990b). Modelling of lengthening muscle. In: J.M. Winters and S.L.-Y. Woo, eds., *Multiple Muscle Systems: Biomechanics and Movement Organization*, pp. 46–56. New York: Springer-Verlag.

Mote, C.D., and Kuo, C.Y. (1989). Identification of knee joint models for varus-valgus or internal-external rotations: Snow skiing experiments. *J. Biomech.*, **22** (3), 245–259.

Ohnishi, T. (1963). Rheology of glycerinated muscle fibers. *Biorheology*, **1**, 83–90.

Plonsey, R. (1969). In: *Bioelectric Phenomena*. New York: McGraw-Hill.

Podolsky, R.J., and Nolan, A.C. (1973). Muscle contraction transients, cross-bridge kinetics, and the Fenn effect. *Cold Spring Harb. Symp. Quant. Biol.*, **311**, 219–249.

Pollack, G.H. (1983). The cross-bridge theory. *Physiol. Rev.*, **63**, 1049–1113.

Richmond, F.J.R., MacGillis, D.R.R., and Scott, D.A. (1985). Muscle fiber compartmentalization in cat splenius muscles. *J. Neurophysiol.*, **53** (4), 868–885.

Ritchie, J.M., and Wilkie, D.R. (1958). The dynamics of muscular contraction. *J. Physiol.*, **143**, 104–113.

Robles, S.S., and Soechting, J.F. (1979). Dynamic properties of cat tenuissimus muscle. *Biol. Cyber.*, **33**, 187–197.

Schoenberg, M. (1985). Equilibrium muscle cross-bridge behavior. Theoretical considerations. *Biophys. J.*, **48**, 467–475.

Sherif, M.H., Gregor, R.J., Liu, L.M., Roy, R.R., and Hager, C.L. (1983). Correlation of myoelectric activity and muscle force during selected cat treadmill locomotion. *J. Biomech.*, **16** (9), 691–701.

Shue, G-H. (1990). Multiplicative models of stimulated muscle for FNS control. *M. S. Dissertation*. Cleveland: Case Western Reserve University.

Smith, D.A. (1990). The theory of sliding filament models for muscle contraction. III. Dynamics of the five-state model. *J. Theor. Biol.*, **146**, 433–466.

Soechting, J.F., and Roberts, W.J. (1975). Transfer characteristics between EMG activity and muscle tension under isometric conditions in man. *J. Physiol. [Paris]*, **70**, 779–793.

Solomonow, M., Baratta, R., Zhou, B-H., Shoji, H., and D'Ambrosia, R.D. (1987). The EMG-force model of electrically stimulated muscle: Dependence on control strategy and predominant fiber composition. *IEEE Trans. Biomed. Eng.*, **34** (9), 692–703.

Squire, J.M. (1986). In: *Muscle: Design, Diversity, and Disease*. Menlo Park, CA: Benjamin/Cummings.

Stein, R.B., and Wong, E.Y. (1974). Analysis of models for the activation and contraction of muscle. *J. Theor. Biol.*, **46**, 307–327.

Stein, R.B., and Oguztoreli, M.N. (1976). Tremor and other oscillations in neuromuscular systems. *Biol. Cybern.*, **22**, 147–157.

Tirosh, R., Liron, N., and Oplatka, A. (1978). A hydrodynamic mechanism for muscular contraction. In: H. Sugi and G.H. Pollack, eds., *Cross-Bridge Mechanisms in Muscle Contraction*, pp. 593–609. Baltimore: University Park Press.

Tozeren, A., and Schoenberg, M. (1986). The effect of cross-bridge clustering and head-head competition on the mechanical response of skeletal muscle fibers under equilibrium conditions. *Biophys. J.*, **50**, 873–884.

Tozeren, A. (1987). The influence of doubly attached crossbridges on the mechanical behavior of skeletal muscle fibers under equilibrium conditions. *Biophys. J.*, **52**, 901–906.

Truong, X.T. (1972). Viscoelastic wave propagation and rheologic properties of skeletal muscle. *Am. J. Physiol.*, **226** (2), 256–264.
Truong, X.T. (1972). Visco-elastic propagation of longitudinal waves in skeletal muscle. *J. Biomech.*, **5**, 1–10.
van Ingen Schenau, G.J., Bobbert, M.F., Ettema, G.J., de Graaf, J.B., and Huijing, P.A. (1988). Simulation of rat EDL force output based on intrinsic muscle properties. *J. Biomech.*, **21**, 815–824.
Volterra, V. (1930). *Theory of Functionals*. Glasgow: Blackie and Sons, Ltd.
Wilkie, D.R. (1954). Facts and theories about muscle. *Prog. Biophys.*, **4**, 288–324.
Williams, W.J., and Edwin, A.I. (1971). An electronic muscle stimulator for demonstration and neuromuscular systems modelling. *Med. Biol. Eng.*, **22**, 29–74.
Winters, J.M. (1985). Generalized analysis and design of antagonistic muscle models: Effect of nonlinear muscle properties on the control of fundamental movements. *Ph.D. Dissertation*. Berkeley, CA: University of California.
Winters, J.M. (1990). Hill-based muscle models: A systems engineering perspective. In: J.M. Winters and S.L-Y. Woo, eds., *Multiple Muscle Systems: Biomechanics and Movement Organization*, pp. 69–93. New York: Springer-Verlag.
Woledge, R.C., Curtin, N.A., and Homsher, E. (1985). In: *Energetic Aspects of Muscle Contraction*. New York: Academic Press.
Wood, J.E. (1976). Theoretical formalism for kinesiological trajectories of a computer simulated neuro-musculo-skeletal system, *Ph.D. Dissertation*, Massachusetts Institute of Technology, Cambridge, MA.
Wood, J.E., and Mann, R.W. (1981). A sliding-filament cross-bridge ensemble model of muscle contraction for mechanical transients. *Math. Biosci.*, **57**, 211–263.
Zahalak, G.I., and Heyman, S.J. (1979). A quantitative evaluation of the frequency-response characteristics of human skeletal muscle in-vivo. *J. Biomech., Eng.*, **101** (1), 28–37.
Zahalak, G.I. (1981). A distribution-moment approximation for kinetic theories of muscular contraction. *Math. Biosci.*, **55**, 89–114.
Zahalak, G.I. (1983). Predictions of the existence, frequency and amplitude of physiological tremor in normal man based on measured frequency-response characteristics. *J. Biomech. Eng.*, **105**, 249–257.
Zahalak, G.I. (1986). A comparison of the mechanical behavior of the cat soleus muscle with a distribution-monment model. *J. Biomech. Eng.*, **108**, 131–140.
Zahalak, G.I. (1990). Modelling muscle mechanics (and energetics). In: J.M. Waters and S.L-Y. Woo, eds., *Multiple Systems: Biomechanics and Movement Organization*, pp. 1–23. New York: Springer-Verlag.
Zahalak, G.I., and Ma, S.-P. (1990). Muscle activation and contraction: Constitutive relations based directly on cross-bridge kinetics. *J. Biomech. Eng.*, **112**, 52–62.
Zajac, F.E. (1989). Muscle and tendon: Properties: Models, scaling, and application to biomechanics and motor control. *CRC Crit. Rev. Biomed. Eng.*, **17**, 359–411.
Zhou, B-H., Baratta, R., and Solomonow, M. (1987). Manipulation of muscle force with various firing rate and recruitment control strategies. *IEEE Trans. Biomed. Eng.*, **34** (2), 128–139.

3
Model Identification in Neural Prosthesis Systems

WILLIAM K. DURFEE

Motor neural prostheses are complex engineering systems which place the human musculoskeletal system under the control of artificial stimulation input to the muscles. In designing a neural prosthesis, the engineer attempts to develop a mathematical description of the system to predict its mechanical behavior under a variety of specified inputs and external loading. This is an analysis problem whose success at prediction depends on the accuracy of the mathematical model. The engineer will also use models during the process of control system design and testing through simulation. Here the accuracy of the model is a critical factor in the ability to design effective controllers. This chapter discusses model structure and identification of model parameters for stimulated muscle in the context of neural prostheses. The chapter opens with an overview of model-based control for neural prostheses. Next, established engineering methods for system identification are discussed. Following that, basic musculoskeletal system models are reviewed with particular emphasis on model identification. Finally, an overview of the author's own research in muscle model identification is provided.

The task of model identification is intimately tied to the task of control, as is made clear if one consults Chapter 14 of this book. Simple neural prosthesis controllers can be designed and tuned with no models and therefore have no need for parameter identification. An example is the four-channel, "withdrawal-reflex" paraplegic gait restoration paradigm which was initiated by the research group in Ljubljana, Yugoslavia (Kralj et al., 1980, 1983), and replicated by many others around the world (Peckham, 1987). Here, stimulation parameters are set through trial-and-error tuning while the subject walks, with either subjective or objective measures of gait quality serving as the controller performance indicator. It is also possible to tune basic proportional-derivative (PD) closed-loop controllers in much the same manner (Durfee and Hausdorff, 1990), since a skilled practitioner can iterate rapidly to values of the two feedback gains which are near optimum. In this case, one treats the musculoskeletal system as simply a black box that produces a force or motion output for a stimulus input.

The practice of designing control systems without the use of models breaks down when anything other than rudimentary performance is required. Functional electrical stimulation (FES) aided quadriplegic grasp restoration systems which seek to restore fine grasp, or FES-aided gait systems which aim to achieve acceptably fast walking velocities can only be realized through the implementation of advanced control strategies which depend on accurate models for their success. A feedback controller with more than two gain settings cannot be tuned by trial-and-error iteration but must be set through analytical methods, saving only the final tuning for the implementation stage. Likewise, a feedback linearization controller, which cancels nonlinearities by inverting the plant, requires a model of the plant to invert. All advanced controllers can be designed more effectively if simulations are conducted in advance to predict the performance of the neural prosthesis system before the hardware is implemented.

Neural prosthesis systems are complex. The stimulated musculoskeletal system has multiple degrees of freedom with nonlinear, time-varying dynamics. Further, gait restoration neural prostheses must work to control a statically unstable plant. Clearly, success in synthesizing control designs or in creating an accurate control system analysis requires the use of musculoskeletal models, and the assignment of parameters to those models.

Parameter identification of models cannot be conducted in isolation from a set of overall objectives which, in the context of this book, are the design and analysis of neural prosthesis controllers. Here, we are not concerned with elucidating the biophysics of muscular contractions or with understanding the mechanics of skeletal structure, but rather in defining and using models suitable for control. The discussion of identification techniques and experimental results presented in this chapter is therefore driven by the application.

BASIC IDENTIFICATION METHODS

This section reviews basic methods for system identification, while the remaining sections demonstrate the use of these methods in neural prosthesis applications. Because this is an overview chapter which seeks to reach a wide audience, mathematical rigor will be set aside in favor of intuitive reasoning. The references provide a resource for the interested reader to explore further.

Parametric and Nonparametric Model Descriptions

There are two approaches to developing models for predicting the behavior of a given physical system. Figure 3–1 shows a basic, single-input, single-output (SISO) system where $u(t)$ describes the input as a function of time and $y(t)$ the output. One

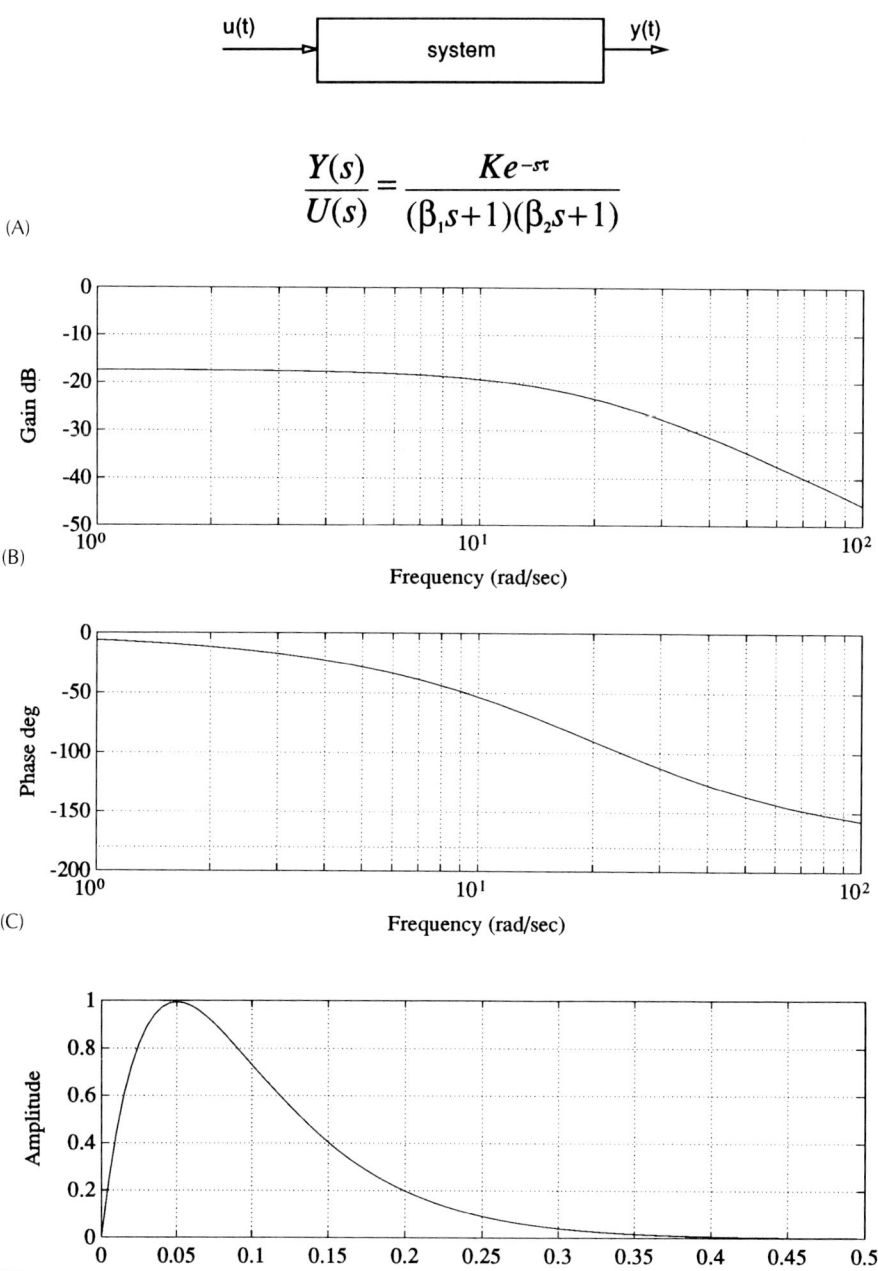

Figure 3–1 Single-input, single-output (SISO) systems. (A) Block diagram form. (B) Parametric model in transfer function form. (C) Nonparametric description in frequency (magnitude and phase plots) response form. (D) Nonparametric description in impulse response form.

example of such a system might be a model of isometric muscle producing force in response to electrical stimulation. The first approach to modeling such a system is to work from basic physical principles; that is, to use the available knowledge of the underlying physics to develop a set of static or dynamic equations which describe the system behavior. As described in Chapter 2 of this book, for the muscle system, this might be a Huxley-type model based on what is known about the sliding-filament theory of muscle contraction (Huxley, 1974). It might also be a model whose equation structure is developed by observing the basic input-output mechanical behavior of activated muscle, leading to Hill-type model forms (Hill, 1938, Winters, 1990). These forms are known as *parametric* models because the structure of the model (and therefore the equations) is fixed, while the parameters of the equations are free to be adjusted to fit the particular muscle of interest.

In many cases, the physical system is so complex, or so little is known, that model building from first principles is ineffective. Here, one can still gain considerable insight into the behavior of the system through *nonparametric* modeling, where no assumptions are made about the structure of the system. Instead, the system is viewed as a "black box" described by one or more functions which completely characterize the input-output behavior. For linear systems, these functions are usually either the impulse response of the system (a function of time) or the frequency response of the system (a function of frequency), both of which describe the system completely (Ogata, 1990). Nonparametric models are also known as "black-box models" or "functional models."

Figure 3–1 shows an example of these model representations. In Figure 3–1B, a parametric model of the system is given, represented as a second-order transfer function with an added constant delay (it could just as easily be represented by a set of two, coupled linear differential equations). The parameters which must be fit are the two time constants β_1 and β_2, the time delay τ, and the DC gain K. This model has been shown to be effective in describing the response of cat hind limb muscle to a sinusoidally varying stimulation input (Baratta and Solomonow, 1990). An equivalent nonparametric model is shown in Figure 3–1C, which displays the frequency response; and another nonparametric form is shown in Figure 3–1D, which displays the impulse response. Although parametric model forms may be more satisfying because they nominally reveal the inner construction of a system, either form can be used for the prediction of system behavior and for the design of controllers.

Linear System Identification

Methods for identifying parameters of linear system models are highly developed and are used throughout many fields of engineering. Software which implements reliable algorithms is readily available. The relative ease of parameter identification is one reason why musculoskeletal systems have often been represented by linear models in neural prosthesis modeling and control-design studies. Experimentally, a lengthy, pseudorandom sequence is applied to an input of the system of interest, and the resulting output measured for off-line analysis by the algorithm. The SISO systems are the simplest to handle, although some work has been done on methods for multiple-input, multiple-output (MIMO) systems. The standard identification algorithms are particularly well suited for models which neglect the underlying physiology and anatomy of the musculoskeletal system and instead represent its behavior with simple models described by a handful of linear coefficients. Although one could argue convincingly that these models cannot possibly represent the full complexity of the musculoskeletal system, they still deserve careful consideration simply because they are backed with powerful, reliable methods for identification.

Nonparametric linear models are developed using one or more sets of input-output data to generate estimates of the system frequency response functions using spectral methods. If necessary, these can then be transformed into time-domain impulse response functions. For parametric linear models, a model structure is chosen by specifying the order of the system based on expectations of system complexity and on how much detail is required of the model. Parametric algorithms generally use least-squares minimization or maximum likelihood methods to fit the parameters so that when the input excitation sequence is applied to the model, its output represents the best match to the experimentally determined output. Examples of software packages which implement these algorithms include the *Systems Identification Toolbox* of MATLAB (MathWorks, 1990) and *Numerical Recipes* (Press et al., 1986).

Nonlinear System Identification

Identification of nonlinear systems is much less developed, and indeed a search of the literature for available methods to handle a particular problem generally ends in disappointment. This is not surprising given the complexity and variety of behaviors which are possible when the constraint of linearity is lifted. Few biological systems are linear, however, forcing the researcher who must simulate or control neural prosthesis systems to either linearize the response about a nominal operating point or to make do with one of the limited choices for nonlinear analysis.

Nonlinear, black-box models can be identified nonparametrically using functional series methods. By exciting a nonlinear system with a white-noise input and measuring the resulting ouput, a set of functionals can be computed which describe the system behavior. The most common form of these functionals are a set of Wiener kernels, an infinite series of functions $\{h_0, h_1, h_2, \ldots\}$ which are the nonlinear equivalent of the linear system impulse response. Given a complete set of kernels, one can predict the response of the system to any input. Further, the Wiener kernel series give the best (in a statistical sense) representation of the system for any state of the series truncation. For example, $\{h_0\}$ is the average DC response of the system, $\{h_0, h_1\}$ is the best linear-system response, and the set $\{h_0, h_1, h_2\}$ provides the best second-order nonlinear representation. Since computation of the kernels is unwieldy, truncation of the series at second order is common. The second-order representation is sufficiently powerful to predict the time-varying response of some biological systems to two impulses spaced by a variable time delay, or the nonlinear response to a continuous sinusoidal input (Marmarelis and Marmarelis, 1978). Wiener methods have also been used to model slow, tetanic potentiation and nonlinear impulse summation in isometric contractions of cat muscles (Parmiggiani et al., 1982). The power of functional series methods are their generality, since no assumptions need

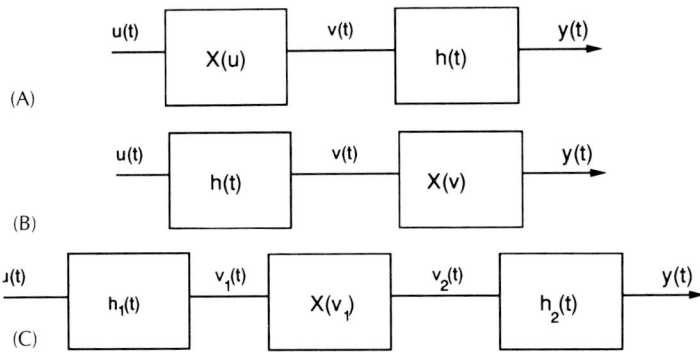

Figure 3–2 Cascaded block structure nonlinear systems. $X(u)$ is a static function relating output to input while $h(t)$ are linear dynamics expressed in impulse response form. (A) Hammerstein form. (B) Wiener form. (C) General form.

be made about the underlying system which produces the set of input-output sequences used for computing the kernel. This power is also the root of the weakness evident in these methods. First, computing the kernels is numerically intensive so that systems containing nonlinearities which require description by higher than second-order kernels (e.g., hard nonlinearities such as dead zones or hysteresis) cannot be accurately identified. Second, interpretation of the kernel functions is nonintuitive. Third, there are no means of relating the kernels to the physical processes underlying the system and also no means of incorporating a priori information about the system into the identification process.

If the system of interest can be represented as a cascaded structure of linear dynamic blocks and nonlinear static blocks, several possibilities for identification arise. Three examples of these block-oriented system representations are displayed in Figure 3–2 where $u(t)$ and $y(t)$ are the input and output functions of time, $X(u)$ is a nonlinear function whose current output depends only on its current input, $h(t)$ is the impulse response of a linear system, and $v(t)$ is an internal (and in many cases fictional) signal which cannot be measured. Depending on the arrangement of the blocks, these representations are known as Hammerstein models (Figure 3–2A), Wiener models (Figure 3–2B), or general block-oriented models (Figure 3–2C). General methods for simultaneous identification of both linear and nonlinear blocks for Hammerstein and Wiener models are presented in a paper by Hunter and Korenberg (1986). Although the class of physiologic systems which can be realistically partitioned into cascaded blocks is limited, isometric, electrically stimulated muscle can be represented effectively by a Hammerstein model where $h(t)$ is a linear system with second-order dynamics, and $X(u)$ represents the nonlinear recruitment curve (Durfee and MacLean, 1989). Two specific cases of isometric-stimulated muscle identification where muscle is represented in this Hammerstein form are presented below in the section on experimental muscle-model identification.

Parametric nonlinear models have a structure described by a set of nonlinear algebraic or differential equations where functions or parameters of the equations are unknown. For nonlinear systems, these equations are generally developed based on a knowledge of or assumptions about the underlying physics which determine the behavior of a system. Unlike linear systems where black-box parameterized models can be developed simply by specifying a system order, some information about the fundamental nature of the system is required for nonlinear systems.

Some nonlinear models can be structured as a linear combination of functions. These models have the form

$$y(x) = \sum_{k=1}^{M} a_k X_k(x)$$

where the set $\{X_1(x), \ldots, X_M(x)\}$ are arbitrary basis functions. For example, one common choice of basis functions are powers of x, which results in polynomial fitting. General linear least-squares methods can be used to identify the parameter set $\{a_1, \ldots, a_M\}$ where the solutions are found using Gaussian elimination or singular value decomposition techniques (Press et al., 1986).

Most model structures relevant to neural prostheses are nonlinear in the parameters. For example, a Hill hyperbolic muscle force-velocity relation is parameterized by three parameters which appear nonlinearly in the equation (Winters, 1990). If the model is in a form where its output can be differentiated with respect to each of the parameters to form a gradient matrix, the parameters can be identified through a nonlinear least-squares algorithm which seeks to minimize the prediction errors between the experimental and model output (Goodwin and Sin, 1984). This method has been applied successfully to the identification of a nonlinear model for electrically stimulated muscle (Shue, 1990), which will be described below in the section on muscle-model applications. A second form of nonlinear least-squares identification is the Levenberg-Marquardt method which is based on a steepest descent process (Press et al., 1986). Another parametric identification method is to replace unknown, continuous nonlinear functions in a model structure with piecewise linear approximations, and then to use a least-squares fitting algorithm to identify the segments, a process referred to as "self-modeling" (Lawton et al., 1972). This approach has been used by the author's group at MIT for stimulated muscle-model identification (Palmer, 1990), a study which will also be described in more detail below.

Model Verification

A danger inherent in the ready accessibility of system identification methods is the ease with which they can be applied without regard for model verification. It is simple to generate a completely parameterized model for a complex physiological system. It is a much more difficult problem to verify that the model is correct. A good identification process will yield not only the model parameters, but also estimates of the parameter errors, and a statistical description of how well the model fits the measured data.

There are two components to model verification. First, the errors between the model and experimental output must be examined statistically using methods established for the particular identification algorithm. If the model is perfect, all of the error should be attributed to noise. The second component of validation is to test the *predictive* capabilities of the model. Here the model output is compared to experimental output using an input-output sequence which is different from that used to generate the model. If the errors are unacceptably large, the methods have only produced data fitting not identification, and the results will be of little value in simulation or control design applications.

MUSCULOSKELETAL SYSTEM MODELS

To design a controller for a motor neural prosthesis, one must develop an accurate model of the musculoskeletal system, the "plant" to be controlled. The neural prosthesis control designer is usually not concerned with modeling or analyzing the behavior of the central nervous system (CNS), which is fortunate, since the complexity of the CNS has yet to lend itself to effective modeling at anything other than a superficial level of detail. Instead, the remnant actions of the CNS on the neural prosthesis (e.g., the spastic reflexes commonly seen in spinal-cord-injured individuals) can be modeled as disturbances. The plant, therefore, consists of the skeletal links, the joints, and the musculotendon actuators[1]. For a review of how this system is modeled by the motor-control community, the reader is referred to the book edited by Winters and Woo (1990) and to Zajac and Gordon (1989). For an example of how the musculoskeletal plant can be modeled to perform simulations of dynamic gait with applications to neural prostheses, see Yamaguchi et al. (1990). Here only a brief overview is given with an emphasis on how models for each component of the system can be parameterized.

The final output of a neural prosthesis is seen through the motion of limb segments. For gait prostheses, the inertial behavior of the lower limb segments in response to gravitational loads, and joint torques exerted by the muscles dominate the dynamic response of the system. An example of the importance of limb dynamics can be found in the work of Zajac's group, which has demonstrated effectively that the action of any lower limb muscle has an effect on all of the lower limb segments due to the inertial coupling properties of the lower limb (Zajac and Gordon, 1989). For grasp prostheses, the inertia of the hand and finger limb segments is small, but the kinematics must be known accurately if precision grasping tasks are to be analyzed.

The necessity for simplification and approximation appears immediately on determining the kinematic degrees of freedom for a musculoskeletal model. Many modeling studies of gait have restricted themselves to a sagittal plane model to retain the simplicity of two-dimensional dynamic equations. Most would agree, however, that hip adduction-abduction, pelvic lateral translation, and ankle inversion-eversion are necessary for a complete description of gait, forcing a three-dimensional model. More complications arise when joint motions are considered. A full analysis of the knee joint requires a description of its motion in six degrees of freedom as well as the addition of motion constraints produced by the ligaments. During swing phase, the motion of the knee joint has been compared to that of a trunk top moving on loose strap hinges (Murphy et al., 1984). More discussion of the degree of freedom problem can be found in Yamaguchi (1990).

Unfortunately, there are few good methods for identifying skeletal geometry and limb inertias, even with simplified limb kinetics. As reviewed in Yamaguchi et al. (1990), most information on link lengths and limb inertias have been obtained from a limited number of cadaver dissection studies. This presents two problems. First, tissue properties begin to change immediately following death (e.g., muscle tissue shrinks as it desiccates), which will change inertial estimates. Second, and more severe, is that insufficient information is available to determine how geometric and inertial parameters scale with size and weight of a particular subject. Intuitively, one might simply scale skeletal link lengths by normalizing to the subject's height, but such uniform scaling methods are bound to contain errors. Recent advances in medical imaging techniques, and particularly in magnetic resonance imaging (MRI) methods, may provide a more reliable means of estimating anatomical data on a subject-by-subject basis (Brown et al., 1987).

Similar difficulties arise when estimating the geometric properties of the musculotendon actuators. In particular, estimation of muscle origins, insertions, path lengths, and joint moment arms can only be achieved through unsatisfying approximations, where the problems result from the inherent complexity of the biological system and inadequate identification methods. To keep models tractable, not all muscles can be modeled, and for those that are, simplifications must be made such as reducing line insertions to one or more point insertions. Muscle path-length information can again come from cadaver studies, which must necessarily neglect the change in path (and therefore joint moment arm) as an active muscle generates tension.

The remaining element of a complete musculoskeletal model are the musculotendon actuators. Muscle has been modeled as a simple torque generator, as a spring, as variants of Hill-type models which combine a force-generating element with a mechanical network of energy storage and dissipation elements, and as variants of Huxley-type models based on biophysical cross-bridge mechanics. The reader is referred to Chapter 2 of this book as well as to several chapters of Winters and Woo (1990) for comprehensive reviews of these models, which will not be repeated here.[2] It should be remembered that muscle has two inputs, neural activation and kinematic configuration. It is convenient to view the kinematic configuration as a muscle length input, and muscle velocity input (although the two are mathematically related), and to describe the muscle as a three-input system. All three of these inputs have a strong influence on muscle input force.[3] Because of this three-input, single-output system, where the output depends nonlinearly on all three inputs, nonparametric identification methods (which are optimized for SISO nonlinear systems) will have limited utility.

Before a musculotendon model can be used in simulation or control design, parameters must be identified and assigned. These can be derived either through scaling values found in the literature or through direct, experimental measures using the methods described in the prior section. An example of the former can be found in the work of Hatze (1977, 1978); who created a series of complex, nonlinear muscle models based on sliding-filament mechanics, and used them to predict the behavior of human motion. Because much of the model is based on experimental evidence derived from frog and cat muscle, one is forced into numerous assumptions and extrapolations to assign values to the many constants contained in the model. Examples of the latter, experimental methods are covered in the next section of this chapter. Here, direct measurements minimize the number of assumptions required to parameterize the model.

In applying musculotendon models to neural prostheses and in planning identification strategies, one must consider the unique features inherent to electrically stimulated muscle. Most importantly, the muscle activation input provided by the stimulation is not the same as the normal input from the CNS. For example, the surface electrodes commonly used in simple, lower limb neural prostheses provide little selectivity over the actual muscle stimulated, particularly in regions where muscles are densely packed. Even if the electrode is placed directly over the muscle, spillover to adjacent muscles is likely to occur as the stimulation activation level is increased. Another possibility with surface electrodes is that the entire muscle bulk may not be activated, even at high stimulus strengths. Nerve cuff electrodes alleviate these difficulties, but the activation is still nonphysiologic. Motor units are stimulated synchronously and at high frequency to generate smooth, fused contractions. Since the stimulation frequency is generally fixed, additional force is generated solely through modulation of current pulse strength rather than by mimicking the combined rate and recruitment strategy used by the CNS. Recruitment of additional motor units depends on the local current densities surrounding the electrodes, and on the diameter and proximity of the motor unit axon. Typically this results in reverse size-order principle recruitment with large motor units activated at low stimulus current levels. With large motor units being fired at artificially high stimulation frequencies, the muscle output force will show rapid fatigue, which presents the experimenter with a time-varying system to identify, or with the prospect of developing fatigue models. Usually, this problem is ignored and the experiment designed with bouts of stimulation surrounded by long rest periods to minimize fatigue. One then can argue that the resulting parameterized model would not be valid for the continous use that is seen in a neural prosthesis.

Some methods do exist to make stimulated muscle more "normal." First, in clinical applications of neural prostheses, the muscles of interest undergo a program of chronic stimulation which both strengthens the muscle contractions and increases the proportion of slow-fatiguing fibers (Peckham et al., 1976). Second, if nerve cuff electrodes are used, methods exist to provide size-order recruitment through either anodal block principles (Fang and Mortimer, 1987) or through high-frequency blocking (Baratta et al., 1989; Zhou and Baratta, 1987). Also, one can build cuff electrodes with multiple contacts and rotate the stimulation so that individual axons are stimulated only once per cycle, but the total contraction remains fused (Petrofsky, 1978; Rack and Westbury, 1969). Third, some work has been done in combined rate and recruitment control to modulate stimulated muscle force (Chizeck et al., 1991; Zhou and Baratta, 1987).

Despite the pessimistic picture which has been painted of modeling and parameter estimation for musculoskeletal systems, one should not lose sight of the objective. Even a crude model of the lower limb can reveal major features of the coupled dynamics, which in turn can lead to new methods and new ideas for the design of gait restoration systems. Models will only fail if they are extrapolated into operating regions beyond their error limits, which will happen if high-performance control systems with extreme sensitivity to modeling error are designed. The appropriate choice for the neural prosthesis control designer is to recognize and accept the errors inherent in musculoskeletal models, and to design robust control systems which explicitly account for those errors. Chapter 14 of this book explores this relation between modeling errors and controllers in some detail.

EXPERIMENTS IN MUSCLE-MODEL IDENTIFICATION

The remainder of this chapter reviews a selection of experimental studies concerned with muscle-model identification. Of the many reports on muscle-model parameters which can be found in the literature, this review will be limited to those studies which have direct application to neural prosthesis control. In particular, only stimulation experiments of isolated muscle in animal models will be discussed. Although the objective of muscle-model verification is to reveal properties of stimulated human muscle (more specifically, paralyzed human muscle), there are several advantages which draw researchers to animal model experiments. Most importantly, well-controlled experiments can be designed using animal models. Single muscles can be surgically isolated and fixed to accurate length, velocity, and force transducers. The muscle tendons (or limb joints) can also be fixed to servomotor systems which can apply controlled length, velocity, or force inputs to the muscle, or which can be set under computer control to present generalized second-order loads such as springs, masses, and dampers to the muscle. Electrodes can be surgically implanted, including cuff electrodes which wrap around the nerve branch leading to the muscle, intrafascicular electrodes which are implanted inside the nerve, epimysial electrodes which are fixed to the surface of the muscle, or coiled-wire intramuscular electrodes which are embedded in the muscle. The ability to place electrodes in precise locations enables the application of stable, controlled stimulation activation to the muscle of interest. Along with accurate measurements and controlled input, animal models allow the design of complete experimental procedures for identification without concern for the overall length of the experiment, often a limiting factor in human subject experimentation.

This section will cover identification work in both linear and nonlinear muscle models. Most neural prosthesis identification studies have been concerned with properties of isometric muscle, although recent work has lifted this important restriction.

Linear, Isometric Models

Several groups have investigated isolated, isometric muscle with the objective of fitting the observed output force in response to stimulation to a linear (typically second-order) model. Partridge (1965) conducted one of the first of these studies. He subjected isolated cat hindlimb muscles to stimulation inputs where the pulse amplitude (PA) was fixed, and the interpulse interval (IPI) was varied sinusoidally. By applying a swept-frequency ramp of IPI sinusoidal variation, the resulting sinusoidal force output was fit to the transfer function of a second-order linear system. Mannard and Stein (1973) repeated these studies in the cat soleus muscle, but this time randomly varied IPI and used efficient, spectral methods to fit the force to a second-order system, one of the standard linear nonparametric identification methods described above. An ideal digital filter was applied to convert the stimulus pulse input to a continuous signal appropriate for the identification algorithm (French and

Holden, 1971a). The parameters describing the second-order system transfer function (gain, natural frequency, and damping ratio) varied with muscle length and number of active motor units. Recently, Baratta and Solomonow (1990) returned to this problem, but this time applied a "physiologically correct" stimulation input where muscle force was modulated through size-ordered recruitment of motor units combined with firing rate modulation which matched that found through electromyographic (EMG) studies of human muscle contraction. For nine cat hindlimb muscles, these authors demonstrated good fits to second-order, critically damped linear transfer functions to which was added a transmission delay. The poles ranged from 1.55 to 2.8 Hz depending on the muscle. That the pole locations were considerably slower than those found by either of the prior studies demonstrates the dependence of the identification study on the particular input used.

When the term "isometric" is used in the context of stimulation experiments, in most cases it does not mean that the contractile element (CE) of muscle is being held constant because of the influence of the series element (SE). The SE is viewed generally as being contained both in the contractile tissue and in the tendon. Fixing the limbs or clamping the end of a tendon does not hold the CE isometric, but rather holds the entire musculotendon actuator isometric. Thus experiments which attempt to determine the force-length properties of the CE by measuring force-length properties of the musculotendon actuator or by measuring joint moment-angle relations are in error because of the SE. Accurate measurement of the SE force-length relation is difficult, and therefore is generally ignored in the identification experiments found in the neural prosthesis literature. The importance of the SE, however, is demonstrated in the simulation studies of Zajac (1989). Further examples which emphasize the necessity of including tendon elasticity in muscle models are provided by the experiments of Griffiths (1987) and the experiments of Hoffer (1989). Both have generated direct, simultaneous measurements of musculotendon length and muscle fiber length, and have showed that large joint angle excursions are possible with almost no muscle fiber length changes.

For more discussion of the importance of the SE, and of existing methods for measuring SE properties, see Winters (1990). One should remember, however, that both the SE and the CE are *conceptual concepts* of the Hill model and are only loosely related to anatomical structures.

Linear, Nonisometric Models

Bawa et al. extended their experimentation with isolated muscle stimulation to cases of contracting against elastic (Bawa et al., 1976a) and inertial (Bawa et al., 1976b) loads, demonstrating reasonable fits to second-order linear models. As shown in Bawa et al. (1976b), the results could be explained by a linearized Hill model with a contractile component consisting of a contractile element in series with a linearized series elastic element. The CE model consisted of a force generator with first-order dynamics in parallel with a linear spring and a linear damper. This model contained no force-length relation and assumed linear force-velocity behavior. The model fit experimental results for the plantaris muscle, but significant nonlinearities were observed for the soleus.

Although linear muscle models may appear oversimplified and therefore inadequate for neural prosthesis applications, identifying the model parameters is considerably simpler than identifying the parameters of nonlinear models. Thus a linear model may be appropriate as a base for controller design. The control strategy must, however, be robust to deviations from linear behavior exhibited by the actual muscle.

Nonlinear, Isometric Models

One of the difficulties with linear models of isometric muscle is their inability to characterize the electrode recruitment properties as reflected in the isometric recruitment curve (IRC). The IRC is defined as the static gain between stimulus activation level and output muscle force when the muscle is held isometric. A typical IRC will exhibit a dead zone, a high-slope, monotonically increasing region, and a saturation region whose shape can be explained by the size and location distribution of individual motor unit axons within the nerve (Crago et al., 1980b; Durfee and MacLean, 1989; Grandjean and Mortimer, 1986; McNeal, 1976). A simple model to explain isometric muscle behavior can be derived by block partitioning the system into a Hammerstein structure (Figure 3–2A), where the static nonlinearity represents the IRC, and all of the muscle dynamics are assumed to be linear. This model ignores the nonlinear dynamics due to differences in twitch contraction time of motor units, ignores neural transmission and excitation-contraction time delays, and ignores time-varying properties such as muscle potentiation and fatigue. Nevertheless, its simplicity dictates its choice in many neural prosthesis applications.

Bernotas et al. (1986) used a recursive least-squares method to identify the dynamic part of this model and found a close fit to a second-order system with two poles and a single zero. By using a pseudorandom binary sequence (PRBS) input which switched back and forth between two stimulus-activation values only, the dynamics could be identified independently from the IRC. On-line recursive algorithms with a variable "forgetting factor" have the advantage of tracking the slow time variations commonly seen in stimulated muscle systems. In a related study this group implemented a direct adaptive controller for control of stimulated muscle force, demonstrating the close relation between system identification and adaptive control methodologies (Bernotas et al., 1987). The nonlinear IRC was modeled as a time-varying linear gain where the gain parameter was tracked by the controller.

Chia et al. (1991) developed a constrained, recursive parameter identification method to simultaneously identify both the IRC and the linear dynamics in a Hammerstein model of stimulated muscle. The recruitment curve was modeled as a shifted, third-order polynomial (to enable a least-squares identification approach), while the dynamics were modeled as second order. A constraint was applied to force the recursive algorithm to restrict the polynomial to be monotonically increasing. A value for the polynomial shift, corresponding to the stimulation dead zone, was identified in an experiment conducted prior to the main identification run. Application of the constraint, which is well justified on physiologic grounds, resulted in considerable improvement in model fits, demonstrating the value of embedding known facts about the system into the identification process.

Another method for simultaneous identification of both the linear dynamics and nonlinear statics of a Hammerstein model has been developed by Hunter and Korenberg (1986). A stochastic input is applied to the system, and an iterative method

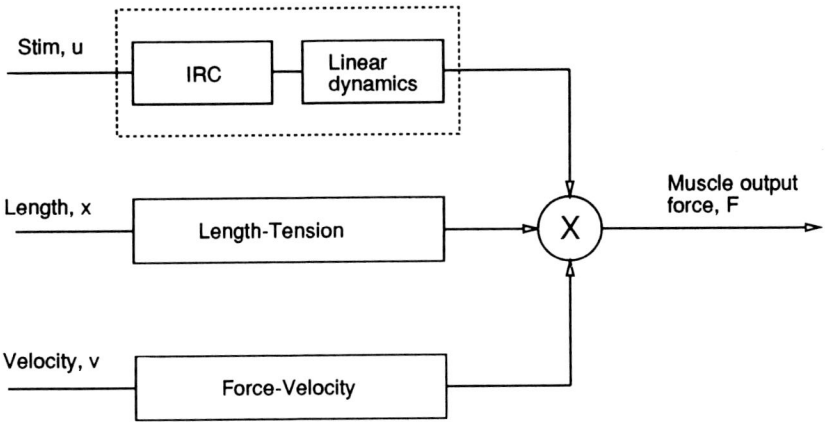

Figure 3-3 Multiplicative model of muscle contraction force. The top block passes the stimulus activation input through a static nonlinearity representing the recruitment characteristics, and a linear dynamic system representing the muscle activation dynamics. The middle box is a nonlinear length-tension relation, and the lower box is a nonlinear force-velocity relation.

used to converge on a polynomial approximation to the statics, and on a nonparametric impulse response description of the dynamics. This method was used by the author's group to identify the recruitment curve and linear dynamics of isometric muscle, achieving excellent results in simulations, but needs further work in noise reduction to produce acceptable results with experimental data (MacLean, 1988).

Nonlinear, Nonisometric Models

Practical applications of electrical stimulation in neural prostheses requires that the limbs, and therefore the muscles, move. Identification methods must be expanded to cover parameterization of muscle models over the complete range of length, velocity, and stimulation activation.

With a full nonlinear, nonisometric system, a model structure must be chosen carefully. As always, there is a tradeoff between a model which adequately describes stimulated muscle behavior, and one whose parameters can be identified through the set of available measurements. In this respect, variations of Hill-type models appear at this time to be the most appropriate for identification.

For neural prosthesis applications, Crago et al. (1990) switched from the traditional, Hill-type model-based picture of the CE as a parallel force generator and nonlinear dashpot, to a block diagram formulation where output force is the product of (1) activation dynamics which take the form of the isometric Hammerstein model described above, (2) the muscle length-tension relation, and (3) the muscle force-velocity relation (Figure 3-3). The features and assumptions of this model will be discussed below in the context of the author's own work. In simulation work by Geng (1989) and related experimental work by Shue (1990), it was demonstrated that a simplified model in this form could be identified by a sequential nonlinear least-squares algorithm (Goodwin and Sin, 1984). The simplified model assumed linear, second-order activation dynamics described by two time constants and a linear gain. The length-tension behavior was modeled as a linear relationship with a single slope, and the force-velocity as a piecewise linear relation with one slope for lengthening and a second for shortening. This model has the advantage of being completely identified by six parameters (the two activation time constants, the activation gain, the slope of the length-tension curve, and the two slopes of the force-velocity curve), which can be recursively identified on-line using random stimulus activation and muscle length records as inputs. The price paid for the reduced model can be seen in the experimental results where force prediction was acceptable (under 18%) for modest length and velocity perturbations, but errors grew rapidly for large length excursions where the assumptions of linear length-tension and a piecewise linear force-velocity relation were no longer valid. If operation of the neural prosthesis remains within a modest range of operating values, and if one assumes that behavior outside of the model can be treated as a disturbance by a robust control algorithm, this simple model is still of great value.

MUSCLE MODEL IDENTIFICATION WORK AT MIT

The muscle model identification work of the author's research group at MIT will now be reviewed briefly. One of the goals of this work is to explore the relation between complexity of the muscle model and the control algorithm used for a neural prosthesis. For example, with sliding-control methods, precise model structure and parameterization are not required, and the control will remain stable to model errors and disturbances if the bounds on the model errors can be determined (Durfee and DiLorenzo, 1990). Another goal of the work is to develop rapid identification methods suitable for fast, off-line calibration of models, or for on-line implementation in conjunction with adaptive controllers. This is important for practical implementation of complex, multichannel neural prostheses where the controller could require daily calibration.

Identification of Isometric Recruitment Curves

Identification of the IRC is important for neural prosthesis applications, both for determining recruitment properties of electrodes, and for control. For example, as shown in Figure 3–4, if the shape of the IRC is known and monotonic, an inverse IRC block can be placed in the feed-forward path of a controller to cancel the nonlinear static gain characteristics.

Three methods of identifying the IRC were implemented and evaluated for use in neural prosthesis applications (Durfee and MacLean, 1989; MacLean, 1988). The experimental preparation involved stimulation of isolated cat medial gastrocnemius and tibialis anterior muscles. The first IRC identification method tested was the *steady-state step response* method, the simplest and most common. Here, the IRC was estimated by stimulating the muscle at a fixed activation level with a stimulus burst of length n, and the force averaged over a period of length m at the end of the stimulation burst. The delay of length $n - m$ before averaging the force allowed the step-response transients caused by the muscle dynamics to settle. To minimize muscle fatigue, long rest periods were inserted between stimulation bouts, resulting in an IRC estimate with coarse resolution and a long identification session.

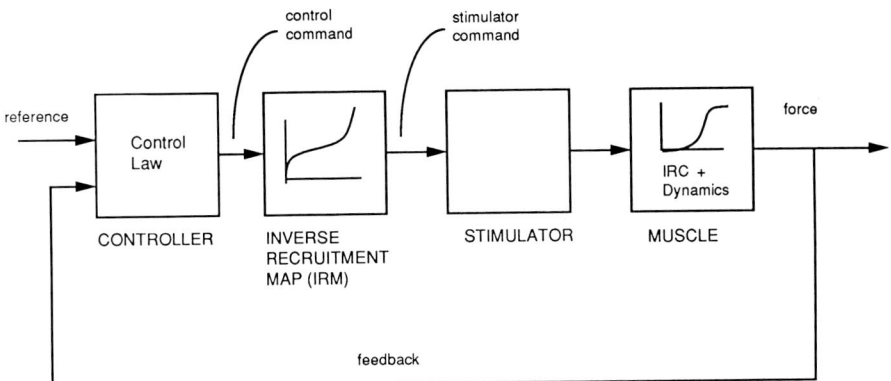

Figure 3–4 Block diagram of a closed-loop neural prosthesis controller using an inverse recruitment map to cancel the IRC nonlinearity.

The *peak impulse response* method estimated the IRC by plotting the peak of the muscle twitch response to a single stimulus pulse against the strength of the pulse. Because single twitches do not fatigue the muscle, many points on the IRC can be established in a brief time period. If the isometric muscle could indeed be modeled as a Hammerstein structure, this method should produce an IRC with the same shape as one generated with the step-response method. Although this was generally the case for our experiments, the presence of the SE implies that twitch and tetanus results will not always match (Zajac, 1989; Parmiggiani and Stein, 1981; Stein and Parmiggiani, 1981).

The *ramp deconvolution* method was a new technique we created to generate high-resolution IRC estimates with a minimum of stimulation and algorithm processing time. Here the muscle was subjected to a ramp of stimulation strength, and the output force was deconvolved back through an estimate of the muscle dynamics to provide an estimate of the output of the static nonlinear block of the Hammerstein structure model. This was cross-plotted against the input to generate the IRC estimate. The muscle dynamics were estimated by fitting the averaged muscle twitch response to the impulse response of a linear, second-order, critically damped system. Details of the identification procedure are provided in Durfee and MacLean (1989). Figure 3–5 shows a comparison between IRCs estimated by this method and those generated by the steady-state step response method. The match is close, with the exception of Figure 3–5D where the two tests were separated by other stimulation tests, resulting in fatigue and stimulation threshold shifts. The advantage of the deconvolved ramp response method was that high-resolution IRCs could be obtained in less than 30 seconds, including only 2 seconds of stimulation time.

Identification of Nonlinear, Nonisometric Muscle Models

In recent work, our group has investigated the problem of parameter identification for a nonlinear, Hill-type model of stimulated muscle. The model we have chosen is shown in Figure 3–6, and is similar in spirit to the model of Crago (1990) that was shown in Figure 3–3. Total force is the sum of passive element (PE) force F_P from joint and muscle tissue, and active force F_{MT} from the musculotendon (MT)

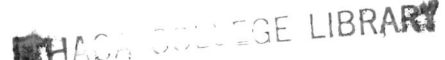

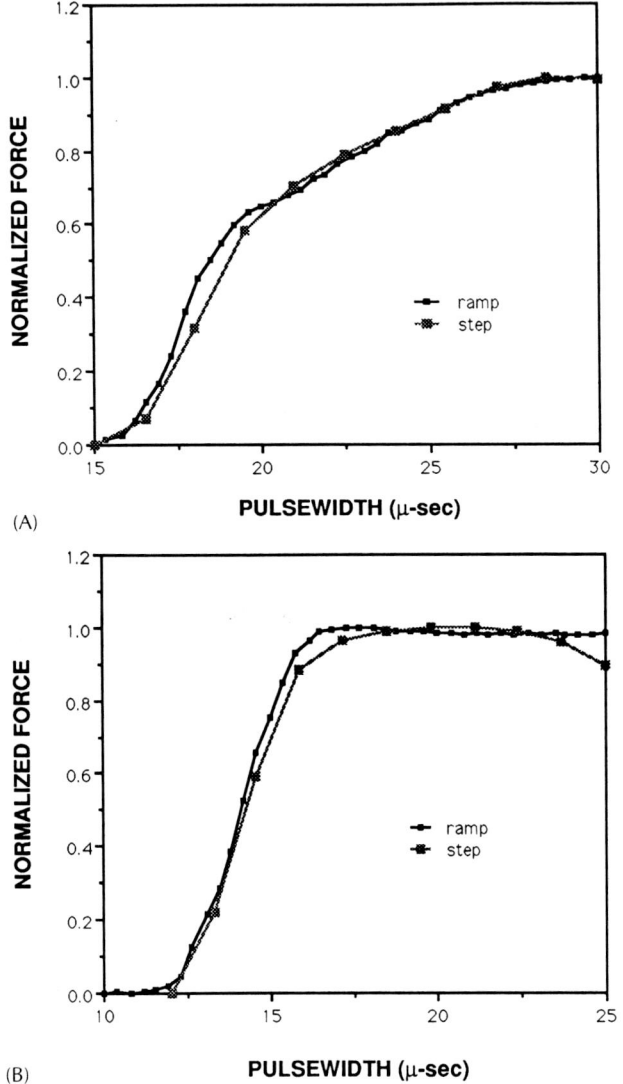

Figure 3–5 Four typical IRCs estimated by the deconvolved ramp response method, compared with IRCs estimated by the step response method. All curves are normalized to their peaks. (A) and (C) are MG muscle, (B) and (D) are TA muscle. The IRCs in (D) do not match because the two stimulation tests were separated by other tests, resulting in muscle fatigue and stimulation threshold shifts.

actuator. The PE force is produced by a parallel nonlinear spring and nonlinear dashpot. The MT force is transmitted by both the CE and the SE, with the CE force generated from the product of four factors, F_{STIM}, F_{LT}, F_{FV}, F_{SCALE}. The CE activation block is modeled as a Hammerstein structure with the IRC cascaded with second-order linear muscle activation dynamics to produce F_{STIM}. A nonlinear CE force-length relation produces F_{LT}, while a nonlinear CE force-velocity relation produces F_{FV}. All of these functions are normalized, and absolute muscle force is regained with the constant scaling factor F_{SCALE}. The SE is modeled as a nonlinear

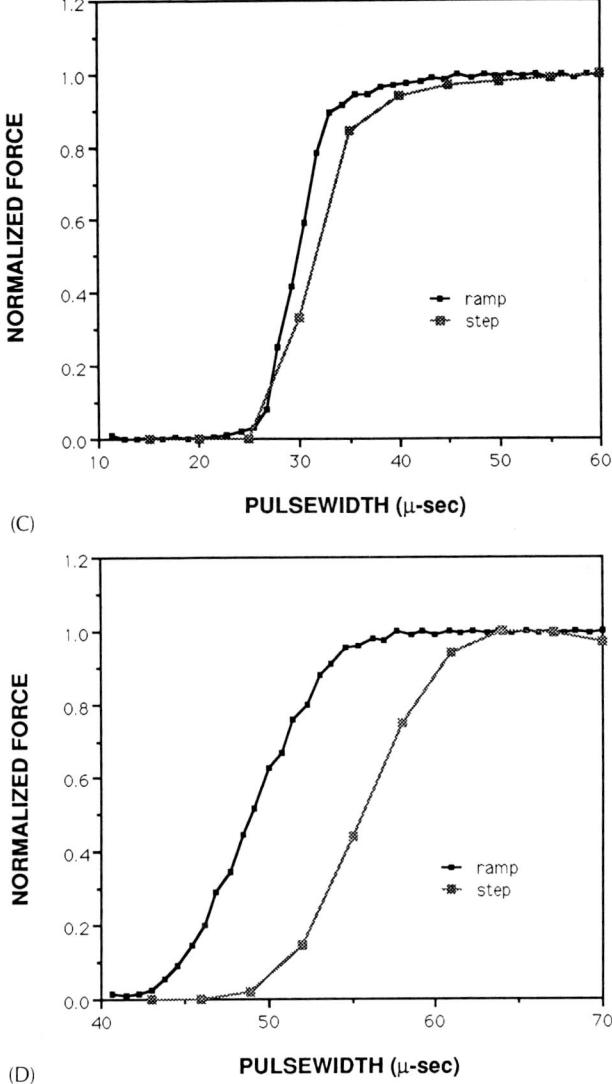

Figure 3-5 (Continued).

spring which relates the length and velocity of the CE to the length and velocity of the full MT actuator through $x_{MT} = x_{CE} + x_{SE}$.

Several critical assumptions are embedded in this model. First, as discussed above, the linear contraction dynamics are modeled as being invariant to the recruitment of motor units with different properties. Second, the CE properties are modeled as *independent* blocks. For example, this assumes that the shape of the CE force-velocity relation remains the same over the full range of muscle activation levels. As demonstrated in the experimental data of Joyce et al. (1969), this assumption does not hold for lengthening muscle, which exhibits yielding at low activation levels. Yielding behavior can be modeled by sliding-filament models, most notably in Zahalak's

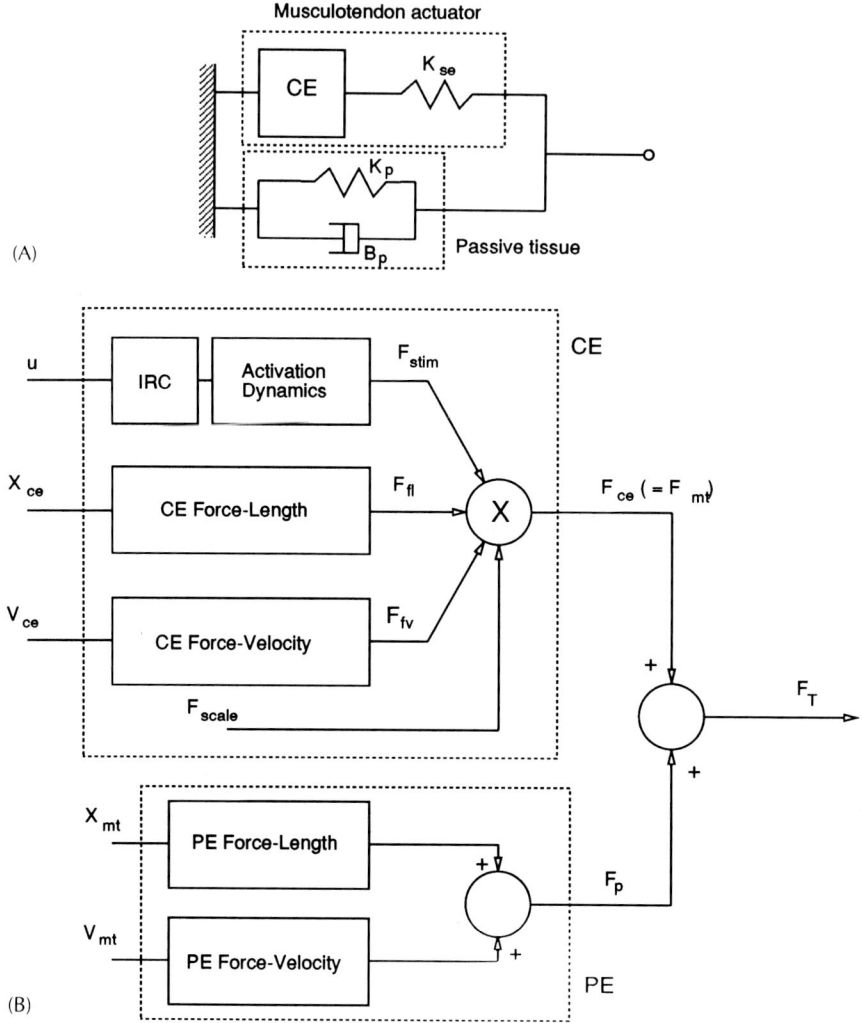

Figure 3-6 Nonlinear, Hill-type model of electrically stimulated muscle. See text for details. (A) Mechanical element form. (B) Block diagram form.

simplified distribution moment model (Zahalak, 1990), but remains beyond the power of standard Hill-type models (Winters, 1990). Third, important time-varying properties such as tetanic potentiation and fatigue are ignored completely in the model. One could possibly model fatigue as a fifth multiplicative factor in the CE block whose input was the prior time history of muscle activation, but little is known about what form this function should take.

We have developed methods for identifying the model described above, and have experimentally tested them in an animal model preparation (Palmer, 1990). In the preparation, the tendons of isolated cat hindlimb muscles were attached through an inline force sensor to a servomotor system which provided controlled length and velocity inputs. Nerve cuff electrodes were used to provide stimulation activation, the third input to the muscle. Where possible, our identification methods followed the strategy of using inputs which were in the normal physiologic range seen by the muscle. For hindlimb muscles, this would mean the length, velocity, and activation levels experienced by the muscles during normal gait.

For all of our identification studies to date, we have neglected the SE by assuming it was infinitely stiff. Although this will contribute to the errors in our ability to predict muscle force, it greatly simplifies the process of identification, since the CE force-length and force-velocity properties can be estimated directly from external measurements. We are currently working on incorporating more realistic estimates of the SE into our identification procedures.

The IRC was estimated using the ramp deconvolution method described above, while the activation dynamics were parameterized by fitting averaged twitch responses to impulse responses of linear, second-order systems. The CE force-length and force-velocity, and the passive force-length and force-velocity relations were modeled as a set of connected line segments whose vertices could be identified through a least-squares procedure (Lawton et al., 1972). No additional constraints were placed on the shapes of these curves, although one could, for example, force the force-velocity curve to fit a Hill-type hyperbola.

First, the passive force characteristics were identified by subjecting the unactivated muscle to a random length trajectory which covered the length and velocity space of interest. The total force was assumed to be the sum of length and velocity dependent functions with

$$F_P(x,\dot{x}) = f_1(x) + f_2(\dot{x})$$

Setting $f_1(x)$ and $f_2(\dot{x})$ to be piecewise linear then enabled the identification problem to be reformulated as a general least-squares equation, which was solved using a singular value decomposition algorithm (Press et al., 1986).

The active force was modeled as

$$F_{MT}(u,x,\dot{x}) = f_3(u) \times f_4(x) \times f_5(\dot{x})$$

The transducer measured total force $F_T = F_P + F_{MT}$. By taking logs and rearranging, one arrives at

$$\log\left(\frac{F_T - F_P}{f_3(u)}\right) = \log[(f_4(x)] + \log[(f_5(\dot{x})]$$

The left side of this equation is known, since $f_3(u)$ can be computed from the stimulation input acting on the estimated IRC and second-order muscle dynamics, and F_P is computed based on the estimate of passive muscle properties. The problem can be formulated in a least-squares format to solve for piecewise linear approximations of the logs of $f_4(x)$ and $f_5(\dot{x})$ which are then inverted to generate the estimates of active force-length and force-velocity relations.

Figure 3–7 displays sample results for fitting the passive characteristics. Passive force-length is shown in Figure 3–7A and passive force-velocity in Figure 3–7B. The actual force output and model force output for the random-length trajectory input is shown in Figure 3–7C, with the model errors in Figure 3–7D. Note that the estimated passive damping is small, justifying the common practice of neglecting passive force-velocity effects in musculotendon models.

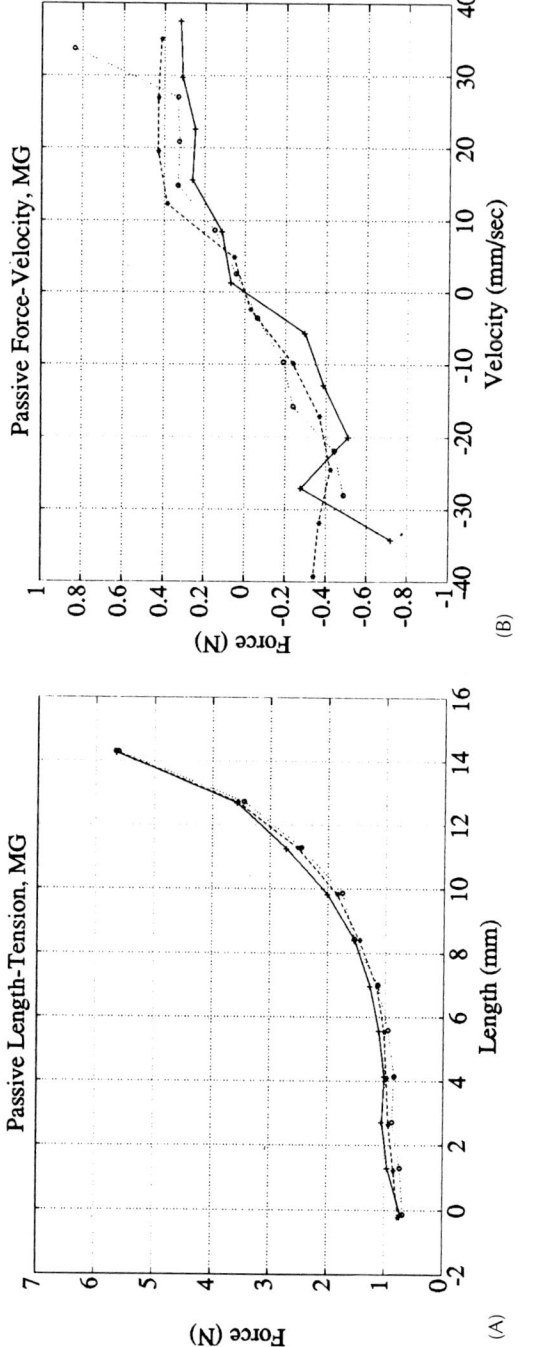

Figure 3–7 Results of passive property fitting for MG muscle. (A) Passive force-length curve for three different trials. (B) Passive force-velocity curve for three different trials. (C) Model (solid) and measured (dotted) passive force output for the identification trial. (D) Error between model and measured passive force.

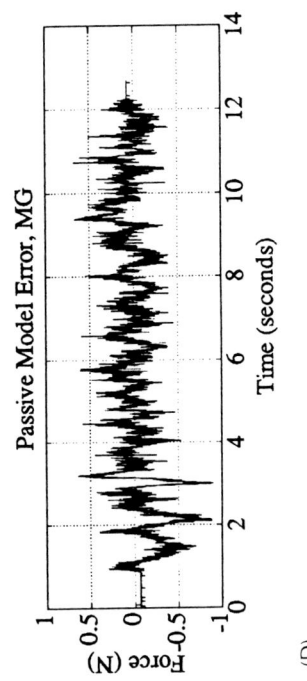

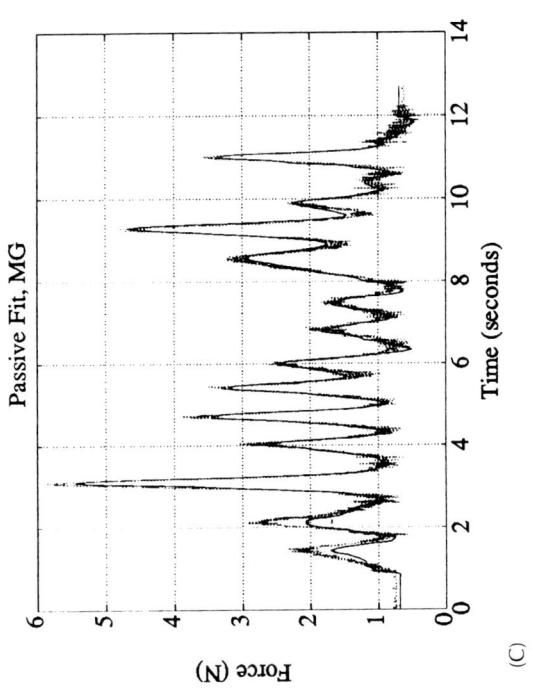

Figure 3–7 (Continued).

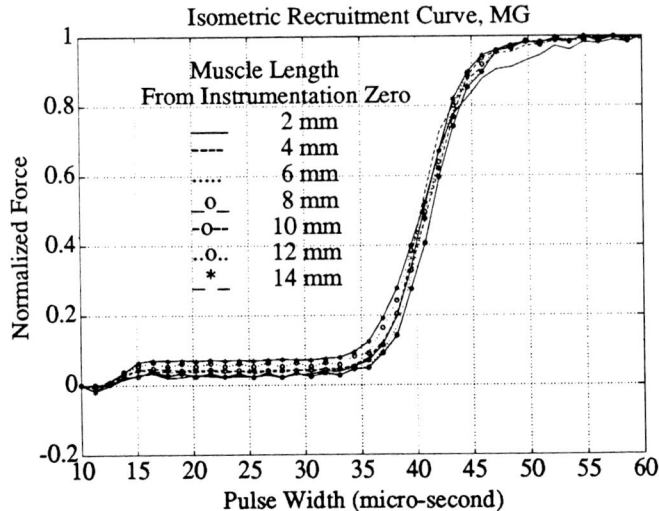

Figure 3-8 Normalized, isometric recruitment curves for several muscle lengths. The test was designed to determine if the IRC shape was a function of muscle length.

Figure 3-8 shows the results of a test designed to see if the shape of the IRC was independent of muscle length, an assumption made in the muscle model. The plot overlays normalized IRCs for the MG where the isometric length varied between 2 mm and 14 mm (the location of 0 mm was arbitrary). The steady-state peak muscle force varied from 0–60 N over these length changes. The results demonstrated IRC shape invariance with length when using nerve cuff electrodes. This shape invariance does not hold for coiled-wire intramuscular electrodes (Crago et al., 1980b) or for surface electrodes (Hausdorff and Durfee, 1991) where the relative distance between motor unit axons and the electrodes changes as the muscle contracts.

Sample results for active force fitting are shown in Figure 3-9, where Figure 3-9A shows the fitted force-length relation, Figure 3-9B shows the fitted force-velocity, Figure 3-9C shows the measured and model forces, and Figure 3-9D shows the error between the measured and modeled forces. The identification test was run with fixed stimulation and a randomly varying muscle length. Several identification runs were performed with force-length and force-velocity properties defined to be single, straight-line sections. This increased the prediction errors greatly in regions where the length excursions were large, confirming the results of Shue (1990) described above.

These results demonstrated that the identification method has the ability to *fit* the measured data, but we were most interested in the ability of the parameterized model to *predict* the muscle force output when it is subjected to a different set of inputs than the ones used for the fitting procedure. Figure 3-10 shows the measured and predicted muscle force for a case where stimulation, length, and velocity inputs to the muscle were all varied randomly. In general, the ability of the model to predict muscle force depended strongly on the accuracy of the IRC estimate since time-varying muscle fatigue was a dominant effect in our experimental preparation.

We also measured force-length and force-velocity properties of the same muscles using "classic" isometric and isovelocity methods to see whether they would match the shapes found in the experiments described above. The results showed some similarities, but significant discrepancies were apparent due to muscle fatigue and because the isometric and isovelocity paradigms subjected the muscle to significantly different loading trajectories than the random methods.

The experiments demonstrated the value of using a full, nonlinear Hill-type muscle model for neural prosthesis applications. Much work remains in refining the model to add SE effects, and in developing more efficient identification strategies. Because of the close relation between identification and adaptive control, the recursive identification methods of Shue (1990) may be effective, although current algorithms limit real-time implementation to the tracking of only a few parameters. Modeling and identification will always entail approximations and errors, given the inherent complexity of stimulated muscle. This brings out the importance of exploring robust control methods for neural prostheses where model structure and parameter uncertainty can be treated as disturbances by the controller.

FURTHER READING

This chapter has presented an overview of identification methods relevant to neural prosthesis applications. The interested practitioner is urged to explore the literature to learn more. An appropriate survey path would start with tutorial descriptions of linear system identification methods which can be found in many textbooks on systems and control. Chapter 8 of the text by Franklin et al. (1990) or Chapter 13 of Astrom and Wittenmark (1990) are suggested. More detail on linear parameter identification is provided in the comprehensive text by Ljung (1987) and the matching *System Identification Toolbox* software package which runs under MATLAB (Mathworks, 1990). For those who wish to write their own identification algorithms, the book by Press et al. (1986) is recommended. Chapter 14 of that source is particularly relevant to system identification.

The literature on nonlinear system identification is less codified, reflecting its continually evolving status as an active research area. An overview of nonlinear identification methods is provided in a review by Billings (1980). From there one can turn to the book by Marmarelis and Marmarelis (1978) for a thorough treatment of the theory behind functional series methods and their application to physiological systems. Another review of functional methods is provided in an article by Hung and Stark (1977). Nonlinear least-squares methods are covered in the text by Goodwin and Sin (1984) and also, briefly, in Chapter 14 of Press et al. (1986). The Goodwin and Sin book is particularly appropriate, with its emphasis on the identification of dynamic systems using both off-line and recursive, on-line algorithms.

For a single-source reference on the biomechanical modeling of motor control systems, the survey book edited by Winters and Woo (1990), which contains several tutorial chapters on musculoskeletal modeling and identification, is recommended. Applications of identification methods to neural prostheses were covered in this chapter and the reader is encouraged to consult the cited literature for specific details.

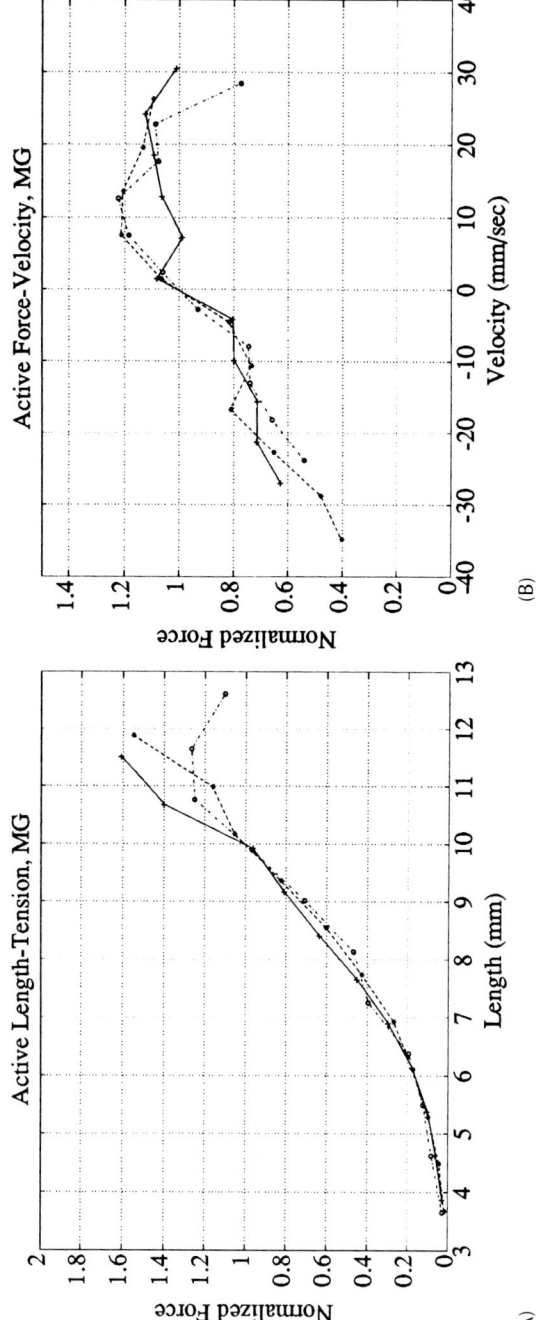

Figure 3–9 Results of active force fitting for MG muscle. (A) MT force-length curve for three different trials. (B) MT force-velocity curve for three different trials. (C) Model (solid) and measured (dotted) total force output for the identification trial. (D) Error between model and measured force.

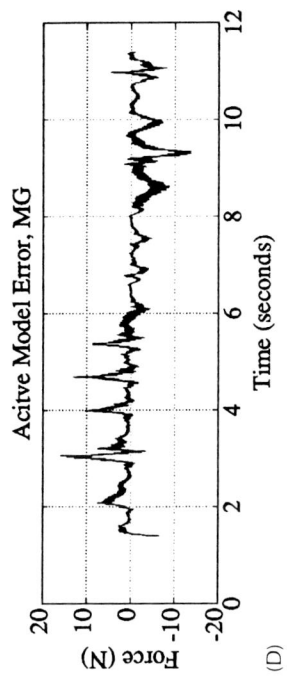

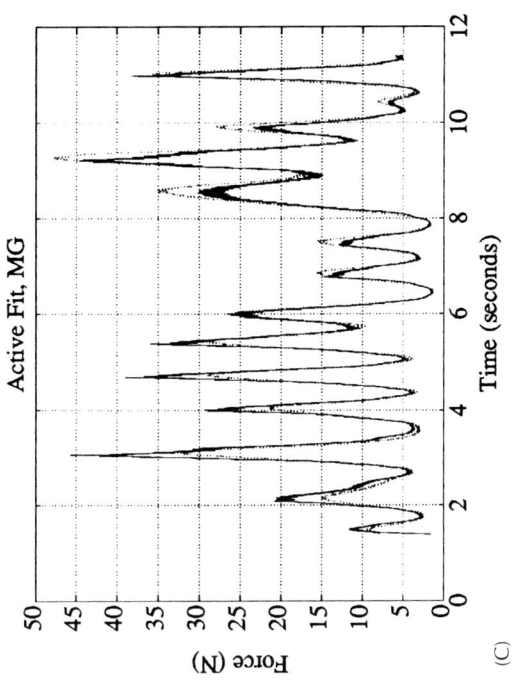

Figure 3–9 (Continued).

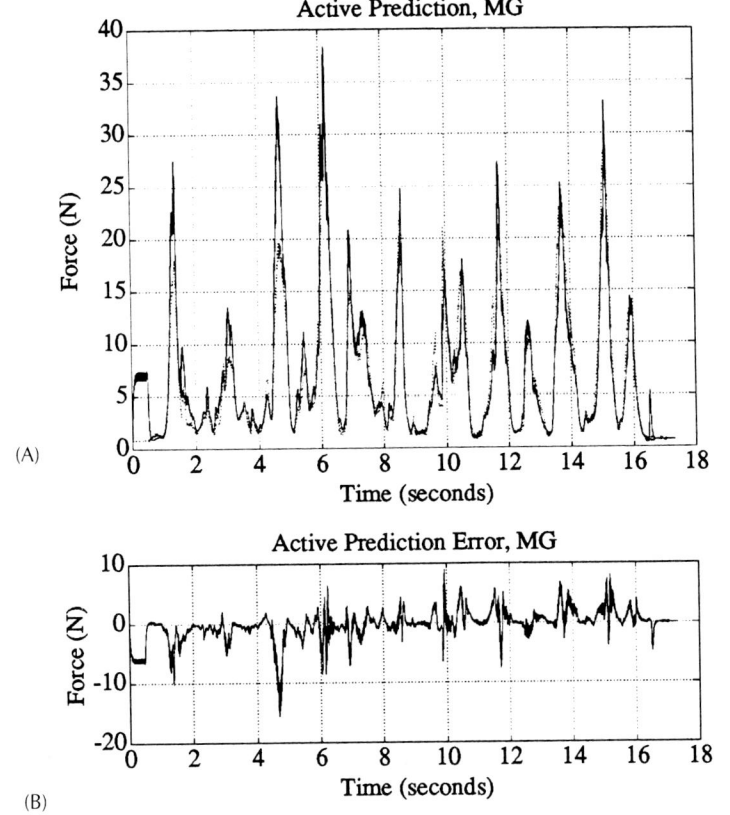

Figure 3-10 Results of a test to demonstrate predictive capability of the model. For this test, both muscle stimulation and muscle length were varied randomly. The model was parameterized in a prior trial using a different input sequence. (A) Model (solid) and measured (dotted) total force output for the trial. (B) Error between model and measured force.

NOTES

1. The term "musculotendon" was coined by Zajac (1989) to reflect the anatomical fact that muscle and tendon are inextricably bound and cannot be treated separately in a model.

2. A recent, interesting development is that treating long, parallel-fiber muscles as a single entity may be an oversimplification. New anatomical data indicates that these muscles are not composed of single fibers which run completely from origin to insertion, but rather are made up of independently controllable short fibers arranged in series (Loeb and Levine, 1990). The implications of this to neural prosthesis control are unclear.

3. Although in this chapter we have made the implicit assumption that the output variable of interest is muscle force, one could just as easily assume an output of muscle length, or an output of muscle-driving point impedance. For a discussion of this tissue as it relates to the biomechanics of motor control, see Stein (1982).

REFERENCES

Astrom, K.J., and Wittenmark, B. (1990). *Computer-Controlled Systems: Theory and Design,* 2nd ed. New York: Prentice-Hall.

Baratta, R., and Solomonow, M. (1990). The dynamic response model of nine different skeletal muscles. *IEEE Trans. Biomed. Eng.*, **37**(3), 243–251.

Baratta, R., Ichie, M., Hwang, S., and Solomonow, M. (1989). Orderly stimulation of skeletal muscle motor units with tripolar nerve cuff electrode. *IEEE Trans. Biomed. Eng.*, **36**(8), 836–843.

Bawa, P., Mannard, A., and Stein, R. (1976a). Effects of elastic loads on the contractions of cat muscles. *Biol. Cybern.*, **22**, 129–137.

Bawa, P., Mannard, A., and Stein, R. (1976b). Predictions and experimental tests of a viscoelastic muscle model using elastic and inertial loads. *Biol. Cybern.*, **22**, 139–145.

Bernotas, L., Crago, P., and Chizeck, H. (1986). A discrete-time model of electrically stimulated muscle. *IEEE Trans. Biomed. Eng.*, **33**(9), 829–838.

Bernotas, L., Crago, P., and Chizeck, H. (1987). Adaptive control of electrically stimulated muscle. *IEEE Trans. Biomed. Eng.* **34**(2), 140–147.

Billings, S.A. (1980). Identification of nonlinear systems—a survey. *IEEE Proc.*, **127d**(6), 272–285.

Brown, G.A., Tell, R., Rowell, D., and Mann, R. (1987). Determination of body segment parameters using computerized tomography and magnetic resonance imaging. *ASME Winter Annual Meeting, Biomechanics of Normal and Prosthetic Gait*, pp. 145–149.

Chia, T.L., Chow, P.C., and Chizeck, H.J. (1991). Recursive parameter identification of constrained systems: An application to electrically stimulated muscle. *IEEE Trans. Biomed. Eng.*, **38**, 429–442.

Chizeck H.J., Lan, N., Palmieri, L.S., and Crago, P.E. (1991). Feedback control of electrically stimulated muscle using simultaneous pulse width and frequency modulation. *IEEE Trans. Biomed. Eng.*, (in press).

Crago, P., Peckham, P., and Thrope, G. (1980). Modulation of muscle force by recruitment during intramuscular stimulation. *IEEE Trans. Biomed. Eng.*, **27**(12), 679–684.

Crago, P.E., Lemay, M.A., and Liu, L. (1990). External control of limb movements involving environmental interactions. In: J.M. Winters and S.L. Woo, ed., *Multiple Muscle Systems*. New York: Springer-Verlag.

Durfee, W., and DiLorenzo, D. (1990). Linear and nonlinear approaches to control of single joint motion by functional electrical stimulation. *Proceedings of the 1990 American Control Conference*.

Durfee, W.K., and Hausdorff J.M. (1990). Regulating knee joint position by combining electrical stimulation with a controllable friction brake. *Ann. Biomed. Eng.* **18**, 575–596.

Durfee, W.K., and MacLean, K.E. (1989). Methods for estimating isometric recruitment curves of electrically stimulated muscle. *IEEE Trans. Biomed. Eng.*, **36**(7), 654–667.

Fang, Z.P., and Mortimer, J.T. (1987). A method for attaining natural recruitment order in artificially activated muscles. *Proc. 9th Ann. Conf. IEEE Eng. Med. Biol. Soc.*, pp. 657–658.

Franklin, G.F., Powell, J.D., and Workman, M.L. (1990). *Digital Control of Dynamic Systems,* 2nd ed. Boston: Addison-Wesley.

French, A., and Holden, A. (1971a). Alias-free sampling of neuronal spike trains. *Kybernetik*, **8**, 165–171.

Geng, K. (1989). *Real-Time Parameter Identification of a Class of Nonlinear Discrete-Time Models of Electrically Stimulated Muscle*, Master's thesis. Cleveland: Case Western Reserve University.

Goodwin, G.C., and Sin, K.S. (1984). *Adaptive Filtering, Prediction and Control*. New York: Prentice-Hall.

Grandjean, P., and Mortimer, J. (1986). Recruitment properties of monopolar and bipolar epimysial electrodes. *Ann. Biomed. Eng.*, **14**, 53–66.

Griffiths, RI. (1987). Ultrasound transit time gives direct measurement of muscle fibre length in vivo. *J. Neurosci. Methods*, **21**, 159–165.

Hatze, H. (1977). A myocybernetic control model of skeletal muscle. *Biol. Cybern.* **25**, 103–119.

Hatze H. (1978). A general myocybernetic control model of skeletal muscle. *Biol. Cybern.*, **28**, 143–157.

Hausdorff, J., and Durfee, W. (1991). Open-loop position control of the knee joint using electrical stimulation of the quadriceps and hamstrings. *Med. Biol. Eng. Comput.*, **29**, 269–280.

Hill, A.V. (1938). The heat of shortening and the dynamic constants of muscle. *Proc. R. Soc. Lond. [Biol.]*, **126**, 136–195.

Hoffer, J.A., Caputi, A., Pose, I., and Griffiths, R. (1989). Roles of muscle activity and load on the relationship between muscle spindle length and whole muscle length in the freely walking cat. *Prog. Brain Res.*, **80**, 75–85.

Hung, G., and Stark, L. (1977). The kernal identification method—review of theory, calculation, application and interpretation. *Math Biosci.*, **37**, 135–170.

Hunter, I., and Korenberg, M. (1986). The identification of nonlinear biological systems: Wiener and Hammerstein cascade models. *Biol. Cybern.*, **55**, 135–144.

Huxley, A. (1974). Muscular contraction. *J. Physiol.*, **243**, 1–43.

Joyce, G., Rack, P., and Westbury, D. (1969). The mechanical properties of cat soleus muscle during controlled lengthening and shortening movements. *J. Physiol.*, **204**, 461–474.

Kralj, A., Bajd, T., and Turk, R. (1980). Electrical stimulation providing functional use of paraplegic patient muscles. *Med. Prog. Technol.*, **7**, 3–9.

Kralj, A., Bajd, T., Turk, R., Krajnik, J., and Benko, H. (1983). Gait restoration in paraplegic patients: A feasibility demonstration using multichannel surface electrode. *J. Rehab. Res. Devel.* **20**(1), 3–20.

Lawton, W.H., Sylvestre, E.A., and Maggio, M.S. (1972). Self-modeling nonlinear regression. *Technometrics*, **14**(3), 513–533.

Ljung, L. (1987). *System Identification—Theory for the User*. New York: Prentice-Hall.

Loeb, G.E., and Levine, W.S. (1990). Linking musculoskeletal mechanics to senorimotor neurophysiology. In: J.M. Winters and S.L. Woo, ed., *Multiple Muscle Systems*. New York: Springer-Verlag.

MacLean, K. (1988). *Estimation of Isometric Recruitment Curves of Electrically Stimulated Muscle*. Master's thesis, Massachusetts Institute of Technology.

Mannard, A., and Stein, R.B. (1973). Determination of the frequency response of isometric soleus muscle in the cat using random nerve stimulation. *J. Physiol.*, **229**, 276–296.

Marmarelis, P.Z., and Marmarelis, V.Z. (1978). *Analysis of Physiological Systems: The White Noise Approach*. New York: Plenum Press.

Mathworks, Inc. (1990). *MATLAB Users Manual*. Mathworks, Inc.

McNeal, D. (1976). Analysis of a model for excitation of myelinated nerve. *IEEE Trans. Biomed. Eng.*, **25**, 329–337.

Murphy, M.C., Zarins, B., Jasty, M., and Mann, R. (1984). In vivo measurement of the three-dimensional skeletal motion at the human knee. In: R.L. Spilker, ed., *1984 Advances in Bioengineering, ASME*.

Ogata, K. (1990). *Modern Control Engineering, 2nd ed*. New York: Prentice-Hall.

Palmer, K. (1990). *Modeling and Identification of Electrically Stimulated Muscle*. Master's thesis, Massachusetts Institute of Technology.

Parmiggiani, F., and Stein, R.B. (1981). Nonlinear summation of contractions in cat muscles: II. Later facilitation and stiffness changes. *J. Gen. Physiol.*, **78**, 295–311.

Parmiggiani, F., Stein, R.B., and Rolf, R. (1982). Slow changes and Wiener analysis of nonlinear summation in contractions of cat muscles. *Biol. Cybern.*, **42**, 177–188.

Partridge, L. (1965). Modifications of neural output signals by muscles: A frequency response study. *J. Appl. Physiol.*, **20**, 150–166.

Peckham, P.H. (1987). Functional electrical stimulation: Current status and future prospects of applications to neuromuscular system in spinal cord injury. *Paraplegia*, **25**, 279–288.

Peckham, P., Mortimer, J., and Marsolais, E. (1976). Alterations in the force and fatigability of skeletal muscle in quadriplegic humans following exercise induced by chronic electrical stimulation. *Clin. Orthop.*, **114**, 326.

Petrofsky, J. (1978). Control of the recruitment and firing frequencies of motor units in electrically stimulated muscles in the cat. *Med. Biol. Eng. Comput.*, **16**, 302–308.

Press, W., Flannery, B., Teukolsky, S., and Vetterling, W. (1986). *Numerical Recipes: The Art of Scientific Computing*. Cambridge: Cambridge University Press.

Rack, P., and Westbury, D. (1969). The effects of length and stimulus rate on tension in the isometric cat soleus muscle. *J. Physiol.*, **204**, 443–460.

Shue, G.H. (1990). *Multiplicative Model of Stimulated Muscle for FNS Control*. Master's thesis. Cleveland: Case Western Reserve University.

Stein, R.B. (1982). What muscle variable(s) does the nervous system control in limb movements? *Behav. Brain Sci.*, **5**, 535–577.

Stein, R.B., and Parmiggiani, F. (1981). Nonlinear summation of contractions in cat muscles: I. Early depression. *J. Gen. Physiol.*, **78**, 277–293.

Winters, J.M. (1990). Hill-based muscle models: A systems engineering perspective. In: J.M. Winters and S.L. Woo, eds., *Multiple Muscle Systems*. New York: Springer-Verlag.

Winters, J.M., and S.L. Woo, eds. (1990). *Multiple Muscle Systems*, New York: Springer-Verlag.

Yamaguchi, G.T. (1990). Performing whole-body simulations of gait with 3-D, dynamic musculoskeletal models. In: J.M. Winters and S.L. Woo, eds., *Multiple Muscle Systems*. New York: Springer-Verlag.

Yamaguchi, G.T., Sawa, A., Moran, D., Fessler, M., and Winters, J. (1990). A survey of human musculotendon actuator parameters. In: J.M. Winters and S.L. Woo, eds., *Multiple Muscle Systems*. New York: Springer-Verlag.

Zahalak, G.I. (1990). Modeling muscle mechanics (and energetics). In: J.M. Winters and S.L. Woo, eds., *Multiple Muscle Systems*. New York: Springer-Verlag.

Zajac, F.E. (1989). Muscle and tendon: Properties, models, scaling, and application to biomechanics and motor control. *CRC Crit. Rev. Biomed. Eng.*, **17**(4), 359–411.

Zajac, F.E., and Gordon, M.E. (1989). Determining muscle's force and action in multiarticular movement. *Exerc. Sport Sci. Rev.*, **17**, 187–230.

Zhou, B., and Baratta, R. (1987). Manipulation of muscle force with various firing rate and recruitment control strategies. *IEEE Trans. Biomed. Eng.*, **34**(2), 128–139.

4
Artificial Sensors Suitable for Closed-Loop Control of FNS

JOHN G. WEBSTER

During neuromuscular stimulation, fixed electric stimulation does not yield fixed muscular force because of fatigue. In the case where sensory function is also lost we require artificial sensors to replace lost natural sensors so we can close the feedback loop. As muscle and tendon organ sensors measure force, so should the artificial sensors measure force. This is difficult at the finger pad because for a fixed force, the pressure distribution varies for small and large objects. Therefore we must use an array of sensors that covers the entire finger pad and the palm. Typically force sensors use a spring to convert force into displacement. This spring should have low hysteresis, so silicon or metal are usually preferred to conductive elastomers. Silicon force sensors are now being developed that have a stop to prevent force overload. Capacitive arrays have been built using latex foam, for which hysteresis is not excessive. Piezoelectric sensors are not effective as they do not respond to steady forces. Optical sensors are currently not made small enough.

If we consider the function of grasp, we need to examine the interaction between cutaneous and proprioceptive sensors in supplying feedback for control of hand exertions. Once we have determined what the body naturally measures, we are in a better position to substitute artificial sensors for control. Then we can determine reasonable numbers of sensors and best locations and select from the variety of possible sensor principles and implementations.

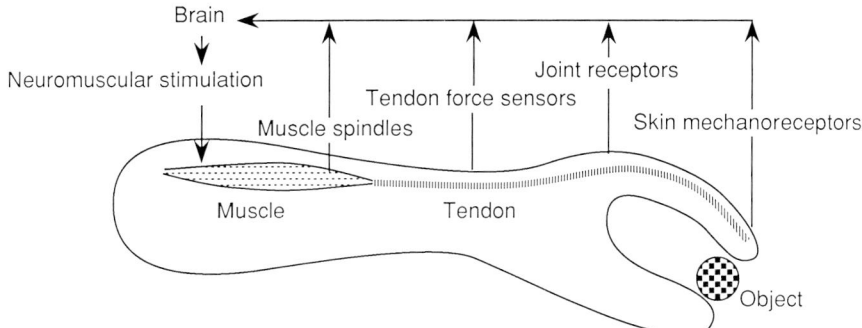

Figure 4–1 In the intact human, the brain transmits action potentials through motor nerves to cause muscle contraction. Sensory nerves transmit muscle-, tendon-, and cutaneous-force information back to the brain.

NEED FOR ARTIFICIAL SENSORS

Spinal cord injury (SCI) can result in a variety of functional deficits. Low level SCI can result in loss of sensory and motor function in the legs and prevent standing and walking. The wheelchair is a common device for restoring support and locomotion. High level SCI can result in loss of sensory and motor function in the arms and prevent adequate grasp.

Benton et al. (1981) describe the placement of conductive rubber electrodes to achieve transcutaneous muscle stimulation. While range of motion may be improved, transcutaneous stimulation is unlikely to be useful for improving grasp because of its lack of spatial specificity. Therefore current research emphasizes percutaneous or implanted intramuscular or nerve cuff electrodes (Peckham, 1988; Marsolais et al., 1990).

Functional neuromuscular stimulation (FNS)—the subcutaneous stimulation of muscle or the motor nerves—has been proposed as a method for restoring grasp. Research on FNS shows that the relation between contraction force and electric stimulation level is not fixed. During a single trial, the electric stimulation is first increased until it exceeds a threshold level. Above this threshold level, the neuromuscular force–stimulation level relationship exhibits a high gain, and at a high level it saturates. During extended trials, the muscle fatigues, and higher electric stimulation is required to achieve the same force. Thus an open-loop control system does not provide satisfactory control and we must resort to a closed-loop control system. A closed-loop control system requires artificial sensors to replace the lost function of the natural proprioceptive and mechanoreceptive sensors. I will consider only the loss of a single function—fingertip pinch grasp—but the reasoning can be extended to other FNS systems.

Normal Feedback Loop

Figure 4–1 shows that in the intact human, a feedback loop improves the control of grasp. Natural sensors return force information to the brain so we neither apply too small a force and drop the object nor too large a force and crush the object.

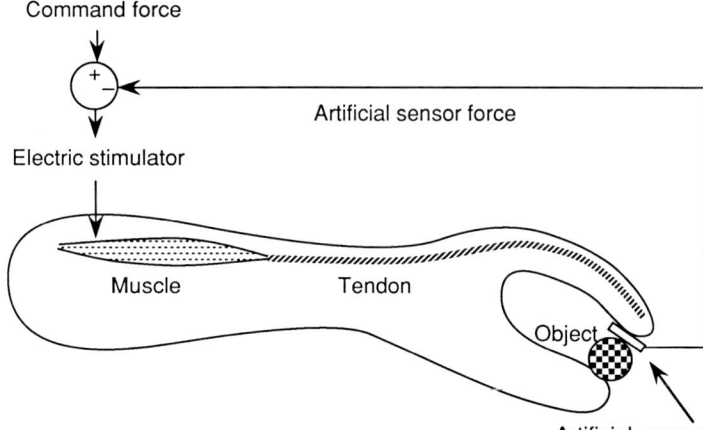

Figure 4-2 In functional neuromuscular stimulation, an electric stimulator causes muscular contraction to increase tendon force. Because a system without feedback has poor control, an artificial sensor to return force information to the brain should improve grasp.

We have two major systems that sense force: cutaneous and proprioceptive. The cutaneous system is composed of touch sensors in the skin. These are most sensitive to small pressures on the skin and provide information about the location of objects on the skin, the distribution of pressure on the skin, and texture of objects. The cutaneous sensors saturate for large forces and then do not return force information to the brain. For large forces, proprioceptive sensors in the tendons and muscles return force information to the brain. Thus we believe there are two complementary overlapping systems that return force information to the brain: cutaneous for small forces, and proprioceptive for large forces.

Artificial Feedback Loop

Figure 4-2 shows that in SCI, motor control is lost and the muscles must be electrically stimulated. Sensory feedback is also lost and must be replaced by an artificial sensor. It would be most desirable to measure the tendon force because it is equal to the muscle force that results from stimulation. But this would require surgery and a complicated implanted sensor system in series with the tendon, which is presently impractical. Therefore, present development concentrates on installing at the location of contact, artificial sensors that have greater range than natural cutaneous sensors. Note that we desire to measure a single force, but are constrained to measure it at a difficult location—the fingertip. We must ensure that the artificial sensor faithfully measures force from a variety of object sizes and locations on the fingertip.

MEASURING FORCE OR PRESSURE?

Artificial sensors can measure force or pressure. Force equals pressure × area. So these variables are closely related, but they are not the same. A force applied to the fingertip by the pointed end of a pencil produces a much higher pressure than

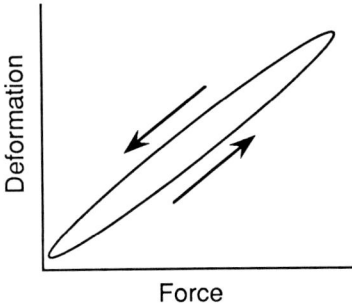

Figure 4–3 All force sensors use a spring to convert force to displacement. We desire small spring hysteresis so the displacement for increasing force is close to the displacement for decreasing force.

the same force applied by the eraser end. Cutaneous sensors let you know that the pressure is much higher using the pointed end. Cutaneous sensors measure pressure, not force. The tendon sensors cannot tell the difference because the force is the same.

Most thin artificial sensors currently suitable for measurement at the fingertip measure pressure. They have been adapted from pressure sensors that use a diaphragm or other large-area device generally used for measuring fluid pressures. If we wished to replace cutaneous sensation, we would need an array of pressure sensors. But since we wish to replace proprioceptive sensation we must devise a system that can convert the output from pressure sensors into a single force produced by the muscle.

Sensor Deformation

Most pressure and force sensors have a spring element that deforms when pressed upon. Figure 4–3 shows that applied force deflects this spring. Ideally, by measuring the deformation of the sensor, we could determine the force that caused it. Unfortunately, springs have hysteresis. For increasing force, the spring tends to stick at its previous level of deformation, so the deformation is less than ideal. The hysteresis loop in Figure 4–3 shows that for a given deformation, we don't really know the force. It might be higher or lower depending upon the previous history of force. So hysteresis causes error.

In general, silicon has very low hysteresis, metals have low hysteresis, latex rubber has moderate hysteresis, and many synthetic polymers have high hysteresis. Because of their ease of use, many tactile sensors have been made of synthetic polymers such as silicone rubber and polyurethane foam. Babbs et al. (1990) measured hysteresis in certain latex foam rubbers and found it lower than other synthetic polymers. Metals have not been used much for miniature sensors because it is difficult to construct these sensors. Most silicon sensors have been of the diaphragm type, which makes mechanical interfacing difficult.

Sensor Contour

Figure 4–4 shows that an artificial sensor must measure force from different sized objects, resulting in different contact areas, and at different locations. Figure 4–4A shows that force from a small object, such as a pencil, would deform an elastomer

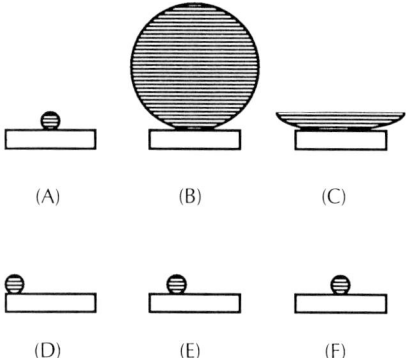

Figure 4–4 A force sensor should yield the same output for (A) small, (B) medium, and (C) large objects. A force sensor should yield the same output for applied forces (D) at the edge, (E) shifted, and (F) centered.

over a smaller area than a medium size object (Figure 4–4B) or large size object (Figure 4–4C). Whereas pressure sensors would give different outputs for each of these different sized objects, we desire the same measured force in each case.

Figure 4–4D, E, and F show that the sensor should yield the same output for different locations of the object. Therefore we cannot use a single diaphragm, which has greater sensitivity at the center than at the edge. Although a diaphragm measures pressures well for a fluid, Figure 4–5 also shows it cannot measure pressures from a flat surface. We can convert a diaphragm pressure sensor to a force sensor by adding a projection on the diaphragm. This concentrates all the force at one particular location on the diaphragm. But then if we measured force from a small object, that object would have to be placed on the projection and not off center.

Most silicon and metal diaphragm sensors are delicate. To achieve maximal sensitivity and minimal temperature drift, they are designed for a stated range plus 100% overload beyond which they will break. It is therefore useful to design them with a mechanical stop as shown in Figure 4–5 to be able to withstand overload.

Single or Multiple Sensors

A single artificial sensor on the finger pad could measure the force when picking up a cup. But it would have to cover the entire 2-cm² cylindrical surface contact area that transmits significant force during this operation. A sensor smaller than the contact area would permit some of the transmitted force to bypass the sensor, so the sensor would measure a force smaller than that transmitted to the supporting bone structures. The sensor should also measure the force when picking up a pencil with an area of 0.5 cm². Figure 4–6A shows a possible clamshell-shaped grasping surface that transmits force through a single beam sensor to a parallel clamshell on the finger pad.

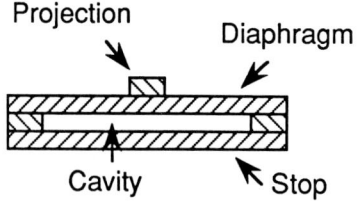

Figure 4–5 A force sensor using a diaphragm requires a projection when contacting planar objects. The cavity must be thin so the diaphragm hits a stop to prevent breakage due to overload.

ARTIFICIAL SENSORS SUITABLE FOR CLOSED-LOOP CONTROL OF FNS

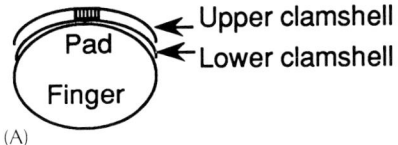

(A)

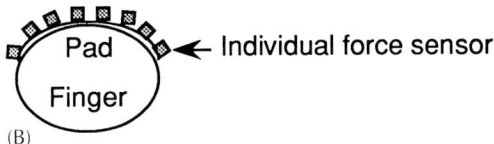

(B)

Figure 4–6 Finger force sensors should integrate pressure over the entire finger pad. These cross sections show possible (A) parallel clamshells with a single force sensor between or (B) a flexible 8 × 8 array of force sensors.

A flexible array might be better than a single sensor. Figure 4–6B shows an 8 × 8 array with elements spaced 2.5 mm apart. It could cover the finger pad and permit measuring force from either a cup or a pencil. The goal would not be to measure pressure distribution, but merely to sum the forces from the 64 elements and yield a single force output. However we may obtain force distribution, or pressure, using this method.

SPECIFICATIONS FOR ARTIFICIAL SENSORS

Harmon (1982) developed a list of desirable characteristics for robotic tactile sensors. These tended to duplicate the cutaneous sensors of the hand and required spatial resolution of 1–2 mm. Crago et al. (1986) listed much more reasonable requirements for FNS. For object contact force they estimated a range of 0.1 to 80 N, a resolution of 0.1 N at threshold and 1 N for high forces, and a frequency response of 100 Hz. We desire an accuracy of a few percent of full scale, which implies low hysteresis and low temperature drift.

FNS Requires a Single Output per Location

When pinching an object as shown in Figure 4–2, we use only a single output from the finger pad. Even though we may choose an array of sensors for the finger pad, we can linearly sum their outputs at the sensor location and thus need only one pair of wires from that location. Note that to pinch the object, we require a second sensor on the thumb pad and a second stimulator for the antagonist muscle.

FNS Requires Multiple Locations

For meaningful hand function we require sensors at multiple locations. It would be difficult to cover the entire hand contact area with sensors because of the wrinkling that occurs when curling the hand. An achievable goal might be to use 16 sensors on the hand. Tan (1988) describes a study of wear patterns of used space-suit gloves

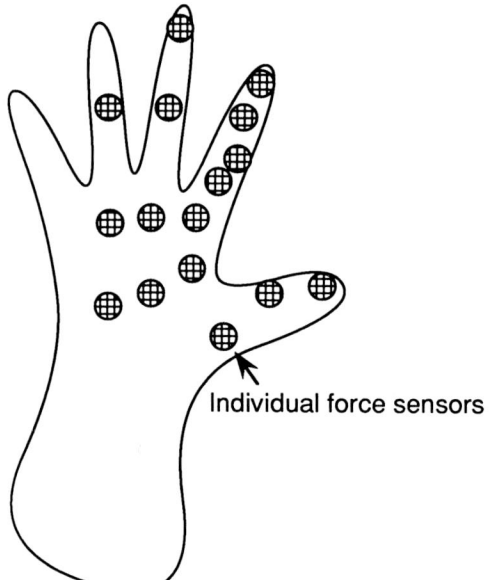

Figure 4–7 Placing 16 force sensors at high-pressure points of the palm would provide much information with reasonable complexity.

and of grip and hand use to yield the location of the sensors as shown in Figure 4–7. A similar study of the likely grasp functions of FNS and the resulting palmar pressure distributions should suggest the high-pressure locations that would yield the maximal feedback information. Note that some forces would bypass the discretely located sensors and yield smaller forces measured by the sensors.

PIEZORESISTIVE FORCE SENSORS

Piezoresistive force sensors are widely used because of their excellent repeatability, low hysteresis, and reasonable manufacture.

Silicon Strain Gages

When silicon is stretched, its resistance increases. The piezoresistive effect is much higher than that for metal, so when silicon strain gages are placed in a bridge, high output results. Because multiple gages can be made using integrated circuit technology, cost is low. Silicon gages have no plastic deformation and are noticeably free of hysteresis effects. Hahm (1988) reviews the available types, which are like Figure 4–5, with gages diffused into the diaphragms, but none have protective stops or suitable packaging. Sorab et al. (1988) used a commercial force sensor of this type to measure fingertip forces applied by obstetricians during delivery. Beebe (1990) is developing a diaphragm silicon sensor with a protective stop using silicon-fusion bonding, micromachining, and novel packaging techniques.

Metal Strain Gages

When metal is stretched, its resistance increases. The piezoelectric effect is small, but the temperature drift is much lower than that of silicon. Metal strain gages must

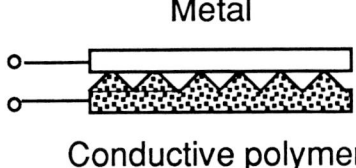

Figure 4–8 Force flattens the peaks of the conductive polymer and increases the area of contact with the metal. This decreases the electric resistance.

be glued on the diaphragm by hand, so the finished gage typically costs $100 and up. Metal strain gages are the choice for highest accuracy, but are difficult to miniaturize and expensive for multiple locations (Hagnar, 1988a).

Elastomeric Strain Gages

Mokshagundam (1988) describes several conductive elastomers and carbon fiber tactile sensors. Figure 4–8 shows the most promising of these, which is commercially available for about $3 per sensor. Pressure applied to the 0.5-mm-thick sensor flattens the peaks of the conductive polymer and decreases the resistance. The pressure-resistance relation is nonlinear, but a look-up table can compensate for this. Also, bending the flexible sensor changes its calibration, so it must be backed with a rigid plate. Its largest defect is a hysteresis that exceeds 10%, so the present gage is not accurate enough for FNS.

CAPACITIVE FORCE SENSORS

Seow (1988) reviews capacitive sensors, which can be discrete or in arrays. Figure 4–9 shows the configuration for a typical capacitive array sensor. All that is required is strips of metal foil separated by a deformable medium. One strip of the array is typically grounded. The other strips may be covered by a driven or grounded shield to reduce or fix the stray capacitance. Unused strips must be grounded to prevent cross-talk through unused nodes. By selecting rows and columns, the number of wires is smaller than the number of nodes.

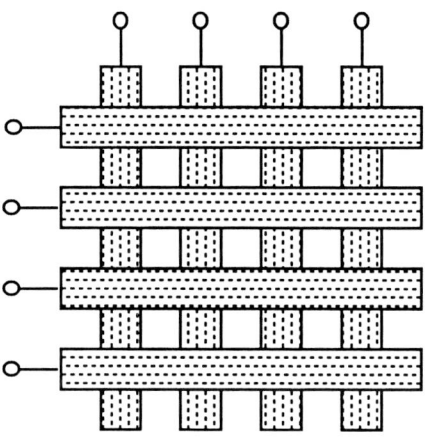

Figure 4–9 Selection of one horizontal and one vertical strip permits measurement of the capacitance between their intersection. Compressible foam rubber or silicone rubber dielectric converts force to capacitor strip separation.

Silicon Capacitive Force Sensors

Capacitive sensors can be fabricated using integrated circuit techniques by placing metal films on the top and bottom of the cavity shown in Figure 4–5. Force bends the diaphragm and brings the metal films closer together, thus increasing the capacitance between them.

Elastomeric Capacitive Force Sensors

Deformable media have been silicone rubber elastomer strips, silicone rubber elastomer containing air channels, and medical pretaping underwrap foam. Most elastomers have an unsatisfactorily high hysteresis. Babbs et al. (1990) developed a 24 × 64 array capacitive mat for measuring pressure distribution on hospital beds and found that natural latex foams exhibit substantially less hysteresis than synthetic polyurethane foams. Precompressing the foam reduced the hysteresis further.

PIEZOELECTRIC SENSORS

Rittler (1988) reviews piezoelectric sensors. Pressure on certain crystals and ceramics generates electric charge, which appears on surface electrodes. Polyvinylidene fluoride (PVF_2) is a flexible polymer that also exhibits the piezoelectric effect. A fundamental defect of all piezoelectric sensors is that they do not respond to a fixed force. The charge generated by a step force is a correct measure of the magnitude of the step. However, the charge leaks off the electrodes over time, although Reston and Kolesar (1990) achieve time constants of about 30 seconds from a 5 × 5 array with integrated amplifiers. Polyvinylidene fluoride is also pyroelectric, so when grasping a warm object we cannot distinguish whether the output is due to force or due to heat.

A time-of-flight force sensor can be made by placing a PVF_2 transmitter and receiver on each side of a compressible silicone rubber pad (Hagnar, 1988b). The transmitter emits an ultrasonic pulse which travels through the pad to the receiver in about 1 μsec. Force decreases the pad thickness and also the time-of-flight. The elastomers have problems with fatigue, hysteresis, and low frequency response. Adequately compressible elastomers were often too porous to conduct the ultrasonic wave. A force near one edge caused a minimal time-of-flight there which was smaller than that for a uniform force.

OPTICAL FORCE SENSORS

Silvermintz (1988) reviews optical tactile sensors. Figure 4–10a shows the reflector type, which is commercially available in a 1.6-mm-thick package. A metal spring must be added to convert force to displacement. Figure 4–10b shows the occluder type. A commercial 8 × 8 array uses an elastomer deformable element, but is 28 mm thick, making it too thick for FNS. Thinner sensors using these principles could

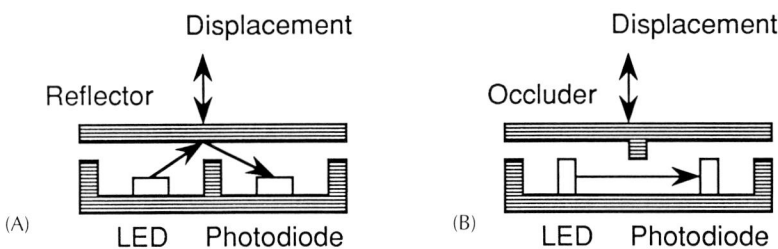

Figure 4-10 Light traveling from a light-emitting diode (LED) to a photodiode can be modulated by (A) changing the distance of a reflector, or (B) moving an occluder to interrupt the light path.

be made by bringing fiberoptics to a deformable element at the sensing location and placing the LED and photodiode at a remote location.

POSITION SENSORS

Antagonistic muscles control the angle of many joints, such as the wrist, elbow, ankle, and knee. To prevent one of the muscles from overpowering the other and yielding awkward angles, position sensors should provide feedback. Crago et al. (1986) note that external angle sensors are bulky and tend to slip. Johnson and Peckham (1990) have extended their experience with nonimplantable Hall-effect angle sensors and bench tested an implantable joint angle sensor. It senses the relative movement between two opposing bones of a joint by using an array of three Hall-effect sensors and a permanent magnet surgically implanted in the bones.

FUTURE DEVELOPMENT OF ARTIFICIAL SENSORS

Many early tactile sensors used elastomers as the spring in pressure and force sensors. Improved elastomers may reduce the large hysteresis in present polymers. Likely, future development will emphasize silicon because of its low hysteresis and potential low manufacturing cost. Packaging on polyimide is attractive because it is flexible and could hold arrays of silicon sensors. Lead wires can be printed on the polyimide and encapsulated in it. Then force can be sensed on the finger pad and the polyimide bent around to the nail side, where wire attachment is less subject to mechanical stress.

ACKNOWLEDGMENT

This work was supported by NIH grant NS-26328.

REFERENCES

Babbs, C.F., Bourland, J.D., Graber, G.P., Jones, J.T., and Schoenlein, W.E. (1990). A pressure-sensitive mat for measuring contact pressure distributions of patients lying on hospital beds. *Biomed. Instrum. Technol.* **24**, 363–370.

Beebe, D.J. (1990). *Tactile sensor packaging and fabrication feasibility studies.* M.S. Thesis, Department of Electrical and Computer Engineering, Madison, WI: University of Wisconsin.

Benton, L.A., Baker, L.L., Bowman, B.R., and Waters, R.L. (1981). *Functional Electrical Stimulation—A Practical Clinical Guide.* 2nd ed. Downey, CA: Rancho Los Amigos Rehabilitation Engineering Center.

Crago, P.E., Chizeck, H.J., Neuman, M.R., and Hambrecht, F.T. (1986). Sensors for use with functional neuromuscular stimulation. *IEEE Trans. Biomed. Eng.*, **33**, 256–268.

Hagnar, D. (1988a). Metal strain gages. In: J.G. Webster, ed., *Tactile Sensors for Robotics and Medicine.* New York: John Wiley & Sons.

Hagnar, D. (1988b). Other pressure sensors. In: J. G. Webster, ed., *Tactile Sensors for Robotics and Medicine.* New York: John Wiley & Sons.

Hahm, G. (1988). Semiconductor strain gages. In: J. G. Webster, ed., *Tactile Sensors for Robotics and Medicine.* New York: John Wiley & Sons.

Harmon, L.D. (1982). Automated tactile sensing. *Int. J. Robotics Res.*, **1**, 3–32.

Johnson, M.W., and Peckham, P.H. (1990). An implantable two-degree-of-freedom joint angle transducer. *Proc. Annu. Int. Conf. IEEE Eng. Med. Biol. Soc.*, **12**, 510–511.

Marsolais, E.B., Miller, P.C., and Chizeck, H.J. (1990). Metabolic energy costs of FNS walking in paraplegic subjects. *Proc. Annu. Int. Conf. IEEE Eng. Med. Biol. Soc.*, **12**, 2262–2263.

Mokshagundam, A.K. (1988). Conductive elastomers and carbon fibers. In: J.G. Webster, ed., *Tactile Sensors for Robotics and Medicine.* New York: John Wiley & Sons.

Peckham, P.H. (1988). Functional electrical stimulation. In: J.G. Webster, ed., *Encyclopedia of Medical Devices and Instrumentation.* New York: John Wiley & Sons.

Reston, R.R., and Kolesar, E.S., Jr. (1990). Robotic tactile sensor array fabricated from a piezoelectric polyvinylidene fluoride film. *Proc. IEEE 1990 National Aerospace and Electronics Conf. (NAECON).* Dayton, OH, III, 1139–1144.

Rittler, C. (1988). Piezoelectric sensors. In: J.G. Webster, ed., *Tactile Sensors for Robotics and Medicine.* New York: John Wiley & Sons.

Seow, K.C. (1988). Capacitive sensors. In: J.G. Webster, ed., *Tactile Sensors for Robotics and Medicine.* New York: John Wiley & Sons.

Silvermintz, L. (1988). Optoelectronic sensors. In: J.G. Webster, ed., *Tactile Sensors for Robotics and Medicine.* New York: John Wiley & Sons.

Sorab, J., Allen, R.H., and Gonik, B. (1988). Tactile sensory monitoring of clinician-applied forces during delivery of newborns. *IEEE Trans. Biomed. Eng.*, **35**, 1090–1093.

Tan, B.T. (1988). Sensor application to the space suit glove. In: J. G. Webster, ed., *Tactile Sensors for Robotics and Medicine.* New York: John Wiley & Sons.

5
Signals from Tactile Sensors in Glabrous Skin Suitable for Restoring Motor Functions in Paralyzed Humans

J.A. HOFFER AND M.K. HAUGLAND

Spinal cord injuries or stroke typically do not affect the peripheral sensory nerves that exit the spinal cord below the level of the lesion. In animal models, electrodes implanted on peripheral nerves have provided sensory feedback signals suitable for the closed-loop control of FES of paralyzed muscles. This chapter presents an overview of: (1) the sensory information normally coded by tactile mechanoreceptors in the human hand; (2) approaches that have been developed to record the activity of, and obtain skin contact force information from, sensory nerves in experimental animals; and (3) approaches that have been recently implemented in experimental animal models, where tactile sensory information has been used for 'closed-loop' control of FES. Permanently implanted, neurally interfaced control systems would be available for use at all times, reliably without need for frequent recalibration, and cosmetically acceptable to users. It is proposed that these neurally interfaced control systems are applicable for the restoration of upper limb motor functions in quadriplegia or hemiplegia, as well as gait and stance in paraplegia or hemiplegia.

An injury to the spinal cord can cause permanent loss of voluntary motor function, as well as loss of sensation. However, the peripheral motor and sensory nerves that exit the spinal cord below the level of the lesion usually remain viable, and so do the muscles. The determination of safe and efficient muscle and nerve stimulation parameters (Mortimer, 1981; Hambrecht, 1985; Grandjean and Mortimer, 1986; Sweeney and Mortimer, 1986) has made possible the restoration of some motor functions with functional electrical stimulation (FES) of paralyzed muscles (e.g., see Chapters 8, 10 and 11). However, the performance of contemporary FES systems is affected by fluctuations in muscle force output that are associated with fatigue, limb movement, and load characteristics (Crago et al., 1980, 1990; Cybulski et al., 1984). It has been proposed (e.g., Crago et al., 1980; Hoffer and Loeb, 1980; Hambrecht, 1985; Hoffer and Sinkjaer, 1986) and shown in laboratory experiments with spinal-cord-injured subjects (Crago et al., 1990), that if feedback from external sensors of force and/or position is used, the resulting "closed-loop" control of FES can significantly improve performance, as well as reduce user dependence on visual monitoring. In paraplegics, feedback about weight distribution, obtained from pressure sensors placed under the feet, improves the control of stance and gait using FES (Cybulski et al., 1984; Crago et al., 1986).

In the intact organism, specialized sensors in the skin, muscles, and joints provide sensory feedback information that is normally used by the central nervous system to regulate and update the motor output. The theme of this chapter is that many sensory functions remain intact after spinal-cord injury or stroke, and can be readily tapped with electrodes implanted in peripheral nerves to provide sensory feedback signals for the closed-loop control of FES.

ACTIVITY OF HUMAN GLABROUS SKIN MECHANORECEPTORS DURING PRECISION GRIP

Tactile mechanoreceptors in the human hand relay detailed information about local deformations and forces that occur at the glabrous skin of the fingertips when textured objects are held or touched (Phillips et al., 1990; Schmidt et al., 1990; Srinivasan et al., 1990). The receptive field properties and activity patterns of tactile mechanoreceptors have been studied in awake volunteers using microneurography, whereby a fine, insulated needle electrode is introduced by hand through the skin and into a peripheral nerve until the uninsulated tip of the electrode comes close to, and records extracellular action potentials from, single sensory axons (Johansson, 1978; Johansson and Westling, 1987; Westling and Johansson, 1987). Four types of mechanoreceptors have been identified that differ in their receptive field properties and characteristic discharge in response to standardized mechanical input to the skin. These types are: fast adapting with small receptive fields (FA I), fast adapting with large receptive fields (FA II), slowly adapting with small receptive fields (SA I), and slowly adapting with large receptive fields (SA II) (Johansson, 1978; Westling and Johansson, 1987). The activity patterns of each receptor type have been characterized during a precision grip task, in which an object is gripped, lifted, held, repositioned, and released with the thumb and fingers (Figure 5–1A). The FA I units become highly active during the initial period of grip-force increase and again, briefly, when the object is released, but fire at low rates or not at all during the hold phase. The SA I units are most active during the early and late phases of a lifting task, but continue firing while an object is held, with a tendency to adaptation. The FA II units are most sensitive to transient mechanical events when the grip force increases and when the object is released. The SA II units have comparatively stronger tonic responses while an object is held statically. The dynamic sensitivity of most glabrous skin mechanoreceptors is highest at low grip forces, because at low

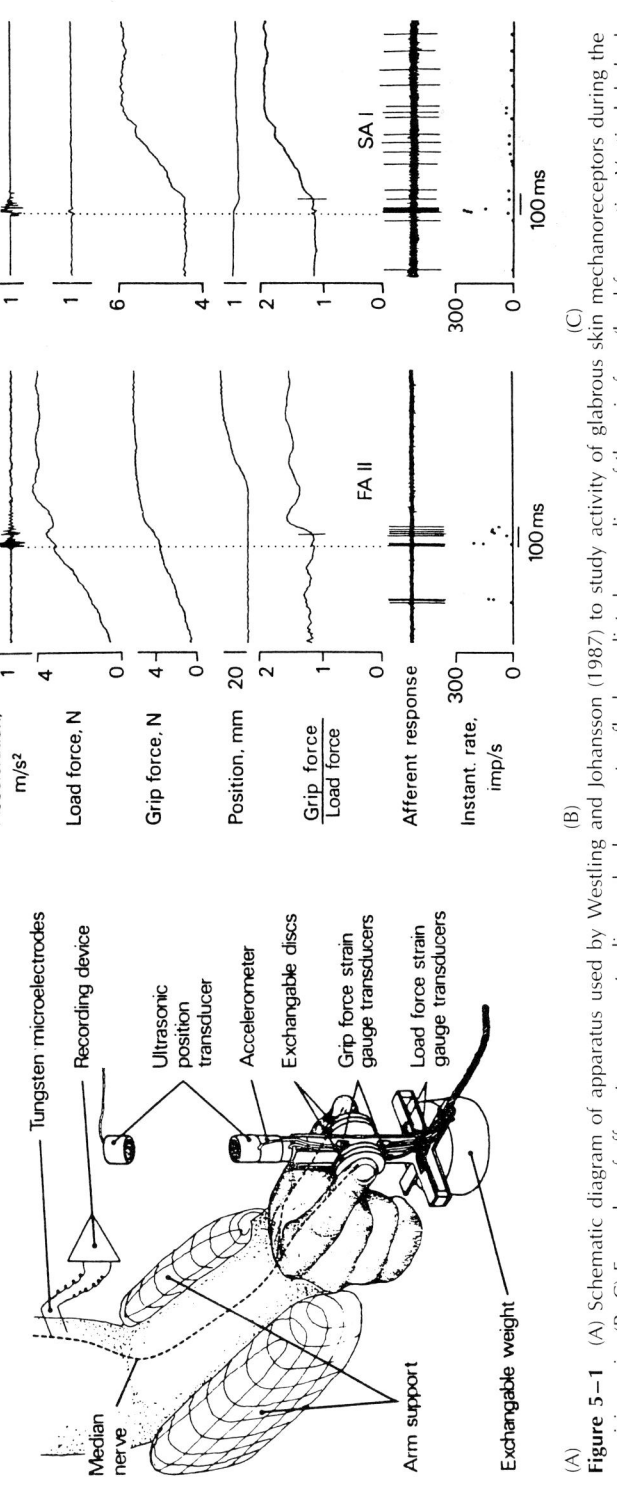

Figure 5–1 (A) Schematic diagram of apparatus used by Westling and Johansson (1987) to study activity of glabrous skin mechanoreceptors during the precision grip. (B, C) Examples of afferent responses to slips and subsequent, reflexly-mediated upgrading of the grip force/load force ratio. Vertical dashed lines indicate the onset of the slips, revealed by the acceleration signal. Short solid lines indicate the onset of the reflexly-mediated upgrading of the force ratio. (B) Shows the response of an FA II unit to a slip during the loading phase. (C) Shows the response of an SA I unit to a slip during the static phase. (From Figure 1A, Westling and Johansson, 1987, and Figure 2A and 2B, Johansson and Westling, 1987).

forces the skin indentation or deformation is relatively greater (Westling and Johansson, 1987; see also Pubols, 1990).

Of part. lar interest are the characteristic response patterns of glabrous skin mechanoreceptors when an object slips with respect to the skin of the fingers. Slips can occur either if the grip force declines below the minimum necessary to hold the object (Johansson and Westling, 1987), or if an unexpected load is added to the object (Johansson and Westling, 1988). During precision tasks, normal subjects produce grip forces just sufficiently larger than the minimum force required to hold an object, which is determined by the weight of the object and the frictional properties of the surface in contact with the fingers. If the grip force is insufficient and the object starts to slip, the type FA I, FA II, and SA I units all exhibit sharp activity bursts. Examples are shown in Figure 5-1B and C.

It has been shown that a short-latency spinal reflex of cutaneous origin is usually elicited by a slip, such that within 80 msec of the start of a slip, the grip force increases and the object is held securely again (Johansson and Westling, 1987; see Figure 5-1B, C). The cutaneous nature of this reflex has been shown by anesthetizing the skin. These rapid corrective responses are automatic, and do not involve conscious participation by the subjects. The reflex action is quite powerful, to the extent that subjects often cannot voluntarily release their grip slowly to let an object fall, because the reflex tends to interfere. The sensitivity of receptors to small slips is so high, that they often fire in response to "microslips" localized to a small area of the skin, in absence of actual movement of the object (Johansson and Westling, 1987).

METHODS FOR RECORDING PERIPHERAL NERVE ACTIVITY IN CONSCIOUS ANIMALS

Over the past 15 years, three main approaches were developed for long-term recording of peripheral nerve activity in conscious, freely-moving animals: (1) nerve cuff electrodes, to record the aggregate activity of nerve fiber populations; (2) intrafascicular "floating, single-unit" microelectrodes, to record the activity of individual neurons; and (3) intrafascicular multiunit electrodes, to record the activity of small groups of neurons. Nerve cuff electrodes have been used to assess the motor and/or sensory traffic in individual peripheral nerves during posture and locomotion, and to monitor the fates, over weeks and months, of motor and sensory axons in cut or regenerating nerves. Floating microelectrodes have been inserted in cat dorsal roots or ganglia to record the activity of individual sensory neurons, in ventral roots to record the activity of motor neurons, and in spinal cord tracts to record the activity of spinocerebellar neurons. See Hoffer (1990) for a review of these approaches. Recently, floating microelectrodes have also been inserted directly in muscle nerves, to record the individual activity patterns of several motor and sensory neurons connected to the same muscle (Hoffer and Weytjens, 1990). Intrafascicular multiunit electrodes have been inserted in cat peripheral nerves to monitor groups of neurons of cutaneous origin. In the following sections, these approaches to record from neuronal populations will be summarized, and their relative advantages and limitations for human applications will be evaluated.

Whole-Nerve Recordings with Nerve Cuff Electrodes

Electrode Design Considerations. Nerve cuff recording electrodes consist of an insulating cuff (usually silicone tubing) that contains several circumferential metal electrodes (usually multistranded, flexible stainless steel wire, Teflon-coated), placed around a length of peripheral nerve. The design, fabrication, and surgical installation of nerve cuff recording electrodes were reviewed in detail by Hoffer (1990). The insulating cuff serves to resolve the small action currents generated by nerve fibers, by constraining the current flow within a long, narrow resistive path. The insulating cuff also reduces the pickup of electromyographic (EMG) potentials generated by nearby muscles as well as signals generated by any other sources outside the cuff. Rejection of unwanted signals is optimized if differential recording from a balanced tripolar electrode configuration is used (Hoffer, 1975; Stein et al., 1975, 1977). Four main parameters—fiber diameter, cuff inside diameter, cuff length, and interelectrode distance—determine the shapes and amplitudes of the axonal potentials recorded (Marks and Loeb, 1976). To obtain maximal signal amplitudes, the length of a nerve cuff should be close to the wavelength of neural action potentials (30–40 mm), and about ten times greater than the I.D. The aggregate electroneurographic (ENG) activity recorded from a nerve depends on the number of active fibers, is usually dominated by the activity of the largest axons, and is biased in favor of superficial axons; in 1- to 4-mm-diameter nerves, action potential amplitudes recorded from deep axons can be attenuated two- or three-fold (Marks and Loeb, 1976; Stein and Oguztöreli, 1978; Hoffer et al., 1981a). Cuff impedances usually range between 3 and 20 kΩ, using a 1-kHz sinusoidal test signal. Electroneurographic amplitudes recorded during walking have ranged from about 5 μV (peak-to-peak) for the cat sciatic nerve (using a 4-mm I.D., 30-mm-long cuff), to up to 90 μV (peak-to-peak) for the much finer rabbit tenuissimus nerve (using a 0.3-mm I.D., 5-mm-long cuff). Since the nerve cuff source impedance is low and the signal amplitude is small, an ultra-low-noise, low-input impedance differential preamplifier should be used (e.g., Leaf Electronics QT-5B; Charles, 1989).

Damage to Nerves. For chronic implantation of a nerve recording cuff, the nerve of interest must be freed from surrounding tissues, as far away from joints as possible, and in a region where local branches or communicating blood vessels are not present. Nerve damage, if it occurs, takes place most commonly in the first 48 hours after surgical implantation. However, if appropriate precautions are taken in mobilizing the nerve, and the nerve cuff is placed so that the nerve is neither pulled nor torqued by the lead-out cable, the long-term prognosis of a nerve preparation is excellent. Following implantation, as connective tissue grows around and into a nerve cuff, the mechanical coupling of the cuff and nerve becomes increasingly stable, and the likelihood of nerve damage diminishes with time. As a bonus, as fluid is replaced by connective tissue inside the cuff the impedance increases, and nerve potential amplitudes increase over a period of weeks (Stein et al., 1978). To prevent compression neuropathy associated with postsurgical edema (Aguayo et al., 1971; Hoffer, 1975; Davis et al., 1978), the cuff I.D. should be about 20% larger than the nerve diameter. Compression affects most severely the largest diameter axons in a nerve, and causes a reduction in axonal conduction velocities (Sunderland, 1968; Gillespie and Stein, 1983). Properly fitted nerve cuffs do not cause compression damage in cats implanted chronically for several months, as evidenced by the normal ranges of axonal conduction velocities measured for group Ia (Hoffer et al., 1981a; Loeb et al., 1985) as well as alpha motor neuron axons (Hoffer et al., 1987).

Functional Longevity. In contrast to transducers that must withstand mechanical deformation for their function (e.g., implantable tendon force or muscle length transducers; reviewed by Hoffer, 1990), nerve cuff electrodes are mechanically passive and robust, contain only biocompatible materials that do not corrode or deteriorate, and cannot migrate. The most common failure, lead breakage, can be reduced by appropriate selection of wire materials, location of connectors, and routing of lead-out cables. Stable signals have been recorded from cat hindlimb nerves for over 1 year (Gordon et al., 1980). Chronic electrical stimulation of human nerves, first attempted over 100 years ago, has been performed on phrenic and peroneal nerves for 25 years. Evidence for the long-term safety and stable performance of nerve cuff electrodes implanted in humans is abundant in the clinical literature (reviewed by Glenn and Phelps, 1985; Hambrecht and Reswick, 1977; McNeal and Bowman, 1985).

Day-to-Day Stability and Reproducibility of Recorded Signals. Unless a nerve is damaged as a consequence of the surgical procedure (Stein et al., 1980), the recorded signals are stable for many weeks and months (Davis et al., 1978; Gordon et al., 1980), and reproducible for matched testing conditions (Hoffer et al., 1989), because nerve cuff electrodes record from a fixed population of neurons. The amplitude of neural potentials tends to increase during the initial weeks after implantation as the cuff impedance rises gradually (Stein et al., 1978). If this impedance change is taken into account, the action current sources can be estimated and the potentials can be calibrated (Hoffer et al., 1981a).

Intrafascicular Recordings from Single Axons

Electrode Design Considerations. In microneurographic recordings in human subjects performing hand tasks, the tip of a microelectrode must be placed in close proximity to axons and remain immobile during a recording session. Since nerves can stretch considerably and bend around joints (Sunderland, 1968), the requirement for stable mechanical coupling between intraneural electrode and nerve is usually only met by: (1) recording from nerve trunks in the mechanically restrained upper arm, far from the hand; (2) limiting the range and velocity of angular motion over which recordings are done; and (3) limiting the range of forces studied. Peripheral nerve studies in unrestrained animals cannot involve conventional microelectrodes, because the electrodes either damage the neural tissue or become dislodged; therefore, floating microelectrodes were developed as an alternative (reviewed by Prochazka, 1984; Hoffer, 1990). Floating microelectrodes usually consist of a short, stiff wire that can penetrate the tissue without bending (usually platinum-iridium or tungsten), attached to a very compliant lead-out wire (usually gold). The electrode is insulated except for a recording tip. Electrodes of this design can remain in close proximity to the same neurons for several days, even during the most vigorous movements performed by conscious animals.

The choice of materials, electrode dimensions, and tip shape determine the amplitude of extracellular potentials recorded from single axons, as well as the background activity recorded from other neurons, movement artifacts, and pickup of noise arising from other sources. Because microelectrodes have higher impedances than nerve cuff electrodes, noise pickup is a more severe problem. Floating microelectrodes with tip impedances between 100 and 200 kΩ have given the best signal-to-noise ratios in cat dorsal (Loeb and Hoffer, 1985; Loeb et al., 1985) or ventral root recordings (Hoffer et al., 1987). Microelectrodes with tip impedance below 50 kΩ rarely resolve unitary potentials larger than background noise in freely moving animals, whereas high-impedance microelectrodes may record larger potentials but, because of the capacitance in lead cables, are also stronger antennas for extrinsic noise pickup and movement artifact (reviewed by Hoffer, 1990). To reduce lead capacitance, microelectrode records are usually current-amplified as close as possible to the source. Coaxial shielding of the implanted lead wires can improve noise rejection (Prochazka, 1984). Depending on the frequency spectrum, noise can often be reduced with bandpass filtering. For myelinated axons, the signal bandpass of interest is 1–10 kHz, whereas electromyographic or electrocardiographic activity picked up by microelectrodes have frequency components mainly below 1 kHz that can be filtered out. Floating microelectrodes usually record potentials from more than one axon in their vicinity. One or a few unitary potentials can often be isolated from background activity, on-line, using threshold and window discriminators. Discriminable unitary potential amplitudes typically range from 25–75 μV, against background activity and peak-to-peak noise of 10 μV or more.

Damage to Nerves. Floating microelectrodes sometimes have caused significant reductions in the axonal conduction velocity of recorded neurons, most likely from focal demyelination and/or local compression near the electrode tip (Hoffer et al., 1987). Nevertheless, floating microelectrodes inserted in peripheral nerves or roots are less likely to disturb the function of axons in their vicinity than similar electrodes chronically implanted near nerve cell bodies in the spinal cord or the brain. This is because the presence of an electrode near a cell body can alter the cell membrane properties, cause damage to dendrites and/or to presynaptic terminal branches, any of which could cause aberrant discharge patterns in the affected neurons. This problem is avoided when electrodes are placed near the axons, far away from the sites of synaptic integration and action potential generation.

Functional Longevity. The survival of intrafascicular fine-wire electrodes depends importantly on the mechanical stresses imposed on the lead wires. Because of the requirement for high compliance, a usual reason for failure has been lead-wire breakage. In the cat spinal cord, roots, or nerves, floating microelectrodes have typically survived only a few weeks after implantation. In electrodes that last more than 3 weeks, a secondary reason for functional failure is encapsulation by fibrous tissue that tends to separate the electrode tip from nearby neurons, by several tens of μm. Evidence for this process has come from histological studies (Schmidt et al., 1976), from the progressively smaller unitary action potentials that are recorded over time, and from the progressively larger currents that are needed to microstimulate units over time (Hoffer, 1990). To be clinically applicable, the functional lifetime of floating microelectrodes must be improved substantially. This will require the use of materials with greater fatigue resistance (to reduce lead breakage) and tissue compatibility (to reduce fibrotic reaction). Approaches under development include implantation of miniature multicontact electrode arrays made of a variety of materials (Weissman and Schwartz, 1981; Edell, 1986; Anderson et al., 1989).

Day-to-Day Stability and Reproducibility of Recorded Signals. Floating microelectrodes implanted in dorsal or ventral roots of cats usually provide stable records from the same axon(s) for several hours, and occasionally for several days. It is therefore possible to study the activity of sensory (e.g., Loeb et al., 1985) as well as motor neurons (e.g., Hoffer et al., 1987) in conscious animals during a variety of conditions, and to identify each neuron rigorously. However, because floating microelectrodes tend to migrate, on any given recording day there is a high probability of losing contact with previously recorded neurons, as well as a chance of encountering new neurons.

Intrafascicular Recordings from Multiple Axons

An intermediate approach to recording from either whole nerves or single axons involves recording the activity of small subpopulations of axons, using flexible monofilament wire electrodes (made of 25-μm platinum-iridium, Teflon-coated, with a 1-mm deinsulated region) inserted in individual nerve fascicles (Malagodi et al., 1989; Goodall et al., in press). A potential advantage of multiunit intrafascicular recordings over nerve cuff recordings is that electrodes implanted in different fascicles of a peripheral nerve could monitor several different modalities and/or sensory fields, and therefore provide several channels of information, instead of the single channel provided by a conventional nerve cuff electrode. As well, even if multiunit intraneural electrodes drift, the summed activity recorded from day to day could be less prone to the large variations that are typical of single-unit microelectrode recordings.

Damage to Nerves. To date there is insufficient evidence on the extent of chronic damage caused by different types of intraneural electrodes. As a minimum, the type of focal damage caused to nearby axons by floating microelectrodes (see previous section) can be expected from any type of intraneural electrode. However, with careful choice of materials and surgical technique, only minor damage should take place, restricted mostly to axons in the nerve in close proximity to the implanted wires.

Functional Longevity. For multiunit intrafascicular recording electrodes followed for up to 6 months in experimental animals, electrode integrity was 100% for the first 2 months, but dropped to 75% by 6 months (Malagodi et al., 1989; Goodall et al., in press). By extrapolation, the functional longevity of these electrodes was predicted to be 18–24 months.

Day-to-Day Stability and Reproducibility of Recorded Signals. In recordings carried out under anesthesia once per month from intrafascicular electrodes implanted for 6 months by Malagodi et al. (1989) and Goodall et al. (in press), an average of ten sensory units were recorded by each surviving electrode, as determined from probing sensory fields, which recorded unitary potential amplitudes up to 12 μV, against background noise of 5–6 μV, in the immobile, anesthetized animal. The modalities, skin field locations, potential amplitudes, and total number of sensory units recorded by individual electrodes were found to change from month to month, indicating migration of the electrodes. Unitary potential signal-to-noise ratios declined after 4 months, suggesting gradual fibrous encapsulation of electrodes, which was confirmed by histological follow-up. The performance of these intrafascicular electrodes with regard to rejection of EMG signals generated by nearby muscles, or presence of movement-associated artifacts in the conscious, moving animal, were not addressed in these studies.

ADVANTAGES AND LIMITATIONS OF NERVE CUFF VERSUS INTRAFASCICULAR ELECTRODES

For the specific purpose of controlling FES systems for restoration of either hand function or gait, the different methods of recording peripheral nerve signals represent compromises among three factors: (1) total number of channels of sensory information required (or available); (2) day-to-day reproducibility of the sensory information recorded; and (3) availability of methods for on-line processing of recorded data.

Whole-nerve recordings with cuff electrodes provide only one channel of information from the aggregate activity of many nerve fibers that represent various sensory modalities and arise from widespread skin areas. On the other hand, nerve cuff signals feature considerable spatial and temporal averaging and are therefore far smoother and less sensitive to the specific location and detailed pattern of the skin input than signals recorded from single mechanoreceptors. The latter properties of cuff signals can be very desirable for feedback regulation of an FES controller. It remains to be shown whether a single channel of feedback information will be sufficient to control the coordinated activation of approximately eight muscles that must be activated with FES to restore grip in paralyzed humans (Peckham, 1987; Kilgore et al., 1989). However, because the several muscles act synergistically, it is not unreasonable that a single channel of sensory information may provide appropriate feedback regulation for the control of grip. This prediction was recently tested in an animal model, where stimulation of four synergistic muscles was controlled securely using tactile feedback from a single nerve cuff electrode (described in a later section).

In contrast to conventional nerve cuff electrodes, intraneural recordings may provide multiple channels of information. In order for intraneural approaches to be clinically useful, however, several practical problems must be solved. First, the functional lifetime of intrafascicular electrodes must be improved, both in regard to lead survival and electrode encapsulation by connective tissue. An appealing potential solution to the lead breakage problem awaits the availability of injectable recording electrodes, akin to stimulating electrodes currently under development (Loeb and Zamin, in press). Second, even if signals could be reliably recorded with intrafascicular electrodes for extended periods of time, it remains to be shown whether the activity recorded from neighboring axons would represent *independent* sensory channels. This is because mechanoreceptors of different modalities vary widely in their receptive field properties (Johansson, 1978), and their afferent fibers are intermingled in the nerve fascicles. In addition, there is considerable, frequent fascicular exchange of axons along peripheral nerves (Sunderland, 1968), with the result that at increasing distances from the skin, the receptive fields of neighboring nerve fibers are increasingly scrambled. Third, intraneural electrodes are known to drift, and the consequent sudden, intermittent changes in the populations of recorded neurons pose formidable problems that will require the development of on-line, adaptive, neural activity recognition and sorting methods, considerably more powerful than currently available methods (e.g., Forster and Handwerker, 1990). For these reasons, a feedback system based on intrafascicular recordings that would be reliable enough to be used by patients without frequent need for adjustment appears to be beyond the capability of present technology. However, given further advances in materials technology, in methods of interfacing that do not require lead wires, and in real-time information processing, these problems may be solvable.

TACTILE SIGNALS RECORDED FROM NERVES IN ANIMAL MODELS OF PRECISION GRIP

The suitability of nerve cuff electrodes for obtaining tactile signals was initially shown by Hoffer et al. (1989), in experiments where the cat footpad served as a model of human glabrous skin. Further studies were carried out by Haugland and Hoffer (unpublished; full reports are in preparation). In this review, the methods used and the main findings are summarized. Four main questions were addressed:

1. How does the ENG recorded from a cutaneous nerve relate to forces applied perpendicularly on the skin?
2. During FES of nearby muscles, can artifact-free tactile signals be recorded from peripheral nerves?
3. How does the ENG recorded from a cutaneous nerve relate to forces applied tangentially on the skin?
4. Can the recorded ENG be used for the closed-loop control of FES in an animal model of grasp?

Surgical Implantation. For this study, ten cats were surgically anesthetized with Halothane gas in a O_2-N_2O mixture. As shown in Figure 5–2, a 30–40-mm-long, 2.2-mm-I.D. silicone rubber cuff with three circumferential stainless steel wire electrodes (Cooner AS 631) was implanted on the left tibial nerve, 2 to 4 cm proximal to the ankle joint. A sciatic nerve recording cuff, 20-mm-long, 4-mm-I.D. with three stainless steel wire electrodes, was implanted in the mid-thigh region. Leads from the cuffs and other implanted devices coursed subcutaneously to an external connector mounted on the cat's back (Hoffer, 1990). After surgery, cats were given analgesics (acepromazine maleate and subcutaneous morphine, 0.10 mg/kg) for at least 24 hours. Recording sessions started 4 to 7 days after implantation.

Nerve Blocking Cuffs. To exclude the participation of motor activity in the ENG recorded from the tibial nerve during walking, in several cats a blocking cuff (Hoffer et al., 1990), 8 mm long, was placed on the tibial nerve between the tibial and sciatic recording cuffs. Axonal conduction was blocked by infusing lidocaine sodium solution (2%) via a catheter that led to the blocking cuff from a port in the external connector. The conduction block was assessed from the progressive reduction of the compound action potential recorded by the sciatic nerve cuff, evoked by stimulation of the tibial nerve at the distal recording cuff. Usually, the tibial nerve was completely blocked

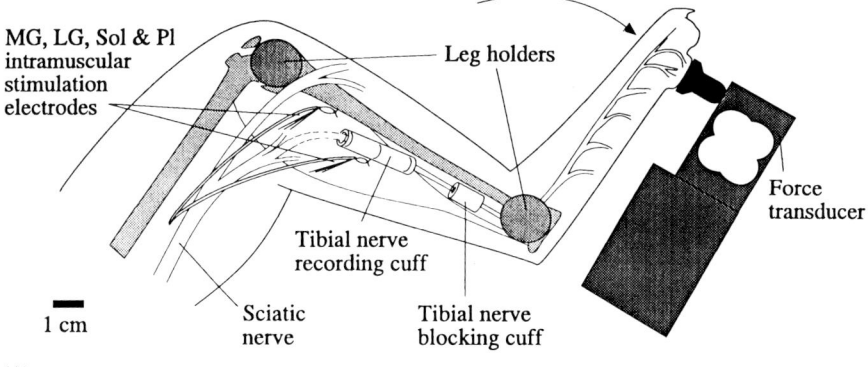

Figure 5–2 (A) Diagram of electrodes implanted in cat hindlimb and apparatus used to measure neural responses to perpendicular forces applied on the footpad. The cat was under anesthesia. The limb was held at the ankle malleoli and knee with atraumatic, cupped clamps. The footpad was in contact with a 1-cm disk in series with a force transducer. Forces were produced either by a servo-controlled printed motor, or be FES via electrodes implanted in the four ankle dorsiflexor muscles (MG, LG, Sol, and Pl). ENG activity in the tibial nerve was recorded with a tripolar nerve cuff electrode. To identify in the recorded signal the contributions from footpad afferents and artifacts caused by the stimulation, a blocking cuff was placed distally on the tibial nerve. Axonal conduction was blocked by infusing 2% lidocaine solution via a catheter that linked the blocking cuff to a port in the backpack connector (Hoffer, 1990). (B) Diagram of apparatus used to measure neural responses during grip. When the plantarflexor muscles were stimulated, the paw moved (curved arrow), until the footpad pressed against an object. The object could slide vertically along a low-friction bearing, was covered with fine sandpaper on the surface contacted by the cat's footpad, and contained two force transducers aligned in the vertical direction and perpendicularly to the footpad (further description in text).

after 20 to 30 minutes. At the end of each experiment the block was reversed with infusion of normal saline solution.

In other cats, a tibial nerve blocking cuff was placed *distal* to the tibial nerve recording cuff (Figure 5–2A, B) in order to identify the contributions from footpad afferents, and the presence in the recording cuff signal or any artifacts caused by the stimuli and/or compound EMG potentials, during FES of nearby muscles.

Data Collection. On average once per week during a 1- to 3-month period, each cat was anesthetized with halothane gas, the left foot was shaved, remaining hair was removed with depilatory cream, and the leg was secured at the ankle malleoli and knee with two pairs of cupped holders (Figure 5–2). In the first series of experiments, a servo-controlled motor was used to push perpendicularly on the central footpad with a 1-cm disc-shaped probe (Figure 5–2A). Applied forces were monitored by a series transducer. The position and compliance of the motor were electronically regulated with position, velocity, and force feedback. Control signals were generated with an IBM-compatible '386 computer. The tibial ENG was analog-rectified and bin-integrated in 1- to 10-msec bins (Bak PSI-1). Electroneurograph, motor position, and force data were digitized on-line (100 Hz/channel) with the same computer (Haugland and Hoffer, in preparation).

PERPENDICULAR FORCE INFORMATION AVAILABLE IN NERVE CUFF RECORDINGS

The ENG signal recorded with cuff electrodes from the tibial nerve has been studied during application of perpendicular, time-varying forces onto the cat footpad, including ramp-and-hold steps of different ramp velocities and amplitudes, sinusoidal or triangular oscillations (0.1–10 Hz) of varying amplitude, and band-limited noise (DC–10 Hz). The impulse response relating rectified ENG to force has been identified using the two-sided linear filter identification method of Hunter and Kearney (1983) for a variety of tasks and data epochs. Estimates of force have been obtained by convolving the impulse response with the ENG (Hoffer et al., 1989; Haugland et al., in preparation).

For descriptive purposes, the properties of the ENG signal are most clearly apparent from the responses to perpendicular force steps. Three reproducible features occur, as seen in the example of Figure 5–3. The first feature is a brief, large-amplitude burst of ENG activity, coincident with the rise in force. The time of occurrence and the magnitude of the ENG peak depend on the rate of rise and amplitude of the force change (Haugland et al., in preparation). After the peak, the ENG signal decreases rapidly.

The second feature is a slow, near-exponential decline in ENG activity during the constant-force phase of a step (Figure 5–3). Because the ENG signal declines with time, the absolute force value can be derived from the ENG signal only if the history of precedent force changes is also known. In particular, when measured at the same time after the onset of a series of individual force steps of varying amplitude, the mean ENG level is linearly related to the amplitude of the step (Haugland et al., in preparation).

The third feature is a brief ENG burst that signals the rapid decline in force at

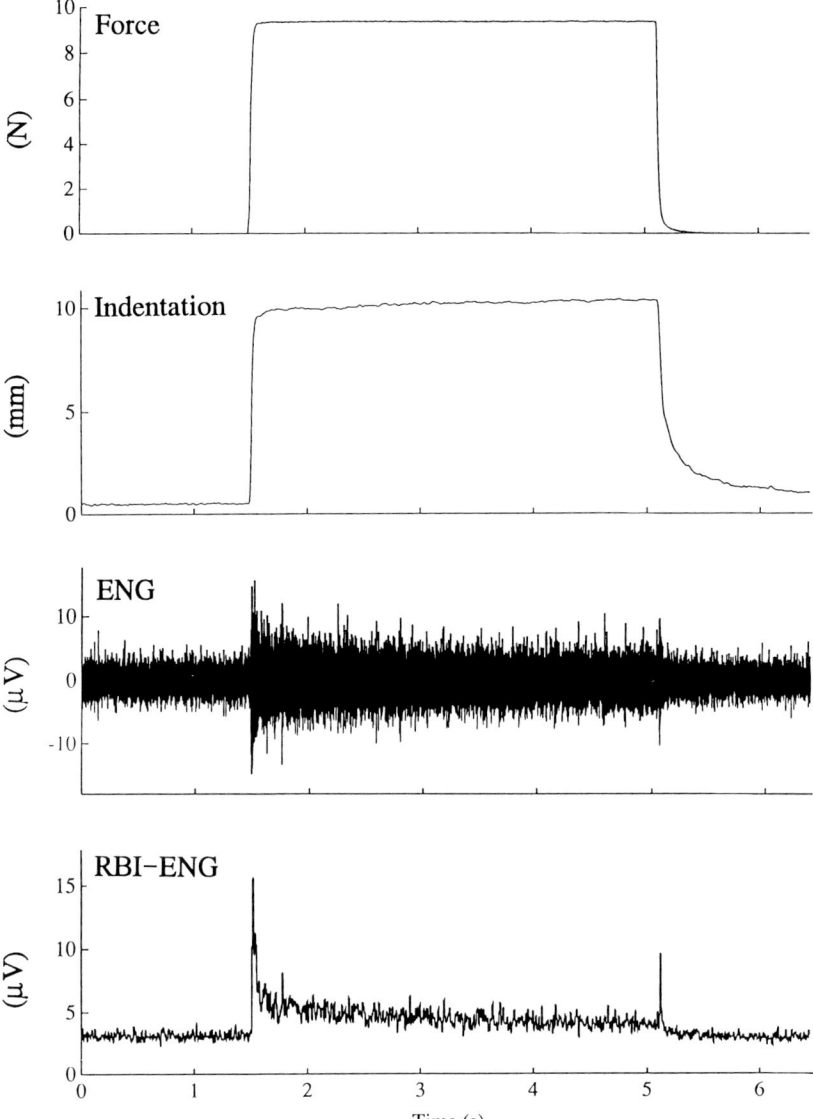

Figure 5–3 Dependence of the tibial nerve cuff signal on the force applied on the footpad. Top trace: External force step applied perpendicularly on the cat footpad by a servo-controlled motor (approximately 9 N, held constant for 3.5 s). Second trace: Resulting indentation of the footpad, where zero corresponds to the probe just touching the uncompressed skin. Third trace: ENG signal recorded by tibial nerve cuff electrode, filtered between 1 and 10 kHz and sampled at 20 kHz. Bottom trace: ENG signal after rectification and bin-integration, sampled at 100 Hz. Three characteristic features are present in the ENG signal: a brief, large activity burst, coincident with the rise in force, a slow, near-exponential decline during the constant-force phase, and a brief activity burst that signals the end of the step.

the end of a step (Figure 5-3). The amplitude of the terminal ENG burst scales with the amplitude of force change, but depends also on the final value of the force. Terminal ENG peaks are largest when the force declines to near-zero values.

In summary, ENG signals recorded from the cat tibial nerve contain reproducible information about the changes in the force applied perpendicularly on the footpad. The ENG responses to force steps recorded from the cat tibial nerve reflect a combination of the characteristic activity patterns of rapidly adapting and slowly adapting tactile receptors described by Westling and Johansson (1987) for human glabrous skin mechanoreceptors during precision grip. Qualitatively similar features have also been observed in ENG recordings during precision grip tasks using a cuff electrode implanted on the median nerve of a monkey (Milner et al., 1989; Milner et al., 1991).

ARTIFACT-FREE NERVE CUFF ELECTRODE RECORDINGS DURING FES

In order for cutaneous ENG signals to be applicable for the control of FES in paralyzed humans, it is necessary to demonstrate that similar ENG signals can be recorded from peripheral nerves during FES. The reason for this concern is that when nearby muscles are stimulated electrically, two kinds of artifacts may contaminate the signals recorded from peripheral nerves: both the electrical stimuli and the large compound EMG potentials that are elicited by FES may be picked up by nerve cuff recording electrodes.

Artifact-free ENG signals have been obtained during electrical stimulation of four calf muscles that surround the tibial nerve, using a specially developed signal processing and sampling method (Haugland and Hoffer, in preparation). In the cat hindlimb preparation described in previous sections, in addition to a recording cuff on the tibial nerve, bipolar intramuscular stimulating electrodes were implanted in the soleus (SOL), medial and lateral gastrocnemius (MG, LG), and plantaris (PL) muscles. In experiments performed under anesthesia, the four plantarflexor muscles were stimulated in turn by the computer, at a fixed stimulation frequency of 25 Hz per muscle. Recruitment was controlled by pulse-width modulation (Crago et al., 1980) in the range between 0 and 255 μsec. For each muscle, the stimulation amplitude was chosen so that the isometric force just saturated for the longest pulse width used. Feed-forward control of these muscles was not reliable, because of ongoing fatigue and the complex geometry and mechanical properties of the muscles, ankle joint, and footpad. Performance was improved considerably with a closed-loop controller that used feedback from an external force sensor (Figure 5-2A).

As could be expected, when the cat plantarflexor muscles were stimulated electrically, large artifacts appeared in the tibial nerve cuff electrode recordings. In addition to stimulus artifacts that lasted about 1 msec, the synchronous activation of motor units in each muscle caused EMG pickup artifacts that lasted up to 6 msec, of shape and amplitude that depended on which of the four muscles was being stimulated. As has been observed before for naturally occurring EMG activity (Hoffer, 1975; Stein et al., 1975, 1977; Gordon et al., 1980), the amplitude of the compound EMG picked up by the nerve cuff electrodes was reduced considerably by bandpass filtering (1-10 kHz). When filtered in this way, the tibial nerve cuff records

SIGNALS FROM TACTILE SENSORS

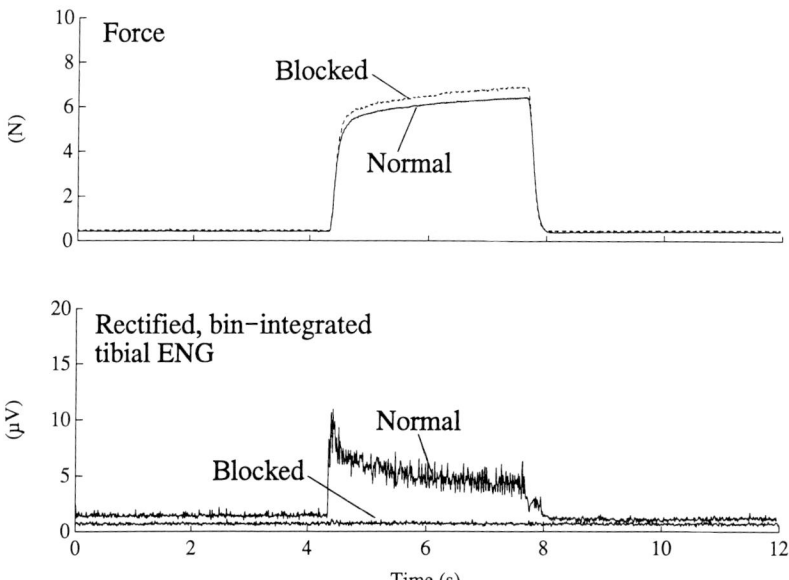

Figure 5–4 Demonstration of tactile origin of cat tibial nerve signals, and absence of artifact contamination, during FES of four plantarflexor muscles. Top: Footpad forces produced by FES when conduction was normal in the tibial nerve (solid line), and after conduction block with lidocaine (dashed line), were similar. Bottom: Tibial nerve cuff signal, sampled after conduction block, was near zero (dashed line), demonstrating that the cuff electrode signal normally sampled (solid line) was produced by sensory fibers and was uncontaminated by artifact associated with FES of nearby muscles (same cat as Figure 5–3).

were again free of stimulation artifact starting 6 to 7 msec after delivery of each stimulus. Because the muscles were stimulated at a cumulative rate of 100 Hz, this meant that for each 10-msec interstimulus interval, the final 3 msec were free of artifact. On this basis, the nerve cuff records were analog-rectified and bin-integrated using a sample-hold integrator (Bak PSI-1) synchronized with the stimulation output, and the computer sampled only the integrated ENG activity that occurred during the 3-msec epoch that just preceded the delivery of each stimulus to the muscles, at a rate of 100 Hz.

The tibial nerve blocking cuff that was implanted distal to the tibial nerve recording cuff (Figure 5–2A) was used to demonstrate the tactile origin, as well as the absence of artifact contamination of the nerve signals that were sampled by the computer during FES of the plantarflexor muscles. An example is shown in Figure 5–4. *Solid lines* show the force produced by FES of the plantarflexor muscles, recorded by the force transducer in contact with the footpad (top trace) and the tibial nerve cuff signal that was sampled by the computer, when conduction was normal in the tibial nerve (bottom trace). The experiment was repeated about a half hour later, after conduction in the distal portion of the tibial nerve was blocked by infusion of lidocaine into the blocking cuff. *Dashed lines* show a comparable force profile, produced again by FES (top trace) and the tibial nerve cuff signal sampled by the computer (bottom trace). When activity in the nerve was blocked, the signal sampled by the computer was always near zero, and was not modulated when the muscles were stimulated and force was applied on the footpad. This demonstrated that the cuff electrode signal normally sampled by the computer was indeed produced by tibial nerve afferent fibers, and was furthermore uncontaminated by artifact associated with FES of nearby muscles.

When conduction in the tibial nerve was not blocked, the activity sampled by the computer resembled the ENG responses to step forces applied to the footpad of anesthetized cats, in the absence of FES (Figure 5-3). The relatively smaller peak ENG amplitudes in Figure 5-4, when compared to ENG responses to step forces produced with the servo-controlled motor (Figure 5-3), reflected the slower rise and fall of the forces attained with FES, compared to the step forces produced by the motor. The force-ENG relations were otherwise comparable in the passive leg and in the FES-activated leg. Therefore, these experiments demonstrated that if appropriate sampling methods are used, it is possible to obtain accurate, artifact-free recordings of tactile afferent activity in peripheral nerves, even during activation of several nearby muscles with FES.

SLIP INFORMATION AVAILABLE IN NERVE CUFF RECORDINGS

The preceding sections have focused on information contained in neural recordings that relates to forces applied perpendicularly to the skin. Records of tactile afferent activity during precision grip in humans have shown that large afferent signals can also occur when a gripped object slips with respect to the skin. In a third set of recent experiments by Haugland and Hoffer, when the cat plantarflexor muscles were stimulated electrically and the cat's paw held an object comparable to that used by Westling and Johansson (1987), the signal recorded by tibial nerve cuff electrodes was found to also contain clear slip-related information.

The experimental apparatus is described in Figure 5-2B. The cat was under anesthesia, with the hindlimb held at the ankle malleoli and knee with atraumatic, cupped clamps. When not stimulated, the foot hung vertically. When the plantarflexor muscles were stimulated, the paw moved slightly until the footpad pressed against an object that could slide vertically with low friction, and that fell out of reach if not held by the paw. On the surface contacted by the cat's footpad, the object was covered with fine sandpaper (300 grit). The weight of the object was 150 grams. Slips were produced in two conditions. In one condition (intended to represent progressive muscle "fatigue"), the force produced with FES was allowed to decline by gradually reducing the pulse durations used to stimulate the muscles until the force was no longer sufficient and the object slipped. An example is shown in Figure 5-5A. In the second condition, the muscles were stimulated at a constant level, sufficient to hold the object. At a certain time, an additional 100-g weight was dropped on the object, that caused the object to slip. An example is shown in Figure 5-5B.

For both experimental conditions, the sampled ENG signal typically shows sharp bursts if one of three kinds of events occur. First, at the start of the electrical stimulation of the plantarflexor muscles, a surge in ENG accompanies the rise in grip force (left-most vertical lines, labeled O in Figures 5-5A, B). Second, when the object (until then held by the experimenter's hand) is released, an ENG burst

SIGNALS FROM TACTILE SENSORS

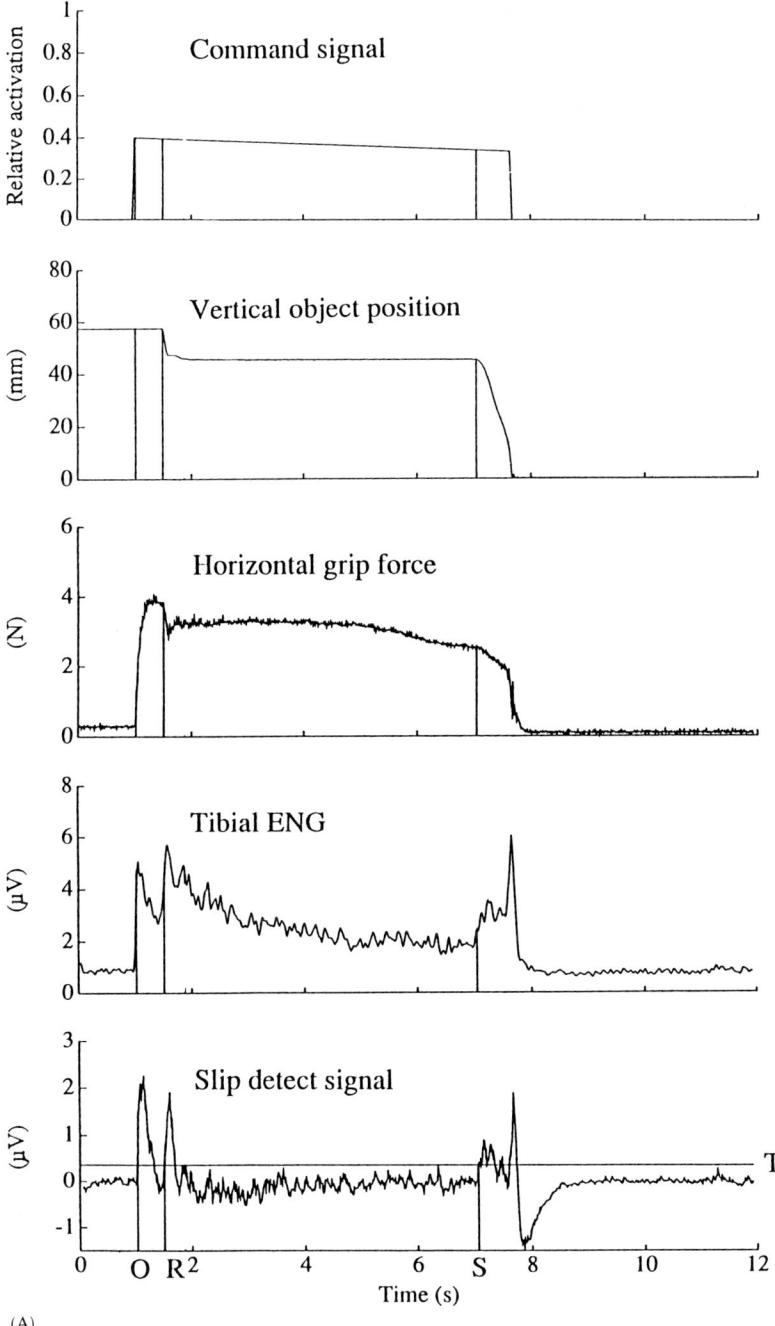

(A)

Figure 5–5 (A) Slip detection from nerve cuff recordings during simulated muscle "fatigue." After start of FES (O) and release of object (R), gradual reduction of the command signal (top panel), caused the horizontal grip force (third panel) to decline until the object slipped and fell (second panel). The differentiated ENG signal (bottom panel) showed a slip-related burst that the computer detected (S) if a threshold value (T) was exceeded.

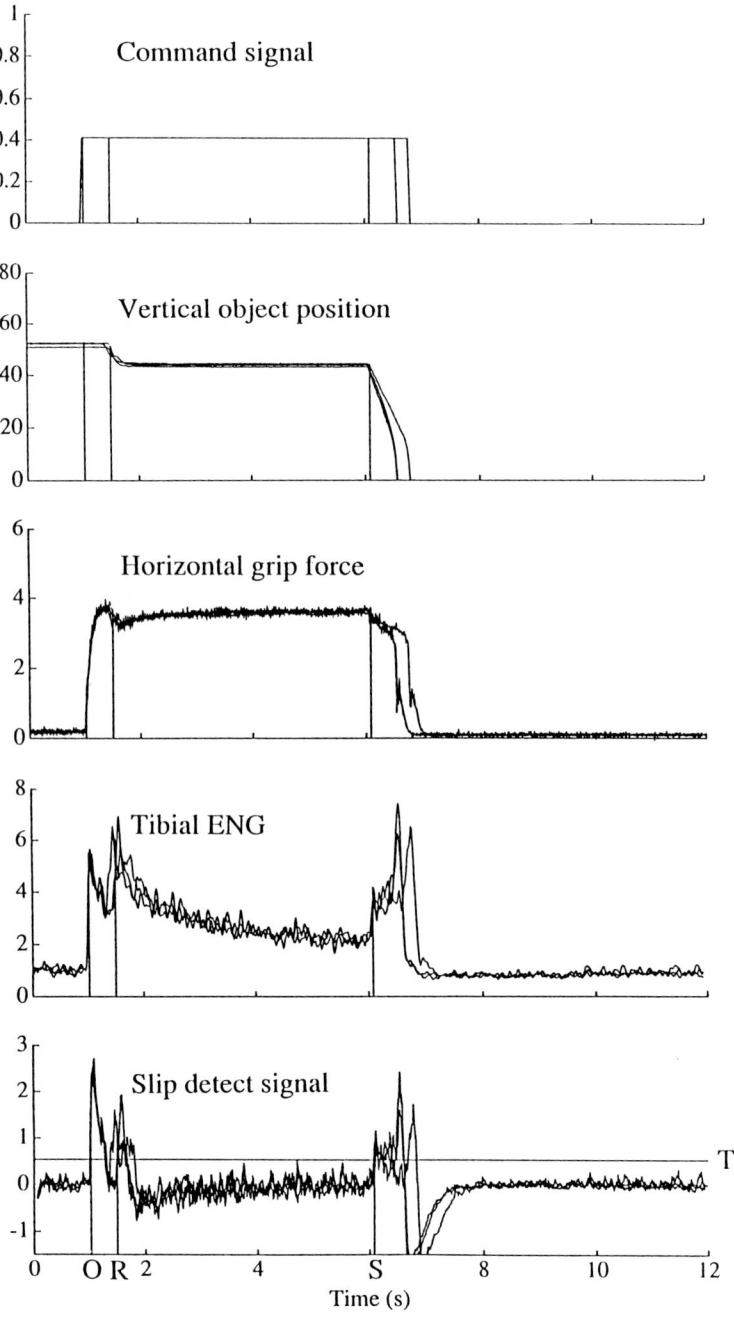

Figure 5-5 (B) Slip detection in response to load increase. Muscles were stimulated at a constant level, sufficient to hold a 150-g object. At time = 6 sec, a 100-g weight was dropped that caused the object to slip. Reproducible slip-related bursts (S) in the differentiated ENG signal (bottom panel) are shown for three similar runs (superimposed traces).

signals a slip associated with the transient fall of the object until it is held by the paw (lines labeled R in Figures 5-5A, B). Third, when an experimentally caused slip occurs, it is signaled immediately by an ENG burst (lines labeled S in Figure 5-5A, B). If the object is allowed to continue to slip, and slides past the cat's paw, the ENG signal can include further activity peaks of variable timing and amplitude.

The ENG bursts that occur at either the start of stimulation, release of the object, or any slips, are quite obvious upon visual inspection of the rectified and smoothed ENG signal (Figure 5-5). However, because slips could occur against variable background ENG activity levels, in these experiments they could not always be correctly detected by the computer on the basis of a simple threshold comparison. To improve the computer recognition of peaks, the ENG signal was low-pass filtered (time constant = 0.07 sec), and a more heavily low-pass filtered version (time constant = 0.2 sec) was digitally delayed (by 2 msec) and subtracted from it. This processing provided a "differential" version of the ENG signal, with peaks of activity that emerged clearly from a nearly constant background level (Figures 5-5A, B, bottom panels). A threshold value was defined that the computer used as reference for automatic detection of activity peaks in the differentiated ENG. Using this approach, a sensitive and robust slip-related signal was reliably detected by the computer as soon as the object started to move (Haugland and Hoffer, in preparation).

NERVE CUFF SIGNALS USED AS FEEDBACK FOR CLOSED-LOOP CONTROL OF FES

Can tactile feedback information derived from nerve cuff recordings be used to control the activation of paralyzed muscles in response to internal changes in the muscles or to changes in the weight or position of a gripped object? In general, in closed-loop control systems, a feedback signal is *continuously* subtracted from a command signal, so that their *difference* is used to control the stimulus intensity. For continuous closed-loop control of FES, an accurate moment-to-moment prediction of grip force or another controllable variable would have to be available from the ENG. Using linear system identification and other linear and nonlinear analytical techniques, contact force could only be predicted from the ENG for particular conditions (Hoffer and Li, 1988; Hoffer et al., 1989; Haugland et al., in preparation). Errors occurred in the prediction of the direction of rapid force changes or the absolute value of slowly varying or constant forces. Implementation of closed-loop controllers using *continuous* feedback from peripheral nerves may only become feasible if substantially improved methods of signal analysis become available.

On the other hand, continuous feedback may not be required for effective control of FES. In analogy to the human precision grip, where a small slip triggers phasic activity in glabrous skin mechanoreceptors that leads to a rapid, reflex correction of grip force by "interrupting" and "updating" the motor program (Johansson and Westling, 1987), the burst that occurs in the whole-nerve ENG during a slip could be used to interrupt and update the command signals produced by an FES controller. This approach was implemented by Haugland and Hoffer in the cat hindlimb model to obtain automatic correction of FES of the four plantarflexor muscles, whenever the held object started to slip.

Two test conditions were studied: simulated muscle fatigue and increased load. Figures 5–6A and 5–6B show examples of feedback-corrected, closed-loop trials. These trials were carried out interleaved in time with the uncorrected, open-loop trials that were shown previously in Figures 5–5A and 5–5B. In Figure 5–6, when a slip-related burst was detected in the differentiated ENG signal, the controller responded immediately with an increase in the activation of all four muscles, starting with the next scheduled stimulus (within 10 msec of slip detection). To speed up the rise in force and so catch the object's fall as soon as possible, the activation update started with either a "doublet" (two stimuli separated by a short interval, usually 5 or 10 msec; viz., Burke et al., 1976; Hoffer et al., 1981b), or by increasing the pulse duration markedly for a short period. Following this brief surge of activation after a slip, the muscles were activated using the same patterns as before the slip occurred, but with 10 to 30% longer pulse durations than before the slip.

In both the fatigue and increased load conditions, the controller responses were highly reproducible. Figure 6–6B shows three consecutive feedback-corrected, closed-loop trials that were carried out interleaved in time with the three "control" trials shown in Figure 5–5B. The tibial ENG responses, slip detection signals, horizontal grip force, and vertical object position overlapped nearly exactly for the three trials. Once an appropriate threshold level was established for the slip-detection signal, misses or false responses by the controller were quite rare. Longer sequences of 10 to 20 paired, interleaved open-loop/closed-loop trials gave similarly repeatable results. In trials that simulated muscle fatigue, the response of the controller allowed the object to fall only about 1 mm upon occurrence of a slip (Figure 6–6A, second panel). In trials where a 100-g weight was dropped on the 150-g object, the object typically fell about 2 mm before it was held securely again (Figure 6–6B, second panel).

FUTURE DIRECTIONS

The studies reviewed in the preceding sections, taken together, provide a basis to suggest a general approach for the automatic regulation of activation of paralyzed muscles with FES, using feedback signals generated by mechanosensors in glabrous skin. Among several restorative applications that can be envisioned, two, in particular, could in principle be implemented readily: control of hand function in quadriplegic or hemiplegic persons, and control of stance and gait in paraplegic or hemiplegic persons.

For hand control applications, tactile information arising from the thumb, index and/or middle fingers could be recorded with nerve cuff electrodes, either from the palmar cutaneous branch of the median nerve proximal to the wrist, or from individual internal digital nerve branches in the hand. Proximal to the wrist, the median nerve is readily accessible in a region appropriate for installation of a nerve cuff. Although at this level, the nerve also includes motor branches to thenar muscles, sensory contributions from the fingers dominate the ENG recorded with nerve cuff electrodes, as was shown in a monkey during precision grip (Milner et al., 1989; Milner et al., 1991). If installed distal to the wrist, cuff electrodes could provide sensory information from single-digit nerves, but surgery would be more demanding,

SIGNALS FROM TACTILE SENSORS

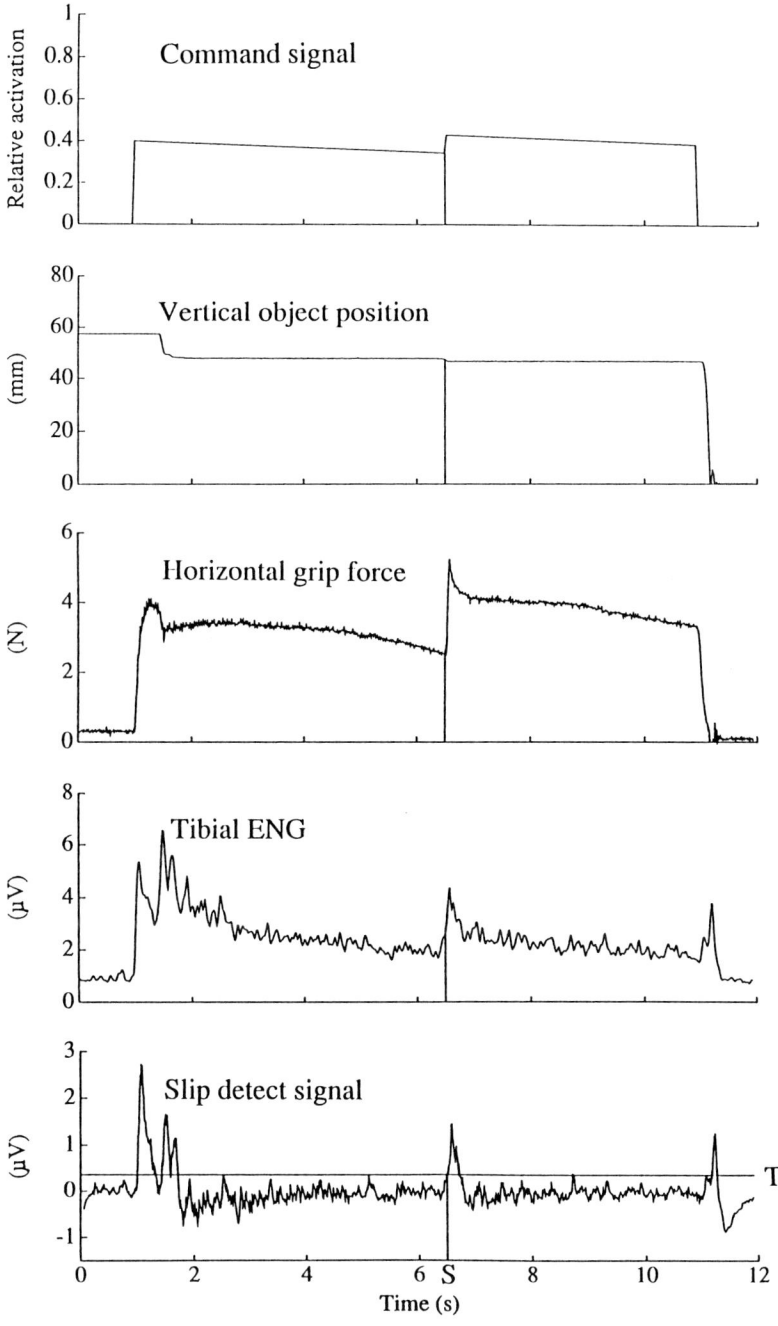

(A)

Figure 5-6 Feedback correction of grip force after slips, for conditions of simulated muscle fatigue (A) and increased load (B). Within 10 msec of slip detection in the differentiated ENG signal (S, bottom panels), the controller responded with a step increase in muscle activation that allowed the object to fall only about 1 mm during "fatigue," or about 2 mm when a 100-g weight was dropped on the 150-g object.

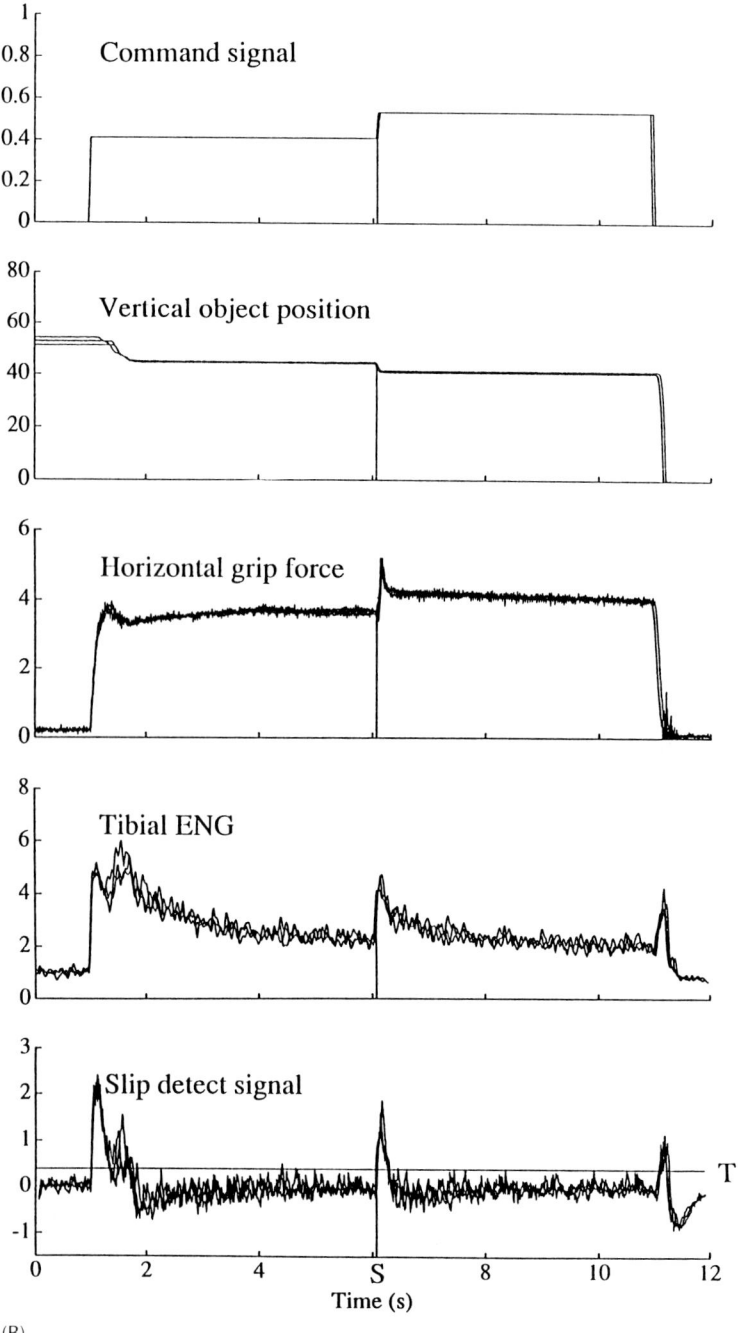

Figure 5–6 Tibial ENG responses, slip-detection signals, horizontal grip force, and vertical object position overlapped nearly exactly for the three trials shown in (B), which took place interleaved in time with the three uncorrected, open-loop trials shown in Figure 5–5.

and it remains to be determined whether the integrity of the nerves and cuff electrodes would be endangered by their superficial location.

The tactile feedback recorded from the median nerve or from its branches would regulate the output of a portable multichannel FES system (Buckett et al., 1988) to control several types of grip (Peckham, 1987) by stimulating forearm and hand muscles via permanently implanted epimysial electrodes (Keith et al., 1988). To avoid risks associated with transcutaneous passage of leads (Stein et al., 1980a; Haugland et al., 1991), both the nerve recording and the muscle stimulation information would be telemetered across the skin (Buckett et al., 1988; Charles and Stein, 1984; Charles, 1989). The command signals for the FES system would be generated by the user, using unaffected motor functions (Peckham, 1987; Kilgore et al., 1989). In initial applications, regulatory feedback would be implemented to use slip information to automatically update the stimulation parameters. To also implement continuous regulatory feedback, appropriate algorithms would have to be available to extract moment-to-moment information on grip force, or other relevant parameters from the ENG signal.

For the restoration of gait and stance in persons impaired by paraplegia or stroke, cutaneous feedback information originating from mechanoreceptors in the soles of the feet could be recorded with nerve cuff electrodes implanted on the internal and external plantar branches of the posterior tibial nerve, and on the sural nerve. The tibial nerve branches contain afferents from the medial and lateral aspects of the ball of the foot, and the sural nerve contains afferents from the heel. To avoid mechanical damage to the nerves or cuff electrodes, the electrodes would best be installed proximal to the ankle rather than in the foot.

In stroke patients who may require electrical stimulation of only the peroneal nerve, to control ankle dorsiflexion during the swing phase (McNeal and Bowman, 1985), a single tibial nerve cuff would be sufficient to monitor whether or not the affected foot is supporting weight. In complete or incomplete paraplegic patients, where the coordinated activation of both legs must be restored, three cuff recording electrodes in each leg would provide information on mediolateral and anteroposterior weight distribution on each leg, as well as on timing of foot contact and interlimb load distribution, considered essential for successful restoration of gait with FES (Cybulski et al., 1984; Hambrecht, 1985). Although such information can be obtained with external pressure sensors placed inside shoes, inherent problems of calibration, mechanical and electrical drift, lead breakage, and sensitivity to environmental factors like moisture and temperature, that affect external transducers, would be avoided if nerve cuff electrodes were used. Additional signals useful for the control of walking (e.g., on joint position) could also be obtained using implanted Hall-effect goniometers (Troyk, et al., 1986). Because satisfactory restoration of gait often cannot be achieved using FES alone, individual solutions are likely to involve FES-based hybrid systems (Mayagoitia and Andrews, 1990; Popovic et al., 1989; Yamaguchi and Zajac, 1990) tailored to the specific pattern of sensorimotor deficit presented by each patient.

In the examples mentioned above, tactile sensory feedback would influence the output of the controller automatically, but this action would be transparent to the user (viz., Cybulski et al., 1984). However, it would be technically possible, and very desirable, to also provide some form of supplementary feedback (Cybulski et al., 1984), where the recorded tactile information is appropriately coded and fed back to the subject's own nervous system via an unaffected sensory modality; for example, cutaneous stimulation in an area where it can be perceived by the subject (Szeto and Riso, 1990).

In summary, sensory signals recorded from peripheral nerves present a feasible option for feedback regulation of implanted FES systems, suitable to restore hand function in quadriplegia or hemiplegia, as well as gait and stance in paraplegia or hemiplegia. By correcting automatically the muscle activation levels provided with FES, tactile feedback would assist the user in the demanding task of activating paralyzed muscles when joint angles and load distributions change, and when fatigue develops. In addition, by virtue of being permanently implanted, a neurally interfaced system would be available for use at all times, reliable without need for frequent recalibration, and cosmetically acceptable to users.

ACKNOWLEDGMENTS

We thank T. Li, K. McLeod, T. Sinkjaer, and M. Stemler for their participation in early experiments, and J. Groves, T. Leonard, and T. Razniewska for training and caring after the cats. This work was funded by the Spinal Cord Research Foundation. U.S.A., (grant No. 623), a personnel salary award from the Rick Hansen "Man in Motion" Legacy Fund, and the Canadian Network of Centres of Excellence for Neural Regeneration and Functional Recovery. M.K. Haugland was a visiting graduate student from Aalborg University, supported in part by the Danish State Education Fund.

REFERENCES

Aguayo, A., Nair, C.P.V., and Midley, R. (1971). Experimental progressive neuropathy in the rabbit. *Arch. Neurol.*, **24**, 358–364.

Anderson, D.J., Najafi, K., Tangue, S.J., Evans, D. A., Levy, K.L., Hetke, J.F., Xue, X., Zappia, J.J., and Wise, K.D. (1989). Batch-fabricated thin-film electrodes for stimulation of the central auditory system. *IEEE Trans. Biomed. Eng.*, **36**, 693–704.

Buckett, J.R., Peckham, P.H., Thorpe, G.B., Braswell, S.D., and Keith, M.W. (1988). A flexible, portable system for neuromuscular stimulation in the paralyzed upper extremity. *IEEE Trans. Biomed Eng.*, **35**, 897–904.

Burke, R.E., Rudomin, P., and Zajac, F.E. (1976). The effect of activation history on tension production by individual motor units. *Brain Res.*, **109**, 515–529.

Charles, D., and Stein, R.B. (1984). Bioelectric control of powered prosthesis: Development of a practical implant. In: H.P. Kimmich, ed., *Proc. VIII Intl. Symp. Biotelemetry, Dubrovnik*, pp. 77–81.

Charles, D. (1989). Neural and EMG biotelemetry implant for control of powered prostheses and functional electrical stimulation. In: C.J. Amlaner, ed., *Biotelemetry X, Proc. X Intl. Symp. Biotelemetry*, pp. 544–551. Little Rock, AK: University of Arkansas Press.

Crago, P.E., Chizeck, H.J., Neuman, M.R., and Hambrecht, F.T. (1986). Sensors for use with functional neuromuscular stimulation. *IEEE Trans. Biomed. Eng.*, **33**, 256–268.

Crago, P.E., Lemay, M.A., and Liu, L. (1990). External control of limb movements involving environmental interactions. In: J.M. Winters and S.L. Woo, eds., *Multiple Muscle Systems: Biomechanics and Movement Organization*, pp. 343–359. New York: Springer-Verlag.

Crago, P.E., Mortimer. J.T., and Peckham, P.H. (1980). Closed-loop control of force during electrical stimulation of muscle. *IEEE Trans. Biomed. Eng.*, **27**, 306–312.

Cybulski, G.R., Penn, R.D., and Jaeger, T.J. (1984). Lower extremity functional neuromuscular stimulation in cases of spinal cord injury. *Neurosurgery*, **15**, 132–146.

Davis, L.A., Gordon, T., Hoffer, J.A., Jhamandas, J., and Stein, R.B. (1978). Compound action potentials recorded from mammalian peripheral nerves following ligation or resuturing. *J. Physiol.*, **285**, 543–559.

Edell, D.J. (1986). A peripheral nerve information transducer from amputees: Long-term multichannel recordings from rabbit peripheral nerves. *IEEE Trans. Biomed. Eng.*, **33**, 203–214.

Forster, C., and Handwerker, H.O. (1990). Automatic classification and analysis of microneurographic spike data using a PC/AT. *J. Neurosci. Methods*, **31**, 109–118.

Gillespie, M.J., and Stein, R.B. (1983). The relationship between axon diameter, myelin thickness and conduction velocity during atrophy of mammalian peripheral nerves. *Brain Res.*, **259**, 41–56.

Glenn, W.W.L., and Phelps, M.L. (1985). Diaphragm pacing by electrical stimulation of the phrenic nerve. *Neurosurgery*, **17**, 974–984.

Goodall, E.V., Lefurge, T.M., and Horch, K.W. (1992). Information contained in sensory nerve recordings made with intrafascicular electrodes. *IEEE Trans. Biomed. Eng.*, in press.

Gordon, T., Hoffer, J.A., Jhamandas, J., and Stein, R.B. (1980). Long-term effects of axotomy on neural activity during cat locomotion. *J. Physiol.*, **303**, 243–263.

Grandjean, P.A., and Mortimer, J.T. (1986). Recruitment properties of monopolar and bipolar epimysial electrodes. *Ann. Biomed. Eng.*, **14**, 53–66.

Hambrecht, F.T. (1985). Control of neural prostheses. In: A. Struppler and A. Weindl, eds., *Electromyography and Evoked Potentials*. Berlin: Springer-Verlag.

Hambrecht, F.T., and Reswick, J.B., eds. (1977). Functional Electrical Stimulation: Applications in Neural Prostheses. *Biomed. Eng. Instrum. Ser. 3*, N.Y., Marcel Dekker.

Haugland, M., Hoffer, J.A., and Sinkjaer, T. (1991). Fully implanted transcutaneous connector for nerve or muscle recording and stimulation. *First European Conference Biomedical Engineering, Nice*, (in press).

Hoffer, J.A. (1975). Long-term peripheral nerve activity during behaviour in the rabbit: The control of locomotion. *Ph.D. Thesis*, Johns Hopkins University, Publ. No. 76-8530, University Microfilms, Ann Arbor, Michigan.

Hoffer, J.A. (1990). Techniques to record spinal cord, peripheral nerve and muscle activity in freely moving animals. In: A.A. Boulton, G.B., Baker, and C.H. Vanderwolf, eds., *Neurophysiological Techniques: Applications to Neural Systems. Neuromethods 15*, pp. 65–145. Clifton, NJ: Humana Press.

Hoffer, J.A., Haugland, M., and Li, T. (1989). Obtaining skin contact force information from implanted nerve cuff recording electrodes. *Proc. Intl. Conf. IEEE/EMBS*, **11**, 928–929.

Hoffer, J.A., Leonard, T.R., Cleland, C.L., and Sinkjaer, T. (1990). Segmental reflex action in normal and decerebrate cats. *J. Neurophysiol.*, **64**, 1611–1624.

Hoffer, J.A., and Li, T. (1988). Real-time processing of cutaneous nerve activity to obtain contact force information. *Soc. Neurosci. Abstr.*, **14**, 64.

Hoffer, J.A., and Loeb, G.E. (1980). Implantable electrical and mechanical interfaces with nerve and muscle. *Ann. Biomed. Eng.*, **8**, 351–360.

Hoffer, J.A., Loeb, G.E., Marks, W.B., O'Donovan, M.J., Pratt, C.A., and Sugano, N. (1987). Cat hindlimb motoneurons during locomotion. I. Destination, axonal conduction velocity and recruitment threshold. *J. Neurophysiol.*, **57**, 530–553.

Hoffer, J.A., Loeb, G.E., and Pratt, C.A. (1981a). Single unit conduction velocities from averaged nerve cuff electrode records in freely moving cats. *J. Neurosci. Methods*, **4**, 211–225.

Hoffer, J.A., O'Donovan, M.J., Pratt, C.A., and Loeb, G.E. (1981b). Discharge patterns of hindlimb motoneurons during normal cat locomotion. *Science*, **213**, 466–468.

Hoffer, J.A., and Sinkjaer, T. (1986). A natural "force sensor" suitable for closed-loop control of functional neuromuscular stimulation. *Proc. 2nd. Vienna Int. Workshop on FES*, 47–50.

Hoffer, J.A., and Weytjens, J.L.F. (1990). Alpha-motoneuron activity, afferent activity and muscle fiber movement simultaneously recorded from cat medial gastrocnemius muscle during posture and locomotion. *Soc. Neurosci. Abstr.*, **16**, 891.

Hunter, I.W., and Kearney, R.E. (1983). Two-sided linear filter identification. *Med. Biol. Eng. Comput.*, **21**, 203–209.

Johansson, R. (1978). Tactile sensibility in the human hand: Receptive field characteristics of mechanosensitive units in the glabrous skin area. *J. Physiol.* **281**, 101–123.

Johansson, R., and Westling, G. (1987). Signals in tactile afferents from the fingers eliciting adaptive motor responses during precision grip. *Exp. Brain Res.*, **66**, 141–154.

Johansson, R., and Westling, G. (1988). Programmed and triggered actions to rapid load changes during precision grip. *Exp. Brain Res.*, **71**, 72–86.

Keith, M.W., Peckham, P.H., Thorpe, G.B., Stroh, K.C., Smith, B., Buckett, J.R., Kilgore, K.L., and Jatich, J.W. (1989). Implantable functional neuromuscular stimulation in the tetraplegic hand. *J. Hand Surg.*, **14A**, 524–530.

Kilgore, K.L., Peckham, P.H., Thorpe, G.B., Keith, M.W., and Gallaher-Stone, K.A. (1989). Synthesis of hand grasp using functional neuromuscular stimulation. *IEEE Trans. Biomed. Eng.*, **36**, 761–770.

Loeb, G.E., and Hoffer, J.A. (1985). Activity of spindle afferents from cat anterior thigh muscles. II. Effects of fusimotor blockade. *J. Neurophysiol.*, **54**, 565–577.

Loeb, G.E., Hoffer, J.A., and Pratt, C.A. (1985a). Activity of spindle afferents from cat anterior thigh muscles. I. Identification and patterns during normal locomotion. *J. Neurophysiol.*, **54**, 549–564.

Loeb, G.E., and Zamin, C.J. (1990). An injectable microstimulator for functional electrical stimulation. *Proc. North Sea Conf.-BME 90*, in press.

Malagodi, M.S., Horch, K.W., Schoenberg, A.A. (1989). An intrafascicular electrode for recording of action potentials in peripheral nerves. *Ann. Biomed. Eng.*, **17**, 397–410.

Marks, W.B., and Loeb, G.E. (1976). Action currents, internodal potentials and extracellular records of myelinated mammalian nerve fibers derived from node potentials. *Biophys. J.*, **16**, 655–668.

Mayagoitia, R.E., and Andrews, B.J. (1990). Stability during standing for 30 minutes in a hybrid floor reaction orthosis. In: D.B. Popovic, ed., *Advances in External Control of Human Extremities X*. Nauka, Belgrade.

McNeal, D.R., and Bowman, B.R. (1985). Selective activation of muscles using peripheral nerve electrodes. *Med. Biol. Eng. Comput.*, **23**, 249–253.

Milner, T.E., Dugas, C., Picard, N., and Smith, A.M. (1989). Median nerve recording during grasping. *Soc. Neurosci. Abstr.*, **15**, 52.

Milner, T.E., Dugas, C., Picard, N., and Smith, A.M. (1991). Cutaneous afferent activity in the median nerve during grasping in the primate. *Brain Res.*, **540**, 228–241.

Mortimer, J.T. (1981). Motor Prostheses. In: *Handbook of Physiology, The Nervous System II*, pp. 155–187.

Peckham, P.H. (1987). Functional electrical stimulation: Current status and future prospects of applications to the neuromuscular system in spinal cord injury. *Paraplegia*, **25**, 279–288.

Phillips, J.R., Johansson, R.S., and Johnson, K.O. (1990). Representation of braille characters

in human nerve fibers. *Exp. Brain Res.*, **81**, 589–592.
Popovic, D., Tomoviç, R., and Schwirtlich, L. (1989). Hybrid assistive system—the motor neuroprosthesis. *IEEE Trans. Biomed. Eng.*, **36**, 729–737.
Prochazka, A. (1984). Chronic techniques for studying neurophysiology of movement in cats. In: R. Lemon, ed., *Methods for Neuronal Recording in Conscious Animals*, pp. 113–128. IBRO Handbook Series: Methods in the Neurosciences, Vol. 4.
Pubols, B.H. (1990). Slowly adapting type I mechanoreceptor discharge as a function of dynamic force versus dynamic displacement of glabrous skin of raccoon and squirrel monkey hand. *Neurosci. Lett.*, **110**, 86–90.
Schmidt, E.M., Bak, M.J., and McIntosh, J.S. (1976). Long-term chronic recording from cortical neurons. *Exp. Neurol.*, **52**, 496–506.
Schmidt, R.F., Wahren, L.K., and Hagbarth, K.-E. (1990). Multiunit neural responses to strong finger pulp vibration. I. Relationship to age. *Acta Physiol. Scand.*, **140**, 1–10.
Srinivasan, M.A., Whitehouse, J.M., and LaMotte, R.H. (1990). Tactile detection of slip: Surface microgeometry and peripheral neural codes. *J. Neurophysiol.*, **63**, 1323–1332.
Stein, R.B., Charles, D., Davis, L., Jhamandas, J., Mannard, A., and Nichols, T.R. (1975). Principles underlying new methods for chronic neural recording. *Can. J. Neurol. Sci.*, **2**, 235–244.
Stein, R.B., Charles, D., Gordon. T., Hoffer, J.A., and Jhamandas, J. (1978). Impedance properties of metal electrodes for chronic recording from mammalian nerves. *IEEE Trans Biomed. Eng.*, **25**, 532–537.
Stein, R.B., Charles, D., Hoffer, J.A., Arsenault, J., Davis, L.A., Moorman, S., and Moss, B., (1980a). New approaches to controlling powered arm prostheses, particularly by high-level amputees. *Bull. Prosth. Res.*, **17**, 51–62.
Stein, R.B., Gordon, T., Hoffer, J.A., Davis, L.A., and Charles, D. (1980b). Long-term recordings from cat peripheral nerves during degeneration and regeneration: Implications for human nerve repair and prosthetics. In: D.L. Jewett and H.R. McCarroll, eds., *Nerve Repair: Its Clinical and Experimental Basis*, pp. 166–176. St. Louis. C.V. Mosby.
Stein, R.B., Nichols, T.R., Jhamandas, J., Davis, L., and Charles, D. (1977). Stable long-term recordings from cat peripheral nerves. *Brain Res.*, **128**, 21–38.
Stein, R.B., and Oguztöreli, M.N. (1978). The radial decline of nerve impulses in a restricted cylindrical extracellular space. *Biol. Cybern.*, **28**, 159–165.
Sunderland, S., *Nerve and Nerve Injuries*. London: Livingstone.
Sweeney, J.D., and Mortimer, J.T. (1986). An asymmetric two electrode cuff for generation of unidirectionally propagated action potentials. *IEEE Trans. Biomed. Eng.*, **33**, 541–549.
Szeto, A., and Riso, R. (1990). Sensory feedback using electrical stimulation of the tactile sense. In: R. Smith and J. Leslie, eds., *Rehabilitation Engineering*, pp. 29–78. Boca Raton, FL, CRC Press.
Troyk, P.R., Jaeger, R.J., Haklin, M., Poyezdala, J., and Bajzek, T. (1986). Design and implementation of an implantable goniometer. *IEEE Trans. Biomed. Eng.*, **33**, 215–221.
Weissman, A., and Schwartz, E. (1981). A flexible high density multichannel electrode array for long-term chronic implantation. *Brain Res. Bull*, **6**, 543–546.
Westling, G., and Johansson, R.S. (1987). Responses in glabrous skin mechanoreceptors during precision grip in humans. *Exp. Brain Res.*, **66**, 128–140.
Yamaguchi, G.T., and Zajac, F.E. (1990). Restoring unassisted natural gait to paraplegics via functional neuromuscular stimulation: A computer simulation study. *IEEE Trans. Biomed. Eng.*, **37**, 886–902.

II
Control of Upper Extremities

6
Feed-forward versus Feedback Control of Limb Movements

JOHN M. HOLLERBACH AND DAVID J. BENNETT

A general control structure for arm movement is presented, and applied to a discussion of the relative advantages of feedforward versus feedback control. Different implementations for feedforward control are examined, including global models, local models, and combinations of the two. Load and time scaling properties of dynamics are shown to be important for possible simplifications of local models. Feedback control implementations include active feedback control and equilibrium point control, which is shown to be functionally equivalent to feedback control. For equilibrium point control, it is shown that time scaling properties are required of the musculo-skeletal dynamics to preserve trajectory invariance. To handle gravity, a revised scheme of static feedforward control is examined.

Experimental tests of putative control schemes require determining the joint mechanical properties during movement. Technical considerations include the choice of perturbation type, the time-varying identification method, and high-performance instrumentation. We briefly describe an airjet system for applying high-frequency stochastic perturbations to the wrist, and a time-varying identification technique requiring ensemble averaging for repeated trials. Results indicate that stiffness and viscosity at the elbow joint vary in a complex way during a trajectory, and do not follow simple scaling rules. These results are not consistent with the equilibrium point hypothesis or with the simple use of dynamic scaling laws.

An enduring issue in biological motor control research is the role of feed-forward control versus feedback control. The same issue arises in robotics (An et al., 1988) and in prosthetics (Lan et al., 1989), but there is an interesting interrelationship. In biological motor control, the mechanical system and the control system are natural.

In robotics, the mechanical system and the control system are artificial. In functional neuromuscular stimulation (FNS), the mechanical system is natural and the control system is artificial; hence FNS is a cross between biological motor control and robotics.

This chapter presents one perspective on this issue from a standpoint of robotics, control theory, and recent results in human arm movement studies. To begin, one must distinguish planning from control processes. Planning processes generate movement goals; control processes realize these goals. For natural arm movements, which are the focus here, planning is presumed to result in a trajectory, which defines the arm path plus the time dependence along the path. There is current debate as to whether an explicit trajectory exists and what the planning variables are, but we will assume that an explicit joint-angle trajectory results from the planning processes. This assumption is in line with at least some of the experimental evidence (Hollerbach and Atkeson, 1987; Soechting and Terzuolo, 1988).

Control then involves execution of the planned joint-angle trajectory. The main issue in control is how the dynamics of arm movement are accommodated to generate the required joint torques. There are essentially two ways to control motion: feed-forward control and feedback control. In *feed-forward control*, a prediction is made about the correct joint torques based on a model of the system or on a motor memory derived from learning. In *feedback control*, joint torque is based on an error signal between the actual and intended motion. Combinations of the two are common and are popular in robotics (An et al., 1988).

These concepts are made more precise in the next section through presentation of a general control structure. The discussion is limited to control of single-joint elbow movement, but concepts apply to multijoint movement as well. Different implementations of feed-forward or feedback control will be examined, and their biological relevance will be assessed. Many proposals about biological motor control can be profitably placed into a framework of feed-forward versus feedback control, and we will recast some well-known proposals into this structure.

ARM CONTROL SYSTEM

For modeling the control of elbow joint motion, we suppose the upper arm is fixed to be horizontal and the forearm moves in a vertical plane (Figure 6–1). The elbow angle $\theta(t)$ is measured relative to vertical, and torque is positive in the clockwise direction in the figure. The forearm mass is m, and the rotary inertia about the center of gravity is I. The distance between the forearm center of mass and the elbow is l. A gravity force mg, where g is the acceleration of gravity, acts at the center of mass. The hand and any grasped load are lumped in with the forearm.

The arm control system may take on the general form depicted in Figure 6–2, where it is assumed that the task is to track a desired joint angle trajectory $\theta_d(t)$. In this diagram the transformation P represents the plant dynamics, A the feed-forward dynamics, and R the feedback dynamics.

Nonlinear Operators

The mathematical form of these transformations is as nonlinear operators, which map one whole time sequence into another time sequence (Desoer and Vidyasagar,

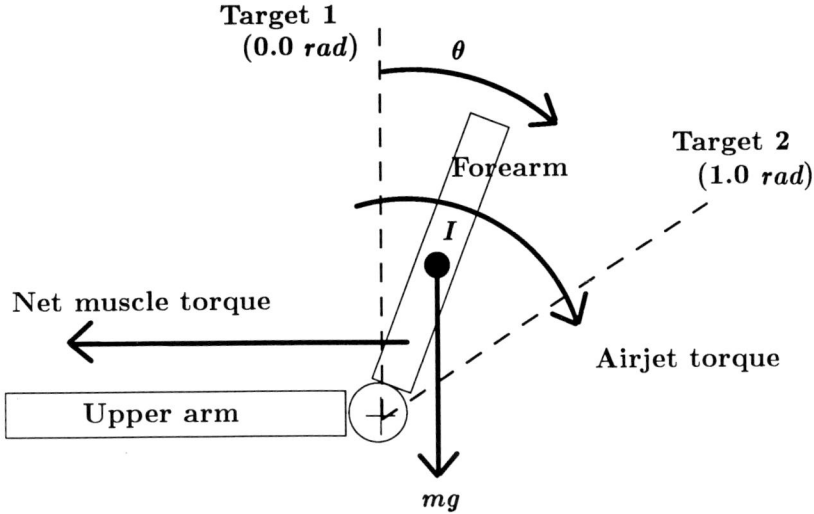

Figure 6–1 Elbow joint model.

1975; Rugh, 1981; Zames, 1961). In contrast to a function, an operator can represent systems with memory. Nonlinear operators have been adopted for two reasons. (1) The human arm system is well known to be nonlinear, and the notation should be able to reflect these nonlinearities as well as any linear approximations. (2) Nonlinear operators act somewhat like Laplace transforms in the linear domain, by providing a mechanism for conveniently deriving input-output relations. For example if $g(\theta(t),\dot{\theta}(t),\ddot{\theta}(t),t)$ is a function not only of the joint angles, velocities, and accelerations, but also of time t (to represent nonstationary systems), then we can write

$$G\theta(t) = g[\theta(t),\dot{\theta}(t),\ddot{\theta}(t),t] \qquad (1)$$

where G is the nonlinear operator representing g. Some mathematically useful properties of operators are now listed, which are required shortly.

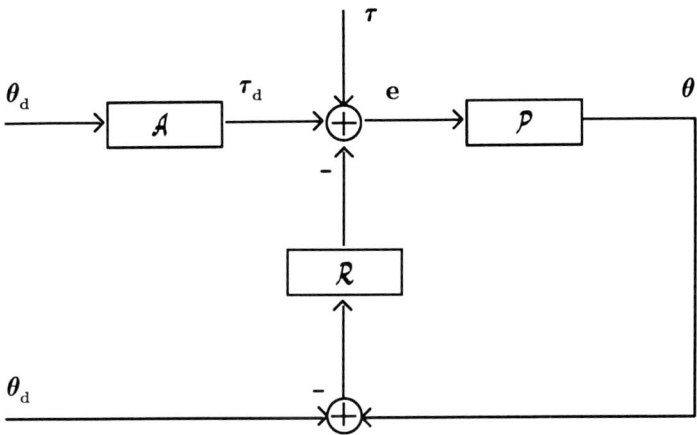

Figure 6–2 General controller for a joint-angle trajectory $\theta(t)$.

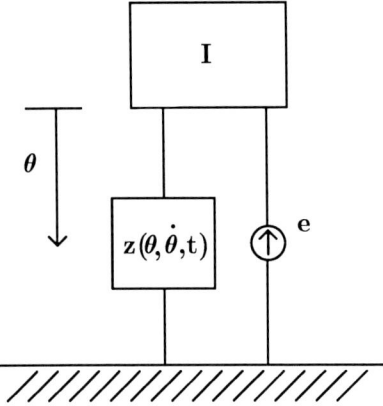

Figure 6-3 Musculoskeletal dynamics.

P1. The additive parallel connection of two systems, A and B, gives the system $A + B$. If $u(t)$ is some time series, then $(A + B)u(t) = Au(t) + Bu(t)$.
P2. The cascade connection of system B followed by system A yields the system AB, or $A[Bu(t)] = (AB)u(t)$.
P3. The cascade connection is distributive with respect to parallel connections, or $A(B + C) = AB + AC$.
P4. The identity operator I has the obvious property that $Iu(t) = u(t)$.
P5. An inverse operator A^{-1} has the property that $A^{-1}A = AA^{-1} = I$. Any physical system that is one to one can always be represented by an operator that has an inverse (Zames, 1961).

Below we discuss elements of the diagram in Figure 6–2 in more detail.

The Plant Operator

The nonlinear operator P represents the musculoskeletal plant being controlled, and combines the dynamics of the elbow joint mechanical properties and the forearm. It produces the actual motion $\theta(t)$ based on an applied torque $e(t)$:

$$\theta(t) = Pe(t) \tag{2}$$

Assume that single-joint musculoskeletal dynamics P can be represented by the general circuit diagram in Figure 6–3 and symbolically as

$$I\ddot{\theta}(t) + z(\theta(t),\dot{\theta}(t),t) = e(t) \tag{3}$$

where $e(t)$ represents the muscle torque generation mechanism and $z(\theta(t),\dot{\theta}(t),t)$ represents the intrinsic parallel force dynamics of the muscles. Here we are not concerned with the exact form of z; more details on the intrinsic muscle dynamics may be found in Chapters 2 and 3. For simplicity, we ignore the series tendon compliance, which can add significant dynamics (Zajac, 1989). Of course, multiple parallel muscles may act on the arm, but their effect can always be reduced to an equivalent form. Define the new operators I and Z:

$$Z\theta(t) = z[\theta(t),\dot{\theta}(t),t] \tag{4}$$

$$I\theta(t) = I\ddot{\theta}(t) \tag{5}$$

where $I = d^2/dt^2$ is in this case a linear operator, and Z is known to be nonlinear. Using property P1, we can write

$$(I + Z)\theta(t) = e(t) \tag{6}$$

The plant operator P requires $e(t)$ as input and $\theta(t)$ as output. Multiply (6) by the inverse operator I^{-1} to obtain

$$(1 + I^{-1}Z)\theta(t) = I^{-1}e(t) \tag{7}$$

where properties P2 to P5 have been employed. Assuming that the operator $1 + I^{-1}Z$ has an inverse, then

$$\theta(t) = (1 + I^{-1}Z)^{-1}I^{-1}e(t) \tag{8}$$

Hence the plant operator is

$$P = (1 + I^{-1}Z)^{-1}I^{-1} \tag{9}$$

This familiar form is analogous to a basic transfer function description of a feedback equation with I^{-1} as the plant and Z as the feedback gain. For an example of a linear analysis of the musculoskeletal plant, see Hollerbach (1990).

The Feed-forward Operator

The nonlinear operator A represents the feed-forward dynamics, which computes a feed-forward torque

$$\tau_d(t) = A\theta_d(t) \tag{10}$$

based on some internal model of the system and on the planned trajectory $\theta_d(t)$. With the operator notation, it is understood that higher derivatives of $\theta_d(t)$ may figure in the computation. In the control literature one can find many examples of feed-forward operators that also take into account the actual trajectory $\theta(t)$, but we will not consider such controllers here.

The Feedback Operator

The reflex system is driven by muscle spindles (or other proprioceptors), which we assume provide position $\theta(t)$ and velocity $\dot{\theta}(t)$ information only. The γ drive system is presumed to set the desired position $\theta_d(t)$ and velocity $\dot{\theta}_d(t)$ and to compute the errors in position and velocity. Let the feedback torque $\tau_r(t)$ be represented by the general function r, which depends on position and velocity errors and which may be nonstationary:

$$\tau_r(t) = r[\theta(t) - \theta_d(t), \dot{\theta}(t) - \dot{\theta}_d(t), t] \tag{11}$$

More specifically, for purposes of discussion we model the reflex loop as a linear proportional-derivative (PD) controller:

$$\tau_r(t) = K_p[\theta(t) - \theta_d(t)] + K_v[\dot{\theta}(t) - \dot{\theta}_d(t)] \tag{12}$$

where K_p is the position gain applied to the position error, and K_v is the velocity

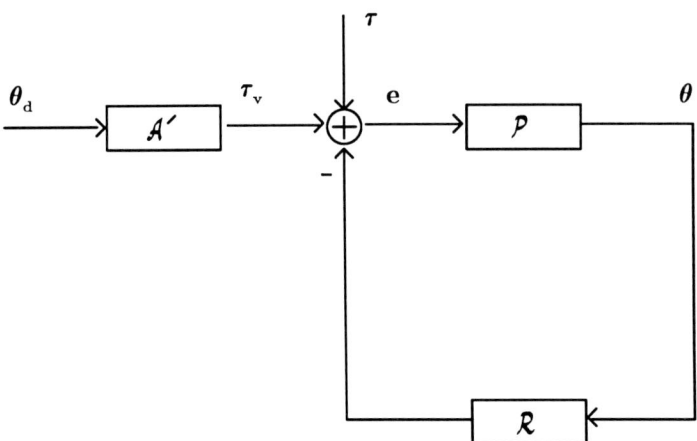

Figure 6-4 Transformational equivalent diagram to Figure 6-2.

gain applied to the velocity error. For the moment, we have ignored the effect of delays. Define the linear operator $R = K_p + K_v d/dt$, so that

$$\tau_r(t) = R[\theta(t) - \theta_d(t)] = R\theta(t) - R\theta_d(t) \tag{13}$$

This distributive property on the input signals holds because R is a linear operator, but does not generally hold for a nonlinear operator.

Equivalent Feedback Model of Joint Mechanical Properties

Next we examine the relation of the feedback operator R to the musculoskeletal dynamics Z identified earlier. As a first step, we transform Figure 6-2 into the functionally equivalent form in Figure 6-4. By use of equation (13), we move that portion of the feedback component depending only on the planned motion, $R\theta_d(t)$, into the feed-forward component by defining a new feed-forward operator

$$A' = A + R \tag{14}$$

Now $\tau_v(t) = A'\theta_d(t)$ is considered to be the commanded (voluntary) torque input to the feedback controller.

Next we explicitly replace the plant operator P by its formulation (8); the result is shown in Figure 6-5. A further transformation of the diagram in Figure 6-5 gives the functionally equivalent Figure 6-6, or symbolically as:

$$0 = I\theta(t) + (R + Z)\theta(t) - \tau_v(t) - \tau(t) \tag{15}$$

This last loop transformation provides an important insight: the intrinsic muscle dynamics can be equivalent to an active feedback system, and effectively provide feedback control. This is the idea behind the equilibrium control theories (e.g, Hogan, 1988). We will refer to the transformation

$$f[\theta(t),\dot{\theta}(t),t] = r[\theta(t),\dot{\theta}(t),t] + z[\theta(t),\dot{\theta}(t),t] \tag{16}$$

and the associated operator $F = R + Z$ as the *effective feedback* system, generated by both intrinsic muscle properties Z and active feedback R.

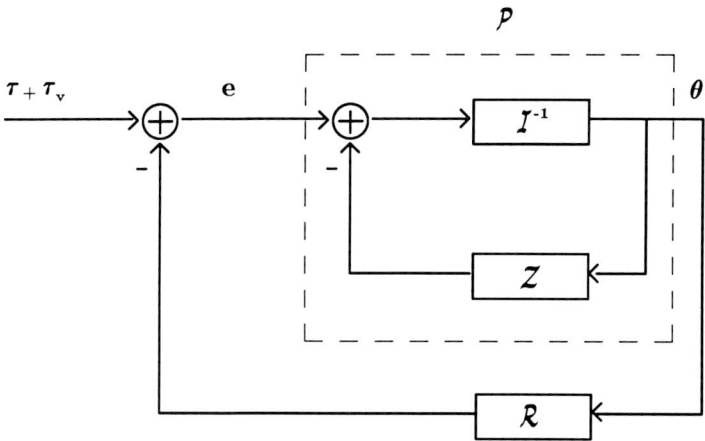

Figure 6–5 Closed-loop dynamics with muscle model explicitly shown.

External Torques

In Figure 6–2 we have introduced a disturbance torque $\tau(t)$, which will be required later to model how the arm dynamics can be identified by external perturbations. Another source of external torque is gravity, with a magnitude of $mgl\sin\theta(t)$. The complete arm dynamics including external torques may now be written as

$$\tau(t) = I\ddot{\theta}(t) + f[\theta(t),\dot{\theta}(t),t] - \tau_v(t) - mgl\sin\theta(t) \qquad (17)$$

where $f - \tau_v$ is the net muscle torque acting on the arm inertia, including parallel connective tissue forces, active feedback, and intrinsic mechanical properties.

FEED-FORWARD VERSUS FEEDBACK CONTROL

In the absence of external perturbations $\tau(t)$, inspection of Figure 6–2 yields the general input-output relation of:

$$(1 + PR)\theta(t) = (PA + PR)\theta_d(t) \qquad (18)$$

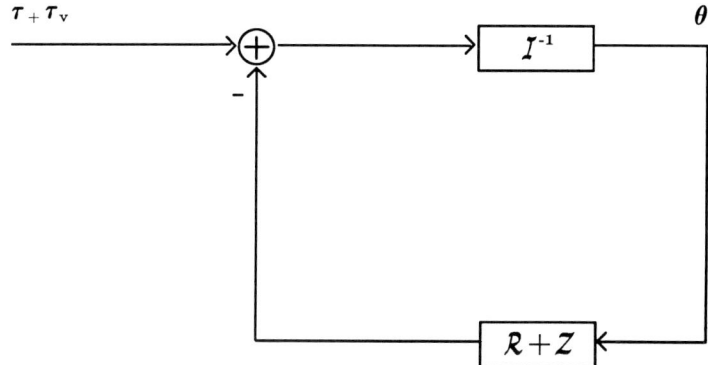

Figure 6–6 Equivalent feedback model of the joint mechanical properties.

Next we consider feed-forward control versus feedback control, and the advantages and disadvantages of each.

Feed-forward Control

Perfect feed-forward control is achieved if A inverts the musculoskeletal plant dynamics:

$$A = P^{-1} = I + Z \tag{19}$$

Then $PA = 1$, and $\theta_d(t)$. With a perfect model, one simply cannot do better than feed-forward control. Nevertheless, there are some serious problems in implementing this solution.

1. *Imperfect models.* Complexity of the real system or difficulties in identifying a model may result in substantial differences between A and P. With no feedback control ($R = 0$), the trajectory error with imperfect feed-forward control would be

$$\theta(t) - \theta_d(t) = P[A\theta_d(t) - \theta_d(t)] = (PA - 1)\theta_d(t) \tag{20}$$

The worse the model, the farther PA diverges from the identity operator I, and the more the actual trajectory will deviate from the desired trajectory.
2. *Wrong initial conditions.* Even with a perfect model, if the arm does not start at an expected position, the resulting trajectory will be in error.
3. *Unmodeled perturbations.* Since no knowledge of the actual state of the arm is present in the feed-forward computation, any deviation from the trajectory caused by an unexpected perturbation will go uncorrected.
4. *Computational difficulties.* The model may be too difficult to compute efficiently, however accurate.

The effect of modeling inaccuracies and unexpected perturbations can be somewhat compensated by adding some form of feedback control.

Feedback Control

In control terminology, PR is referred to as the open-loop operator; its gain or magnitude (Zames, 1961) is denoted $|PR|$. When PR has a much larger effect than either PA or the unit operator I on any signal, then high-gain feedback control is achieved:

$$1 + PR \approx PR \tag{21}$$

$$PA + PR \approx PR \tag{22}$$

and hence $\theta(t) \approx \theta_d(t)$.

The popularity of feedback control arises because accurate control is possible without any knowledge of the plant dynamics; hence it is simple and robust. In practice, sufficiently high gains cannot be achieved for perfect tracking. For the nonlinear case, stability can only be guaranteed if the open-loop gain $|PR|$ is less than unity (Desoer and Vidyasagar, 1975; Zames, 1961). Other limitations follow.

1. *Actuator saturation.* All practical actuators have maximum torques that they can exert, which may be a function of the state. Hence sufficiently high torques cannot always be exerted to correct an error.
2. *Actuator bandwidth limitations.* Real actuators act as low pass filters. Bandwidth limitations can make a system unstable (Eppinger and Seering, 1987).
3. *Noncolocated sensors.* When unmodeled dynamics exist between the actuator and sensor, such as a springy tendon between the muscle and attachment, the gain is limited for stability reasons (Eppinger and Seering, 1980; Jacobsen et al., 1989). With higher gains, the actuator can begin to act out-of-phase with the sensor, and the system will begin to oscillate uncontrollably.
4. *Delays.* The effect of substantial time delays in the feedback loop is to drastically reduce the allowable gains to avoid stability problems (see Chapter 13).
5. *Error driven.* By definition, feedback control is error driven: if there is no error, there is no joint torque. Hence feedback control is suboptimal. Limitations on gains result in significant errors if feedback alone is used.

Linear feedback control will be most effective when the perturbations are not too large. If the plant dynamics, P are treated as a perturbation, then ultimately the controllability of fast movements is limited, because these perturbations increase as the square of movement speed (see below).

IMPLEMENTATIONS OF FEED-FORWARD CONTROL

Two basic ways in which feed-forward control can be implemented are global models and local models. Hybrid models combining the two are possible.

Global Models

Global models characterize a system's dynamics by a few lumped parameters. For example, the mass, center of mass, and moment of inertia completely characterize the rigid-body dynamics of the arm. Global models have two significant advantages.

1. *Trajectory generalization.* The control torques for any movement can be computed accurately from a knowledge of just a small number of model parameters.
2. *Load generalization.* Sudden changes in arm dynamics, such as picking up a load, can be rapidly accommodated by updating the relevant global parameters.

Nevertheless, there are two potential disadvantages.

1. *Nervous system limitations.* Loeb (1983) argues that limitations on the numerical computing ability of the central nervous system (CNS) precludes this form of feed-forward control.
2. *Limitations in representing complex systems.* A more significant disadvantage of global models is that complicated nonlinear systems are hard to model by a few parameters.

What the CNS can compute and whether the CNS has global models are hotly debated questions in motor control research (Hildreth and Hollerbach, 1987; Hollerbach, 1985). Although a global model of the multilink rigid body dynamics of the human arm are complex, computational difficulties have been conquered in robotics (Hollerbach, 1989). Autonomous learning methods have been devised to find an arm's inertial parameters (Atkeson et al., 1986) and kinematic parameters (Bennett and Hollerbach, 1991).

Local Models

Local models involve learning and memorization of individual movements. For example, motor tapes represent fixed sequences of muscle commands or torque profiles that are played out from start to finish without interruption. There are two significant advantages.

1. *Representing complex systems.* Local models are well suited to capture complicated nonlinear systems, since any function can be represented by a table.
2. *Computational speed.* Since memory is substituting for computation, local models produce the proper command torques rapidly.

Yet there are significant disadvantages.

1. *Lack of movement generalization.* If load, speed, or endpoints are changed, then a completely new local model must be learned.
2. *Proliferation of local models.* Consequently there could evolve a proliferation of local models to represent every possible movement and condition.
3. *Laborious learning.* Somehow a local model must be learned for every movement condition.

Neural networks applied to movement dynamics tend to form local models. A review of such neural networks and proposed implementations of local models in the brain may be found in Atkeson (1988).

Dynamic Scaling Properties

Recent results on time- and load-scaling properties of the rigid-body dynamic of arm movements appear to make local models more attractive by allowing some generality in changes in loads and speeds (Atkeson and Hollerbach, 1985). These properties can be illustrated for single-joint motion, although the results generalize to multiple-joint motion. The rigid-body dynamics are:

$$\tau(t) = I\ddot{\theta}(t) - mgl\sin\theta(t) \tag{23}$$

where the $\tau(t)$ contains a speed-dependent inertial term $I\ddot{\theta}(t)$ and a speed-independent gravity term $mgl\sin\theta(t)$.

For the time-scaling properties, suppose the trajectory is time scaled by a factor c to yield a new trajectory $\theta_c(t) = \theta(ct)$. Thus the same trajectory shape is maintained, but the movement speed is changed: if $c > 1$, the movement is sped up; if $c < 1$, the movement is slowed down. By simple differentiation,

$$\dot{\theta}_c(t) = c\dot{\theta}(ct) \tag{24}$$

$$\ddot{\theta}_c(t) = c^2\ddot{\theta}(ct) \tag{25}$$

Replacing t by t/c and substituting into (23) gives

$$\tau_c(t) = c^2 I \ddot{\theta}_c(t/c) - mgl\sin\theta_c(t/c) \qquad (26)$$

where $\tau_c(t)$ is the time-scaled torque. The inertial term scales by c^2, the square of the movement speed, but the gravity term does not scale at all. A more flexible motor tape would contain two subtapes, one for the inertial torques and the other for the gravity torques. By combining these subtapes according to equation (26), the speed of movement could be simply altered.

For the load-scaling properties, each inertial or gravity subtape must be further subdivided into two subtapes, one depending on the load and one independent of the load. The resulting four subtapes can be simply recombined to alter the speed and load, while precisely following the same profile. Details may be found in Atkeson and Hollerbach (1985).

These dynamic scaling laws are probably the only simple relationship between trajectory formation and movement dynamics. They require that a prototype trajectory be followed exactly; namely, the same path and velocity profile shape. Any departure from the prototype trajectory will result in new trajectory dynamics. Hence there is not much hope of further improving the generality of local models.

Experimental results in Atkeson and Hollerbach (1985) show that for one movement task, human arm trajectories seem to show this invariance. Recent research is exploring whether different movement tasks also show such invariances. It is tempting to speculate that each invariant movement represents one of these four-part motor tapes, yet this hypothesis is incomplete because the musculoskeletal dynamics Z must be considered in addition to the rigid-body dynamics.

Let us suppose that the joint mechanical properties can be represented by a quasi-linear second-order system:

$$z[\theta(t),\dot{\theta}(t),t] = K_0\theta(t) + B_0\dot{\theta}(t) \qquad (27)$$

where K_0 is the nominal stiffness and B_0 is the nominal damping for this movement speed. If the trajectory is executed at a new speed $\theta_c(t/c)$, then

$$z[\theta_c(t/c),\dot{\theta}_c(t),t] = K(c)\theta_c(t/c) + cB(c)\dot{\theta}_c(t/c) \qquad (28)$$

where equation (24) has been used. Ignoring gravity, then z would have to scale as c^2 to match the scaling of the inertial torques. This means that it is required that

$$K(c) = c^2 K_0 \qquad (29)$$

$$B(c) = cB_0 \qquad (30)$$

Hence stiffness should scale as the square of the movement speed, and viscosity should scale proportional to movement speed.

Hybrid Local and Global Models

Combinations of local and global models have been proposed. Raibert (1978) has proposed a hybrid approach in which parts of the rigid-body dynamics are tabularized to cut down on the computational requirements.

In robotics, Atkeson (1988) has proposed a scheme for learning a torque profile through repetition. The torque profile is a local model, but it is learned with the aid of an approximately correct global model. The global model converts trajectory errors to torque corrections. The accuracy of the global model determines how many repetitions are required to converge on an accurate torque profile. If the global model is too inaccurate, including having no model at all, then learning may not converge or may take too many repetitions.

There is an intuitive appeal to the notion that a coarse global model is combined with a fine local model in the human motor control system. Our experience is that we have some generality in the movements we are able to produce, but highly skilled movements require a lot of practice.

IMPLEMENTATIONS OF FEEDBACK CONTROL

A previous discussion illustrated that effective feedback control could be achieved either with active feedback R or with joint mechanical properties Z. Both possibilities have had advocates in the literature.

Active Feedback Control

It appears that the neural machinery is in place for possible active feedback control. In the γ *drive hypothesis* (Marsden et al., 1972), also known as the servo-control hypothesis (see Chapter 13), the γ motor neurons set a reference length, and the muscle spindles generate a signal back to the spinal cord that is proportional to the difference in length between the muscle spindle and regular muscle fiber. The spinal cord then generates a feedback torque τ_r. The γ system is thus driving the α motor neurons. The γ drive hypothesis is now discounted, because it was found that the γ motor neurons were activated at the same time as the α motor neurons (Hulliger, 1984; Loeb, 1984). The γ drive hypothesis, on the other hand, would have required that the γ motor neurons fire before the α motor neurons.

Any active feedback scheme for the motor control system will run into the problem of neural transmission delays, which for arm movement are at least 30 msec. Hogan et al. (1987) show how a 30-msec delay limits the usefulness of feedback to a surprisingly low 1.7 Hz; the limit for a 100-msec delay is 0.5 Hz. With a delay the input can get out-of-phase with the output at higher frequencies, and uncontrolled oscillations result. Engineering experience gives a guideline that the maximum allowable frequency is 1/20th the inverse of the delay; hence the 1.7- and 0.5-Hz figures. These frequency responses may be satisfactory for posture or slow movements, but for fast movements active feedback cannot be used and the only alternative is some form of feed-forward control.

Delays are also a serious concern for FNS, because at least the activation delays (duration between onset of stimulation and production of muscle force) must be considered. If biological sensors are tapped as well for control purposes (see Chapter 5), the sensor signal propagation delay must be added. Additional discussion of delays may be found in Chapter 13.

Equilibrium Point Control

Even if $R = 0$, effective feedback control could be provided by the joint mechanical properties, Z. There is a point of terminology here, because control of Z is actually a form of feed-forward control, since Z is part of the plant dynamics. Functionally, though, the control of Z acts like feedback control as previously demonstrated. A potential advantage for the control of Z versus the control of R is avoidance of neural delays associated with the control of R. The control of Z has been advocated as the equilibrium control hypothesis (Bizzi et al., 1982).

Feldman's version of equilibrium control (Feldman, 1986) appears to be different, because both R and Z play a role. Here $f[\theta_d(t),0,t]$ represent the feed-forward torque based on the planned trajectory $\theta_d(t)$, which can be viewed as an equilibrium trajectory in the sense that it can only be achieved when the arm is at rest.

Experimental support is largely indirect for equilibrium control, whose status is uncertain. One problem is that arm movements often show biphasic or triphasic electromyographic bursts, which is consistent with one version of equilibrium point control (Feldman et al., 1990) but not another (Bizzi et al., 1982). Another problem is that very high stiffness would be needed to overcome disturbances caused by ignoring the plant dynamics; such high stiffnesses are seldom observed. Nevertheless, the direct experiments that would be required to test the hypothesis have not been performed in the past due to technical limitations.

Static Feed-forward Control

The influence of gravity has not been adequately addressed in the equilibrium control hypotheses to date. Unless integral control is introduced, gravity would cause a steady-state error in the final position. It is unlikely that the stiffness could be increased enough to compensate. Hence it is necessary in these hypotheses that gravity compensation be included. The feed-forward torque would then be

$$\tau_v(t) = f(\theta_d(t),0,t) - mgl\sin\theta_d(t) \tag{31}$$

where $\tau_v(t)$ is the instantaneous static component of the dynamics. We call this more general form of control by the more precise term *static feed-forward control* (Bennett, 1990).

Consider next the requirement that any form of control should conform to the experimentally observed trajectory invariances with speed (Atkeson and Hollerbach, 1985). Hence f must scale as c^2, as was argued earlier for Z. If f is also represented by a second-order system as in equation (27), where we do not distinguish whether the viscoelasticity arises from feedback or musculoskeletal mechanics, then the stiffness K and viscosity B must scale as in equations (29) and (30). Otherwise, trajectories will differ according to movement speed. For postural tasks involving isometric exertion against a bias force, the viscoelasticity appears to scale as required (Kearney and Hunter, 1990; Xu et al., 1991).

There has been a fair amount of theoretical work on the equilibrium point control that applies static viscoelastic values to a trajectory (Flash, 1987), but the validity of the resultant simulation results is unknown. The variation of B and K during a trajectory is what actually needs to be known, and until recently this information was not available.

TIME-VARYING MOVEMENT DYNAMICS

As previously indicated, a key experimental finding in understanding the control of human arm movements would be the time-varying movement dynamics. Devising appropriate instrumentation and analysis methods have been major difficulties that until recently hindered conducting such experiments.

Perturbation Analysis

We begin by addressing how to experimentally study the closed-loop dynamics represented in equation (17). Since the internal forces [e.g., $\tau_v(t)$] that act in addition to the known external forces cannot be controlled or measured, only the local behavior of the closed-loop dynamics about a nominal trajectory, $\theta_0(t)$, may be studied. Applying an external perturbation, $\tau(t)$, during execution of the nominal trajectory gives a new trajectory that is related to the nominal trajectory through the dynamic behavior of the arm. The arm dynamics can be studied by estimating the relationship between the applied perturbations and the deviations from the nominal trajectory.

Specifically, if the applied perturbations are small enough, the closed-loop dynamics may be approximated by differential behavior about the operating point $[\theta_0(t), \tau_0(t), \tau_v(t)]$:

$$\Delta\tau(t) = I(t)\Delta\ddot{\theta}(t) + B(t)\Delta\dot{\theta}(t) + K(t)\Delta\theta(t)$$
$$\Delta\theta(t) = \theta(t) - \theta_0(t) \qquad (32)$$
$$\Delta\tau(t) = \tau(t) - \tau_0(t)$$

where the joint inertia $I(t) = I + \partial f/\partial\ddot{\theta}$, the joint viscosity $B(t) = \partial f/\partial\dot{\theta}$, and the joint stiffness $K(t) = \partial f/\partial\theta - mgl\cos\theta_0(t)$. The second term of $I(t)$ should be zero, as it could only result from high bandwidth force feedback. Also, the negative gravity contribution to the stiffness turns out to be relatively small (Bennett, 1990). θ_0 and τ_0 are the angles and torques measured during an average unperturbed movement. τ_0 may be nonzero.

In the sense that the parameters I, B, and K relate force input to velocity output, they may be referred to as *mechanical impedance* parameters. The relation between force input and position output may be referred to as *complex stiffness*, with *compliance* being the inverse of this relation.

Identification Method

In applying the perturbation analysis, a first issue is what kind of perturbations to use. There are strong arguments for using stochastic perturbations rather than other alternatives such as step, ramp, or sinusoidal inputs (Kearney and Hunter, 1990). Reasons include efficiency (how long it takes to run an experiment), robustness (accuracy in the presence of noise), and generality (whether nonlinear systems can be identified). Pseudorandom binary sequences are a particularly good implementation of stochastic inputs (Marmarelis and Marmarelis, 1978).

A second issue is how the time-varying movement dynamics during a trajectory can be identified. If these dynamics vary slowly, such as in posture or in slow movements, then an exponentially weighted recursive least-squares method can be used to identify the dynamics during a single trajectory (Xu, 1991). Such on-line identification could be particularly useful for FNS. Otherwise, these dynamics cannot be identified for just a single motion, because they are varying too fast for the perturbations to track accurately. There is no alternative but to do ensemble averaging with repeated trials. Experimental difficulties will result in ensuring that every movement is similar and in aligning movement start. One approach involves methodically shifting a stochastic input sequence for every repetition so that along any time slice the response is available for that input sequence (Hunter and Kearney, 1987). This technique has been applied to time-varying isometric contractions in the ankle (MacNeil et al., 1990). A direct ensemble least-squares approach that does not require special input design was proposed in Bennett (1990) and Bennett et al. (1991).

A third issue is the instrumentation to apply the perturbation. Adequate force and frequency content are necessary. For the arm, it has been shown that frequencies up to 100 Hz are necessary given the range of natural frequencies, and that a 4 N force is required at this frequency in order to produce a detectable displacement of 0.2 mm (Xu et al., 1991). This performance is difficult to get with normal actuators. We have devised a pneumatic thruster employing the Coanda effect that attaches to the wrist and meets these specifications (Xu et al., 1991). An additional benefit of this device is that unrestrained arm motions can be perturbed.

Experimental Results

Using the airjet system detailed in Xu et al. (1991) and the time-varying identification method detailed in Bennett (1990) and Bennett et al. (1991), we have identified the time-varying impedance parameters under a variety of movement conditions (Bennett et al., 1990). One of these experiments investigated a 1000-msec repetitive movement between targets spaced at 0° (forearm straight up) and 60°, and the results for one subject are shown in Figure 6–7. The inertia, I, is constant, as should be the case; in this estimate, the inertia of the airjet is included. The viscosity, B, and stiffness, K, vary throughout the trajectory. The viscosity estimates have a large variance and show no consistent pattern. The stiffness estimates have a low variance and show a consistent modulation throughout a movement. They are highest at the movement endpoints and are lowest during the fastest portions of the movements. In addition, the stiffnesses at the targets are lower than stiffnesses during posture. Calculations show that the damping ratio varies throughout the movement.

The effect of movement speed on the stiffness profiles is shown in Figure 6–8. The stiffness profile for a 750-msec movement has the same general shape as the stiffness profile for a 1000-msec movement. However, it is scaled by only around 1.1, much lower than the 1.78 factor that would be predicted by a c^2 scaling.

The results on stiffness scaling with speed are inconsistent with the static feed-forward control hypothesis, which would have required a consistent 1.78 scaling

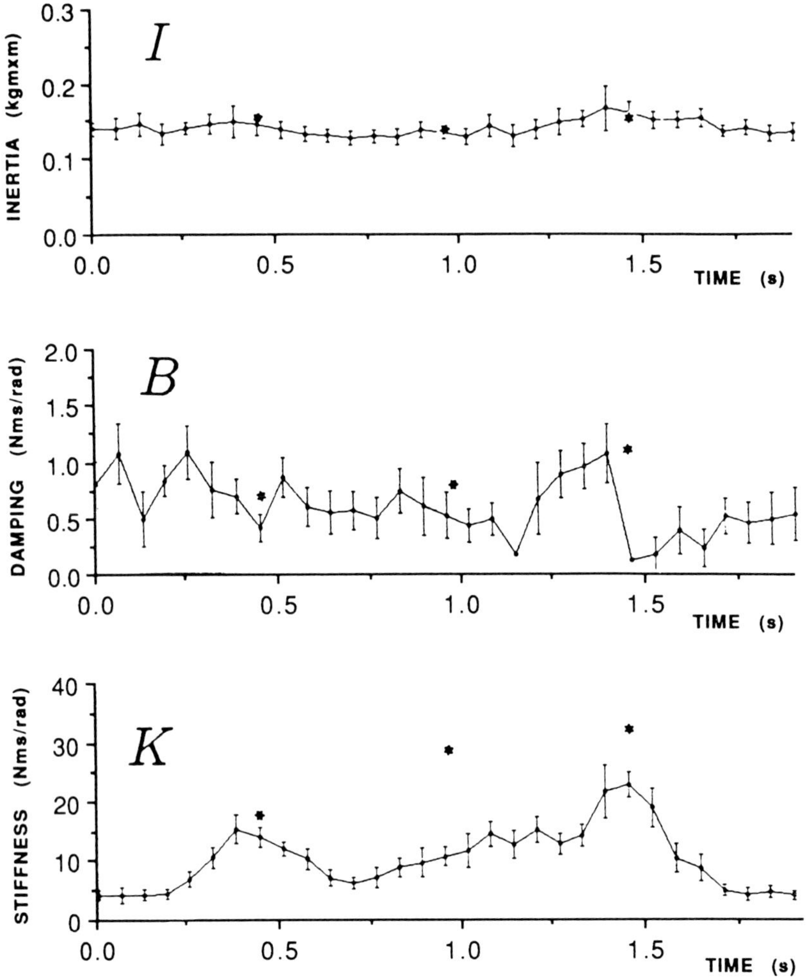

Figure 6-7 Inertia *I*, viscosity *B*, and stiffness *K* during a 1000-msec movement for one subject. Impedances during posture are indicated with an asterisk.

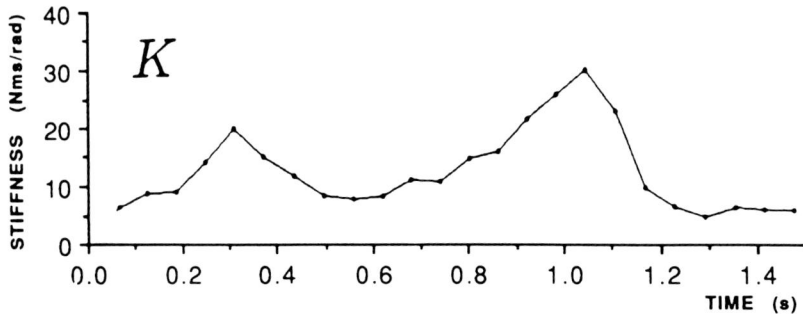

Figure 6-8 Stiffness profile for a 750-msec movement.

factor. If the trajectory had actually been generated by static feed-forward control with a 1.1 scaling, then the trajectory shapes for the two movement speeds would have been different, yet the observed shapes are the same. It remains to be seen whether future modifications of this hypothesis can account for this finding.

DISCUSSION

Full feed-forward control, involving a model both of the rigid-body dynamics and the musculoskeletal dynamics, cannot involve simple use of the dynamic scaling laws, since the musculoskeletal dynamics do not appear to scale appropriately. A more complicated model of the musculoskeletal dynamics would be required. Nevertheless, the musculoskeletal dynamics are confined to a joint, and so are simpler in some sense to model than rigid-body dynamics, where interaction torques act on all joints. The rigid-body dynamic scaling still holds and serves to simplify a significant part of the control task. These considerations also apply to FNS.

It seems quite likely that the motor control system combines feed-forward control with feedback control, to combine advantages of each and to counteract disadvantages of using one type of control alone. The challenge facing researchers is to identify the exact form each type of control takes. Perturbation experiments combined with advanced nonlinear system identification methods will play a vital role in this research endeavor.

ACKNOWLEDGMENTS

This research was supported in part by a Whitaker Foundation Biomedical Engineering Grant. Personal support for JMH was provided by an NSERC/CIAR Chair in Robotics.

REFERENCES

An, C.H., Atkeson, C.G., and Hollerbach, J.M. (1988). *Model-Based Control of a Robot Manipulator.* Cambridge, MA: MIT Press.

Atkeson, C.G. (1988). Learning arm kinematics and dynamics. *Ann. Rev. Neurosci.*, **12**, 157–183.

Atkeson, C.G., An, C.H., and Hollerbach, J.M. (1986). Estimation of inertial parameters of manipulator links and loads. *Int. J. Robotics Res.*, **5**(3), 101–119.

Atkeson, C.G., and Hollerbach, J.M. (1985). Kinematic features of unrestrained vertical arm movements. *J. Neurosci.*, **5**, 2318–2330.

Bennett, D.J. (1990). The control of human arm movement: Models and mechanical constraints. *Ph.D. Thesis.* MIT, Department of Brain and Cognitive Sciences.

Bennett, D.J., and Hollerbach, J.M. (1991). Autonomous calibration of single-loop closed kinematic chains formed by manipulators with passive endpoint constraints. *IEEE Trans. Robotics and Automation*, **7**, 597–606.

Bennett, D.J., Hollerbach, J.M., Hunter, I.W., and Xu, Y. (1991). Time-varying dynamics of human elbow joint stiffness during voluntary movement. *Exp. Brain. Res.*, in press.

Bennett, D.J., Xu, Y., Hollerbach, J.M., and Hunter, I.W. (1990). Mechanical properties of the human arm during voluntary movement. In: *Proc. Can. Med. Biol. Eng. Conf.*, pp. 89–90. Winnipeg: June 9–12.

Bizzi, E., Chapple, W., and Hogan, N. (1982). Mechanical properties of muscles: Implications for motor control. *Trends Neurosci.*, **5**(11), 395–398.

Desoer, C.A., and Vidyasagar, M. (1975). In: *Feedback Systems: Input-Output Properties*. New York: Academic Press.

Eppinger, S.D., and Seering, W.P. (1987). Understanding bandwidth limitations in robot force control. In: *Proc. IEEE Int. Conf. Robotics and Automation*, pp. 904–909. Raleigh, NC: March 31–April 3.

Eppinger, S.D., and Seering, W.P. (1989). Three dynamic problems in robot force control. In: *Proc. IEEE Int. Conf. Robotics and Automation*, pp. 392–397. Scottsdale, AZ: May 14–19.

Feldman, A.G. (1986). Once more on the equilibrium-point hypothesis (λ model) for motor control. *J. Motor Behavior*, **18**, 17–54.

Feldman, A.G., Adamovich, S.V., Ostry, D.J., and Flanagan, J.R. (1990). The origin of electromyograms—explanations based on the equilibrium point hypothesis. In: J.M. Winters and S.L.-Y. Woo, eds., *Multiple Muscle Systems: Biomechanics and Movement Organization*, pp. 195–213. New York: Springer-Verlag.

Flash, T. (1987). The control of hand equilibrium trajectories in multi-joint arm movements. *Biol. Cybern.*, **57**, 257–274.

Hildreth, E.C., and Hollerbach, J.M. (1987). Artificial intelligence: Computational approach to vision and motor control. In: F. Plum, ed., *Handbook of Physiology, Section 1: The Nervous System, Volume V: Higher Functions of the Brain, Part II.*, pp. 605–642. Bethesda, MD. American Physiological Society.

Hogan, N. (1988). Planning and execution of multijoint movements. *Can. J. Physiol. Pharmacol.*, **66**, 508–517.

Hogan, N., Bizzi, E., Mussa-Ivaldi, F.A., and Flash, T. (1987). Controlling multijoint motor behavior. In: K.B. Pandolf, ed., *Exercise and Sport Sciences Reviews*, pp. 153–190. New York: Macmillan.

Hollerbach, J.M. (1985). Computers, brains, and the control of movement. In: E.V. Evarts, S.P. Wise, and D. Bousfield, eds., *The Motor System in Neurobiology*, pp. 140–146. Amsterdam: Elsevier Biomedical Press.

Hollerbach, J.M. (1989). Kinematics and dynamics for control. In: M. Brady, ed., *Robotics Science*, pp. 378–341. Cambridge, MA: MIT Press.

Hollerbach, J.M. (1990). Fundamentals of motor behavior. In: D. Osherson, S.M. Kosslyn, and J.M. Hollerbach, eds., *Visual Cognition and Action: An Invitation to Cognitive Science, Vol. 2.*, Cambridge, MA: MIT Press.

Hollerbach, J.M., and Atkeson, C.G. (1987). Deducing planning variables from experimental arm trajectories: Pitfalls and possibilities. *Biol. Cybern.*, **56**, 279–292.

Hulliger, M. (1984). The mammalian muscle spindle and its central control. *Rev. Physiol. Biochem. Pharmacol.*, **101**, 1–110.

Hunter, I.W., and Kearney, R.E. (1987). Quasi-linear, time-varying, and nonlinear approaches to the identification of muscle and joint mechanics. In: *Advanced Methods of Physiological Modeling*, pp. 128–147.

Jacobsen, S.C., Smith, C.C., Biggers, K.B., and Iversen, E.K. (1989). Behavior-based design for robot effectors. In: M. Brady, ed., *Robotics Science*, pp. 505–539. Cambridge, MA: MIT Press.

Kearney, R.E., and Hunter, I.W. (1990). System identification of human joint dynamics. *CRC Crit. Rev. Biomed. Eng.*, **18**, 55–87.

Lan, N., Crago, P.E., and Chizeck, H.J. (1989). Feedback control of end-point stiffness in a multi-joint limb by FNS. In: *Proc. 11th Annual Intl. Conf. IEEE Engineering in Medicine and Biology Society*, pp. 971–972. Seattle: Nov. 9–12.

Loeb, G.E. (1983). Finding common ground between robotics and physiology. *Trends Neurosci.*, **6**(6), 203–204.

Loeb, G.E. (1984). The control and responses of mammalian muscle spindles during normally executed motor tasks. In: R. L. Terjung, ed., *Exercise and Sport Sciences Reviews*, pp. 157–204. Lexington, MA: Collamore Press.

MacNeil, J.B., Kearney, R.E., and Hunter, I.W. (1990). Identification of the time-varying stiffness of the human ankle. In: *Proc. Canadian Medical & Biological Engineering Conf.*, pp. 177–178. Winnipeg: June 9–12.

Marmarelis, P.Z., and Marmarelis, V.Z. (1978). In: *Analysis of Physiological Systems*. London: Plenum Press.

Marsden, C.D., Merton, P.A., and Morton, H.B. (1972). Servo action in human voluntary movement. *Nature*, **238**, 140–143.

Raibert, M.H. (1978). A model for sensorimotor control and learning. *Biol. Cybern.*, **29**, 29–36.

Rugh, W.J. (1981). In: *Nonlinear System Theory. The Volterra/Wiener Approach*. Baltimore: Johns Hopkins University Press.

Soechting, J.F., and Terzuolo, C.A. (1988). Sensorimotor transformations underlying the organization of arm movements in three-dimensional space. *Can. J. Physiol. Pharmacol.*, **66**, 502–507.

Xu, Y. (1991). Design and application of an airjet system for studying mechanical properties of human and robot arms. *Ph.D. Thesis*. MIT, Aeronautics and Astronautics.

Xu, Y., Hunter, I.W., Hollerbach, J.M., and Bennett, D.J. (1990). An airjet perturbation device and its use in elbow posture mechanics. In: *Proc. 12th IEEE Intl. Conf. Engineering in Medicine and Biology*, pp. 2116–2117. Philadelphia: Nov. 1–4.

Xu, Y., Hunter, I.W., Hollerbach, J.M., and Bennett, D.J. (1991). An airjet actuator system for identification of the human arm joint mechanical properties. *IEEE Trans. Biomed. Eng.*, **38**, 1111–1122.

Zajac, F.E. (1989). Muscle and tendon: Properties, models, scaling, and application to biomechanics and motor control. *CRC Crit. Rev. Biomed. Eng.*, **17**, 359–411.

Zames, G. (1961). Nonlinear operators for system analysis. *MIT Res. Lab of Electronics*. Tech. Rept. 370.

7

What Transcranial Stimulation of the Brain Can Reveal About the Control of Arm Movements in Man

JOHN C. ROTHWELL

Electrical and magnetic methods are now available for stimulation of the human brain through the scalp. Stimulation over motor areas appears to activate the large diameter component of the corticospinal tract. Experiments in animals indicate that this pathway is used preferentially during the performance of fine manual movements. The same appears to be true in man. In patients with multiple sclerosis it has been shown that abnormal conduction in the corticospinal tract correlates with poor performance in tests of fine finger function. Transcranial stimulation has been used to study both children and adults after damage to the central nervous system in order to document the degree of remaining corticospinal function. Such tests can also provide information on how the corticospinal system reorganises after injury.

Stimulation of the brain is not only useful when producing excitatory responses of the muscles. The same stimulus also appears to be able to interrupt brain function for a short period. Stimuli given just before the onset of a reaction time task can delay the expected movement without changing its form. Such results indicate that the brain may be able to store a program for movement during the period of the delay. They also suggest that the brain can monitor the progress of a voluntary motor act by some form of internal feedback system.

An electrical stimulator was developed by Merton and Morton (1980), that uses a high-voltage capacitative discharge applied through two electrodes on the scalp. A small fraction of the applied current penetrates through the skull into the brain and stimulates excitable cells. The disadvantage of the technique is that the remainder of the current flows across the scalp, causing local discomfort and contraction of underlying scalp muscles. The magnetic method, developed by Barker et al. (1985), discharges a capacitor through a coil of wire. This produces a large and rapidly varying magnetic field, which can induce electric current to flow in any conductive structure nearby. Placed over the head, electric currents are induced in the brain and stimulate excitable cells. The method is painless because the currents induced on the scalp are only a little greater than those induced in the brain, and do not cause a large muscle contraction such as that produced by electrical stimulation.

At threshold intensities, electrical and magnetic stimulation of the motor cortex activate the pyramidal tract output cells in different ways. The critical observation is that the latency of electromyographic (EMG) responses evoked in hand muscles can be 1 to 2 msec earlier after electrical stimulation of the cortex than after magnetic stimulation. Day et al. (1989) suggested that the difference was due to the direction of current flow induced in the brain by the two forms of stimulation. Currents induced by magnetic stimulation flow parallel to the surface of the scalp, with little or no vertical component of flow. In contrast, electrical stimulation produces currents which have both horizontal and vertical components. Since pyramidal tract axons are oriented predominantly perpendicular to the surface of the brain, they are best activated by a vertical current flow. Day et al. (1989) suggested that electrical stimulation could activate these pyramidal tract axons directly, whereas magnetic stimulation, with its horizontal current flow could not. Instead, the currents induced by magnetic stimulation were thought to be more likely to activate interneurones or afferent fibers in the cortex running parallel to the surface. These would then excite pyramidal tract cells transynaptically. Thus, the latency difference between responses evoked by magnetic and electric stimulation would be due to transynaptic versus direct activation of the pyramidal tract output cells. A different hypothesis to explain the difference between magnetic and electric stimulation was put forward by Edgley et al. (1990). From data collected in monkey experiments, they suggested that magnetic stimulation would activate the pyramidal tract axons directly at the initial segment. In contrast, electric stimulation was thought to spread deep into the white matter and activate the pyramidal tract axons at the level of the brainstem. The difference in latency between responses evoked by the different methods of stimulation was ascribed to proximal versus distal activation of the output axons.

PATHWAYS ACTIVATED BY MOTOR CORTICAL STIMULATION

The motor areas of the human cerebral cortex are connected to the spinal cord via two main pathways: the direct, corticospinal tract, and indirect projections via the reticular formation and the reticulospinal tracts. Four lines of evidence suggest that transcranial stimulation activates the large-diameter, fast-conducting component of the corticospinal tract which has monosynaptic connections with spinal motor neurones.

1. The latency of EMG responses evoked by transcranial stimulation is very short. After anodal electric stimulation, responses occur after about 20 msec in hand muscles, and about 14 msec in forearm muscles. Since the peripheral conduction time from spinal cord to muscle is about 15 and 9 msec, respectively, the central conduction time from cortex to cord is only of the order of

5 msec. This figure includes the time taken for transmission through at least one synapse between the corticospinal tract and the spinal motor neurones. The conclusion is that the conduction velocity in the pathway activated by magnetic stimulation is rapid, and that the number of interposed synapses is small.

2. Studies of single motor unit behavior in hand muscles also confirm that only a few synapses are interposed between cortex and spinal motor neurone. The variability of discharge of a single motor unit, or of a single muscle fiber within a motor unit, after a cortical stimulus is very small. It is of the order of 1.5 msec for single units (Day et al. 1989), and 250 μsec for single fibers (Zidar et al., 1987). Such low variability is similar to that seen after testing with a known predominantly monosynaptic input to the motor neurones such as the H-reflex.

3. Responses evoked by cortical stimulation are larger (with respect to the maximum peripheral nerve M-wave) in distal than in proximal muscles (Rothwell et al., 1987; Brouwer and Ashby, 1990). Such preferential accessibility of distal muscles is consistent with the known preferential projection of the corticomotoneuronal component of the corticospinal tract to these muscles in higher primates.

4. The final piece of evidence favoring the idea that transcranial stimulation excites the monosynaptic component of the corticospinal system comes from comparing cortical excitability during different types of voluntary movement. Muir and Lemon (1983) have shown in the monkey that corticospinal neurones with monosynaptic connections onto motor neurones supplying hand muscles fire more during the performance of a precision grip using just the thumb and index finger, than they do during performance of a power grip involving the whole hand. This reflects the preferential role of the corticospinal system in the production of fine, discrete movements of the digits. In humans, Datta et al. (1989) have shown that magnetic stimulation of the brain produces larger responses in the first dorsal interosseous muscle when subjects perform a precision grip than it does during performance of a power grip, even though the levels of ongoing EMG activity in the muscle are the same in the two tasks. The larger responses obtained during a precision movement are consistent with heightened excitability of corticospinal neurones during that task. Responses to anodal electric stimulation of the brain were the same during the two tasks, presumably because the electric shock activates corticospinal axons directly, within the white matter, and is therefore uninfluenced by changes in the level of cortical excitability.

The large diameter, monosynaptic component of the corticospinal tract which is activated by transcranial stimulation appears to be of particular importance in humans. This component of the corticospinal tract increases in size as we ascend the phylogenetic scale from cat to monkey to humans. In the monkey, it represents only about 3% of the total tract, and projects primarily to distal muscles, with no projections to proximal or axial muscles such as the biceps or deltoid. In humans, transcranial stimulation suggests that this component of the corticospinal tract may be more widespread and powerful than it is in the monkey. Latency measurements show that a rapidly conducting pathway exists from motor cortex to virtually all muscles of the body, including the first dorsal interosseous of the hand, the deltoid muscle, and even the external anal sphincter.

HOW DO RESULTS OF CORTICOSPINAL STIMULATION CORRELATE WITH ASSESSMENTS OF MOTOR FUNCTION IN HUMANS?

Cortical stimulation has now been used to evaluate corticospinal function in many different disease states, and has revealed transmission deficits in several conditions. However, is the technique of any use in the practical assessment of motor function?

The simplest and most reliable measurement to take after transcranial stimulation is the central motor conduction time. This is obtained by subtracting peripheral latency from spinal cord to muscle from the total latency from cortex to muscle. In any one subject, this measurement is extremely reliable. Across a group of normal subjects, the total variation in central motor conduction time is only of the order of 2 to 3 msec. The relationship between the central motor conduction time and motor function in hand and arm muscles has been studied most extensively in patients with multiple sclerosis. Early papers on the subject were not promising. Central motor conduction time appeared to have no relationship with clinical estimates of hand strength, although increases in conduction time were associated in a proportion of patients with an increased frequency of finger flexor jerks (Hess, et al., 1987). However, Van der Kamp et al. (1991) recently showed that this apparent lack of correlation may have been the result of examining the wrong aspect of motor function. As described above, the corticospinal tract appears to be preferentially involved in control of independent finger movements rather than tonic muscle strength. Work in the monkey by Hepp-Reymond et al. (1973) suggested that another important function of the corticospinal tract was in production of rapid phasic contractions rather than in tonic muscle strength. Monkeys with pyramidal lesions failed to produce changes in muscle force as rapidly as normal, although the maximum force output was within the normal range.

Van der Kamp et al. (1991) assessed the ability of patients with multiple sclerosis to perform independent finger movements, and also measured the speed at which these patients could produce rapid voluntary muscle contractions of a small hand muscle. They found a clear correlation between these measures of corticospinal function and measurements of central motor conduction times. Patients with the longest central conduction times were worst at making independent finger movements, and produced the slowest voluntary contractions. However, none of the patients was classified clinically as being weak. The implication is that simple measures of central conduction time can give some objective indication of functional deficit in corticospinal pathways.

Motor symptoms which are not mediated by the corticospinal tract show no correlations with physiological assessments of corticospinal integrity. A good example of this is the clinical phenomenon of spasticity and heightened tendon reflexes. Patients with hereditary spastic paraplegia have spastic legs, but their central motor conduction times to leg muscles lie within the normal range (Thompson et al., 1987a).

Many reasons probably combine to explain why central motor conduction estimates correlate well with measurements of corticospinal function in patients with multiple sclerosis. The demyelination produced by the disease causes slowing of conduction in myelinated fibers. On its own, pure slowing of conduction should produce little effect on motor function. However, demyelination also is accompanied by failure to transmit repetitive trains of impulses, and in some cases causes conduction block. It is these deficits which are thought to contribute most to the disorder of corticospinal function exhibited by patients with multiple sclerosis.

In addition to measuring central motor conduction time, it is also possible to gain some insight into the total number of active fibers within the corticospinal tract by measuring the size of muscle responses evoked by cortical stimulation. In normal subjects, this measurement has a very high standard deviation, because several factors influence the size of EMG responses evoked by a single cortical shock. One of the most important of these is the level of spinal cord excitability at the time when the cortical stimulus was given. Because of the synapse between corticospinal fibers and the spinal motor neurones, the response to a given size of descending volley depends upon the background level of excitation in the motor neurones. Responses are large if spinal cord excitability is high, and they are small if the spinal cord excitability is low. It is possible to standardize spinal cord excitability to some extent by asking subjects to exert a tonic voluntary contraction of known force, but this technique cannot be used in patients with minimal or no remaining voluntary muscle power.

THE USE OF CORTICAL STIMULATION IN TESTING INTEGRITY OF LONG SPINAL CORD PATHWAYS

Until the advent of transcranial stimulation, conventional electrophysiological techniques were unable to probe the lesions responsible for the major clinical deficit (i.e., paralysis) in patients with spinal cord injury. Indeed, Lesser et al. (1986) drew attention to the failure of somatosensory-evoked potential (SEP) monitoring during spinal cord surgery to alert the clinician to impending damage to the spinal motor pathways. They described four patients who awoke from surgery with paraplegia or quadriplegia and two who developed similar deficits immediately postoperatively, but in whom SEP monitoring had given no warning of the disaster.

The combination of motor cortex stimulation with SEP studies provides a powerful method for testing the integrity of both sensory and motor tracts in the spinal cord. Thompson et al. (1987b) compared the techniques in six awake patients with spinal cord damage. Three had cervical cord trauma and three had cervical myelopathy caused by cervical spondylosis. They found abnormal corticospinal conduction in five of these patients, yet in four of them, SEPs evoked from the same limb were of normal latency (see example in Figure 7–1).

These results emphasize that physiological techniques are capable of detecting differential damage to central sensory and motor pathways in the spinal cord. More importantly, they show that conventional testing of sensory pathways may fail to document cord damage. For example, in conditions like cervical spondylosis in which the major symptoms are produced by involvement of anterior and lateral quadrants of the spinal cord, examination of corticospinal function with motor cortex stimulation should be of considerable value.

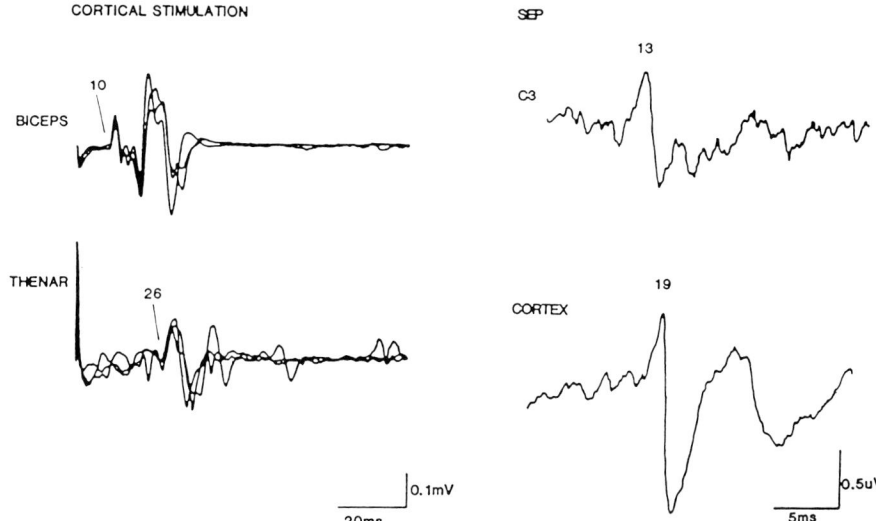

Figure 7-1 Electromyographic responses (three trials superimposed) in the right biceps and thenar (abductor pollicis brevis) muscles after stimulation of the left motor cortex (left traces). Also, the cortical and spinal somatosensory evoked potentials (SEPs) (average of 1024 trials) from stimulation of the median nerve of the same arm in a patient with cervical spondylosis and myelopathy (right traces). The thenar responses at 26 msec was delayed after stimulation of the motor cortex, but the SEP latencies were normal. (From Thompson et al., 1987a, with permission.)

USE OF CORTICOSPINAL TESTING IN THE EVALUATION OF MOTOR FUNCTION IN PATIENTS WITH CENTRAL NERVOUS SYSTEM DAMAGE

Apart from providing information on the integrity of long spinal pathways, there are two situations where corticospinal testing may provide useful prognostic information about motor function in patients with acute injuries of the central nervous system (CNS). MacDonnell et al. (1989) examined whether corticospinal testing could provide an indication of future motor recovery in 19 patients after stroke. The patients underwent their initial corticospinal testing between 1 and 30 days after the ictus and were followed-up for 1 to 6 months. Cortical stimulation produced muscle responses in nine of ten patients who went on to make some degree or full recovery. Responses were absent in eight of the nine patients who made no recovery or died. The suggestion is that if corticospinal pathways remain intact after a stroke, then the patient is more likely to make some functional recovery.

Corticospinal function has also been tested in some detail in children by Eyre et al. (1989). During normal development, the threshold for obtaining motor responses after cortical stimulation is high over the first two years of life, and then declines progressively to reach adult values by 16 years of age. The central motor conduction time declines slowly over the first 6 months (averaging about 21 msec to arm muscles) and then reduces rapidly from 6 to 15 months of age until adult values (4–8 msec) are obtained at about 18 months. These values have been compared with those obtained in children with abnormal motor development. Eyre and colleagues found that children with spastic hemiplegia have absent or prolonged central motor conduction times. In contrast, children with spastic quadraplegia, and poor voluntary motor control have relatively normal corticospinal transmission. This fits with the observation that children with spastic hemiplegia are likely to have some form of focal brain damage to one hemisphere, and that this may interfere with corticospinal function. The children with cerebral palsy and spastic quadraplegia often have diffuse brain damage, and it may be that the problem which they experience with voluntary motor control results from abnormal input to a functioning corticospinal system. If so, then it may be possible, with appropriate physiotherapeutic techniques, to assist the motor system to make full use of the normal pathways available.

REORGANIZATION OF THE CORTICOSPINAL MOTOR SYSTEM AFTER INJURY

Recent work has provided insight into the extent to which the corticospinal system can reorganize after injury. Cohen et al. (1991) examined patients with either acquired or congenital amputation of one arm. They mapped the area of scalp from which they could evoke EMG responses in the deltoid muscles on each side of the body. Contralateral to the intact side, responses could be obtained only from a very small area of the scalp, and then only at high threshold. In contrast, responses could readily be evoked in the deltoid of the amputated side from a large area of contralateral scalp with a significantly lower threshold than that on the opposite side. Reorganization of scalp motor maps was also seen by Levy et al. (1990) in two cases of traumatic paraplegia (Figure 7–2). These patients also had a greatly increased area of representation of muscles spared above the level of the spinal lesion. Both studies emphasize the ability of the corticospinal system to reorganize after peripheral nerve injury, even in fully mature adults. However, there is one report by Hall et al. (1990) which suggests that reorganization in adults may be less effective than that in children. They studied four patients with amputation of one arm. Two patients were congenital amputees, the two others lost their arm at age 10 and 50, respectively. Reorganization of the motor map contralateral to the missing arm was seen in both of the congenital amputees, and in the patient amputated at age of 10. They did not see any change in the corticospinal projections in one subject who had lost his arm in adult life.

The level at which the reorganization occurred in the patients described above could not be addressed directly in these studies. Changes in both cortical and spinal cord circuitry could lead to a change in the area from which muscle responses could be obtained by scalp stimulation. However, since spinal reflexes appeared to be normal in some of these patients, it is tempting to suggest that the reorganization occurred at a cortical level. Such reorganization may improve voluntary control of remaining musculature.

INTERRUPTION OF MOVEMENT BY TRANSCRANIAL STIMULATION

As described by neurosurgeons many years ago, stimulation of the motor areas not only evokes movement, but can also interrupt or stop ongoing voluntary movement.

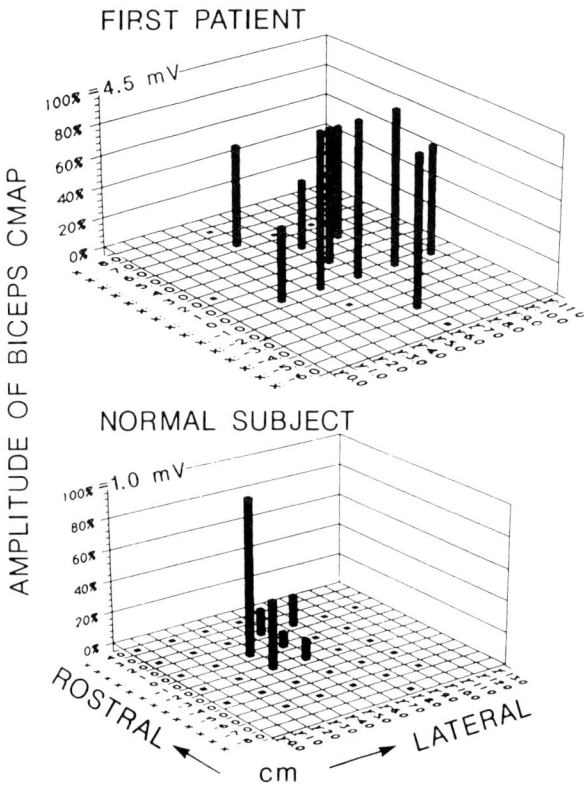

Figure 7−2 Map of excitable scalp positions for evoking responses in biceps in a 27-year-old patient with cervical cord injury sustained 2 years earlier. The patient was quadriplegic except for some biceps function in the arm, implying a level close to C5. He had had extensive physiotherapy, resulting in a current strength of 4/5 in this muscle. The graph plots the amplitude of the EMG response (as a percent of the maximum) evoked by stimulating with a figure-of-eight magnetic coil centered on the positions shown. The size of responses at each point is represented by the height of the bar. (From Levy et al., 1989, with permission.)

It is possible to make use of the latter effect to investigate how the brain programs certain types of voluntary movement. Day et al. (1989b) studied the effect of giving transcranial stimulation prior to a reaction-time wrist-flexion movement. Subjects were trained to flex their wrist through an angle of about 30° as rapidly as possible in response to an auditory tone. Electromyographs recorded from surface electrodes over the flexor and extensor muscles of the forearm showed the typical triphasic EMG activity pattern beginning with a burst in the agonist muscle followed by a burst in the antagonist and then a second burst in the agonist. After several practice trials, the reaction time became relatively stable, and the duration and latency of the EMG bursts quite constant. At this point, the experimenter introduced transcranial stimulation in random trials timed to occur just before the expected time of onset of EMG activity. The effect is shown in Figure 7–3. The stimulus produced an artifact, followed by a direct muscle twitch. This was then followed after a short period of silence by the voluntary triphasic EMG pattern. What appears to happen is that the cortical shock delays the onset of the voluntary movement without dis-

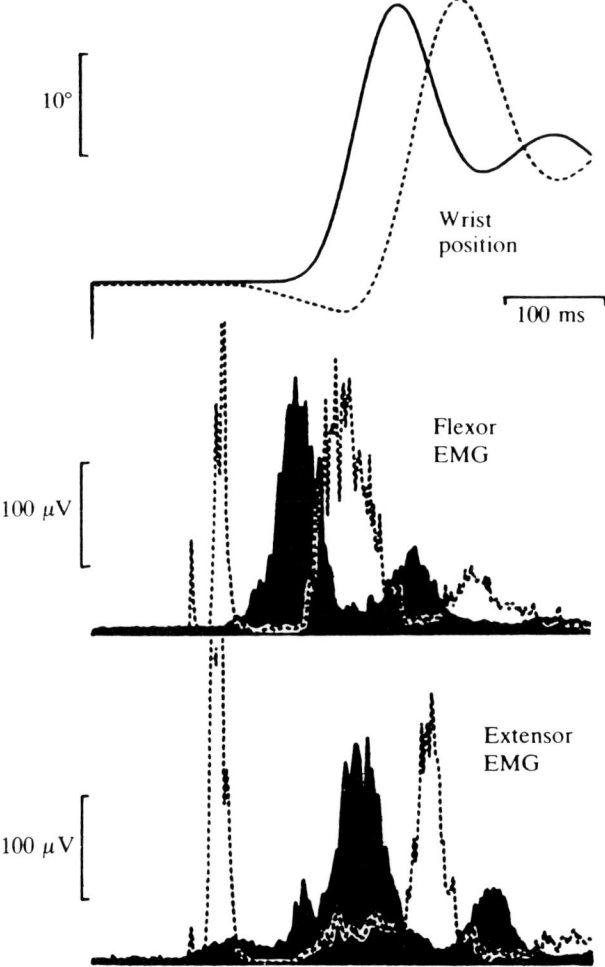

Figure 7–3 Rapid wrist flexion movements in a single normal subject in response to an audio signal given at the start of the sweep, with (dotted lines) and without (solid traces) magnetic cortical stimulation delivered 100 msec after the start of the sweep. Shown are average wrist position (upper traces, flexion upwards), wrist and finger flexor (middle traces), and extensor (lower traces) rectified EMG activity. The control movement (average of 26 trials) is characterized by alternating bursts of activity in the flexor and extensor muscles. In those trials in which a cortical stimulus was given (70% magnetic stimulation, average of 10 trials) the movement and associated pattern of muscle activities are the same but delayed by some 60 msec. Note the direct muscle responses in the flexor and extensor muscles occurring some 15 msec after the stimulus artifact producing, in this case, a small extension movement seen in the wrist position trace. (From Day et al., 1989b, with permission.)

rupting its form. The duration and size of the EMG burst in the triphasic pattern is unchanged from that seen in control trials.

This effect of the cortical shock was quite different from that seen after stimulation of peripheral nerve. Figure 7–4 shows what happened when a single supramaximal stimulus was given to the combined ulnar and median nerves in the axilla in the same task. The stimulus artifact is followed by a large M-response, and a silent

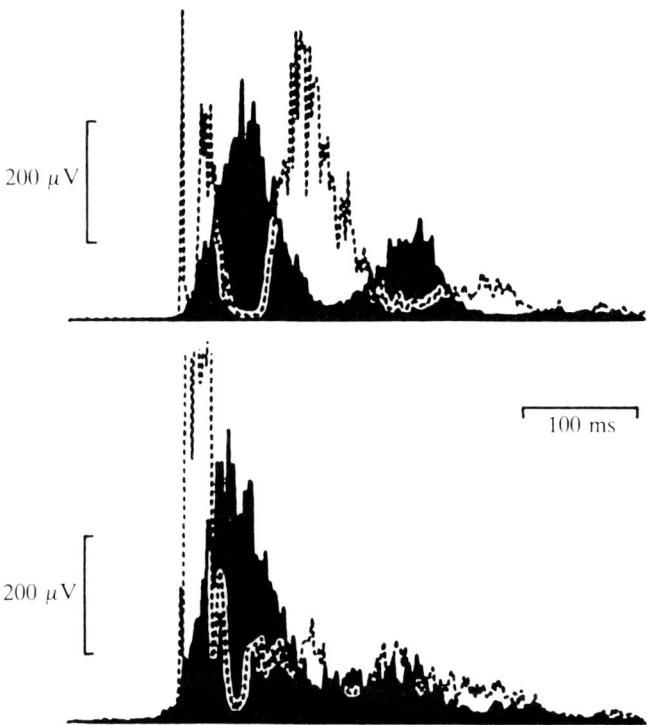

Figure 7–4 Comparison of the effect of brain stimulation with peripheral nerve stimulation on a rapid wrist flexion movement in response to an auditory signal at the beginning of the sweep in a single subject. Shown is the average rectified EMG from the agonist wrist flexor muscles. The average control EMGs are shown by solid traces (top, $n = 23$; bottom, $n = 13$). The dotted lines show the average EMG when a stimulus was delivered 100 msec after the auditory tone, before the expected onset of the first agonist burst. The brain was stimulated electrically at 70% intensity (top trace, $n = 16$) and the median nerve was stimulated with three supramaximal stimuli separated by 4 msec (bottom trace $n = 15$). The movement EMG pattern is delayed only when a brain stimulus is given. The peripheral nerve stimulus has the effect of reducing the size of the movement EMG bursts. (From Day et al., 1989b, with permission.)

period. After the silence, voluntary EMG activity emerges. However, the onset latency of each of the bursts within the triphasic pattern is the same as in the control trials. The peripheral nerve silent period has "eaten into" the onset of the first agonist EMG burst, but has had no effect on the timing or size of the antagonist or second agonist bursts.

The effect of the cortical shock is maximum in the hand contralateral to the stimulated hemisphere. In a bimanual reaction time task, in which subjects had to flex the right and left wrists simultaneously in response to the reaction tone, stimulation of the left hemisphere only delayed movements of the right wrist. The movement of the left wrist was virtually unaffected. In all tasks, the amount by which the movement was delayed depended on both the relative timing and the intensity of the cortical shock. The larger the stimulus, the larger the delay. Very large shocks produced delays of more than 100 msec. However, these delays are difficult to interpret, since voluntary reaction can influence responses within such long time

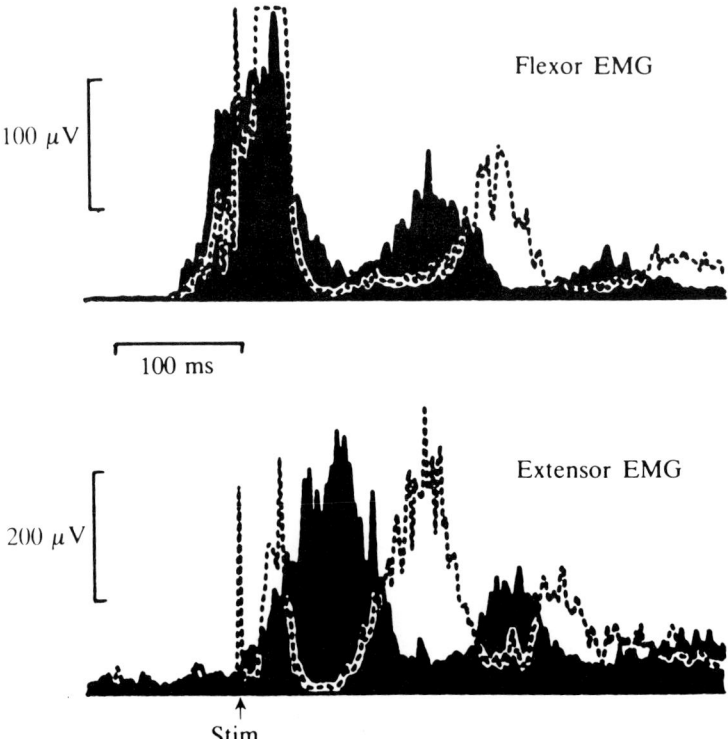

Figure 7–5 Effect of giving a 65% magnetic cortical stimulus 120 msec after the auditory signal (which occurred at the beginning of the trace), during the occurrence of the first agonist EMG burst associated with a rapid flexion movement in a single subject. Shown is the average rectified EMG from the agonist wrist flexor (upper traces) and the antagonist wrist extensor muscles (lower traces). The average of the control ($n = 24$) is shown by the solid traces and those trials in which a cortical stimulus was given ($n = 10$) dotted lines. Although the cortical stimulus was given too late to affect the timing of the first agonist burst, the first antagonist (and later) burst is delayed by the stimulus. (From Day et al., 1989b, with permission.)

intervals. For a given size of stimulus, a large effect was seen if the stimulus was given nearer to the expected time of onset of movement. If given early in the reaction period, then the delay was much shorter. Thus, reaction time increases when the cortical stimulus is given later within the reaction period. Finally, it is also possible to give cortical stimuli during, rather than before, the execution of the wrist movement. Figure 7–5 shows what happens when the cortical shock was timed to occur in the middle of the first burst of agonist EMG activity. The result is that the antagonist burst and the second agonist burst are delayed, but their form remains intact.

Since the greatest delay in reaction time occurred when the cortical stimulus was given later in the reaction period, we assume that the shock interferes with execution of the movement rather than with the perception of the stimulus or the intention of the subject to respond. Although we do not know precisely what parts of the brain were activated by the stimulus, nor the precise mechanism by which the effects occurred, several important conclusions can be drawn from the data as they stand.

The most important is that the brain must be able to store temporarily during the period of the delay some of the information necessary for voluntary reaction. If this is true, then a further implication follows. The brain must have had some internal knowledge that the voluntary reaction had been interrupted in order to detect the failure to deliver a motor command at a specified time. It is not possible to deduce the nature of this feedback from the present experiments. For example, the brain might check the progress of the motor command by some form of internal reafference. Alternatively, the brain might check the readiness of downstream sites to respond to impending instructions. An example of how the latter possibility could be applied might go as follows. Assume that the motor cortex receives motor commands for the movement from some other site within the brain, and that these signals are delivered to the motor strip only when it has signaled to the upstream brain areas that it is ready to respond. The scalp stimulus might produce its delay by activating elements within the motor cortex, making them unavailable to mediate a voluntary motor command. The "ready" signal to upstream brain areas would be removed, and only reinstated when the motor cortex had recovered. The delivery of the motor commands would be postponed until the ready signal was active again, and the reaction would have been delayed.

More recently, two other groups have investigated the effect of cortical stimulation on more complex movements. Amassian et al. (1990) examined sequential movements of the fingers and gave stimuli over the supplementary and premotor areas. The results were quite different from those seen if the motor cortex itself was stimulated. The task consisted of sequential opposition of the thumb to each finger in turn at a rate of about once every 300 to 400 msec. If the motor cortex was stimulated, there was a delay in the onset of the next movement of the sequence, but no other change. In contrast, stimulation of the supplementary motor area had little effect on the movement immediately following the stimulus. Later components of the sequence were affected much more. There appeared to be a minimum interval of about 200 msec after the supplementary motor area stimulus before any part of the task was affected. If was as if the supplementary motor area was operating "upstream" of the motor cortex, planning movements in advance of the one currently being executed.

The movements examined by Amassian et al. (1990) were relatively slow, but Berardelli et al. (1991) examined a more rapid sequential arm movement. They asked subjects to draw out an equilateral triangle on a horizontal pad before them as rapidly as possible after an audio tone. They reasoned that in such rapid movement, more of the program would have to prepared before the movement than in the more slowly executed task of Amassian et al. (1990). In the latter, the program might be updated continuously throughout the course of the movement. After subjects had learnt the task, Berardelli et al. used transcranial magnetic stimulation to try to interrupt the movement by giving stimuli in random trials during or before the task. They used a large coil centered at the vertex so that the precise area of stimulation was unclear. When they stimulated during the course of the movement, then the trajectory was disrupted, but most subjects found it possible to continue the movement to its conclusion with only a slightly prolonged movement time. The effect was quite different if the stimulus was given during the reaction period, before the onset of movement. If the stimulus was given some 200 msec after the reaction tone, most subjects found it impossible to complete the task. They would draw one side of the triangle, and then stop several seconds at the apex. If they continued, then the movement time increased dramatically over the control values. Berardelli et al. (1991) suggested that this stimulus interfered with processes linking together different parts of the movement which had been prepared during the reaction period.

REFERENCES

Amassian, V.E., Cracco, J.B., Cracco, R.Q., and Maccabee, P.J. (1990). Magnetic coil stimulation of human premotor cortex affects sequential digit movements. *J. Physiol.*, **424**, 65P.

Barker, A.J., Jalinous, R., and Freeston, I.L. (1985). Non-invasive stimulation of human motor cortex. *Lancet*, **II**, 1106–1107.

Berardelli, A., Inghilleri, M., Cruccu, G., and Manfredi, M. (1991). Effect of cortical stimulation on the execution of fast complex arm movements in man. *J. Physiol.*, **438**, 30P.

Brouwer, B., and Ashby, P. (1990). Corticospinal projections to upper and lower limb spinal motoneurones in man. *Electroencephalog. Clin. Neurol.*, **76**, 509–519.

Cohen, L.G., Bandinelli, S., Findley, T.W., and Hallett, M. (1991). Reorganization in the map of motor cortex outputs after upper limb amputation in humans. *Brain*, **114**, 615–628.

Datta, A.K., Harrison, L.M., and Stephens, J.A. (1989). Task-dependent changes in the size of responses to magnetic brain stimulation in human first dorsal interosseous muscle. *J. Physiol.*, **418**, 13–23.

Day, B.L., Dressler, D., Maertens de Noordhout, A., Marsden, C.D., Nakashima, K., Rothwell, J.C., and Thompson, P.D. (1989). Electric and magnetic stimulation of the human motor cortex: Surface EMG and single motor unit responses. *J. Physiol.*, **412**, 449–473.

Day, B.L., Rothwell, J.C., Thompson, P.D., Maertens de Noordhout, A., Nakashima, K., Shannon, K., and Marsden, C.D. (1989b). Delay in the execution of voluntary movement by electrical or magnetic brain stimulation in intact man. *Brain*, **112**, 649–653.

Edgley, S.A., Eyre, J.A., Lemon, R.N., and Miller, S. (1990). Excitation of the corticospinal tract by electromagnetic and electrical stimulation of the scalp in the macaque monkey. *J. Physiol.*, **425**, 301–320.

Eyre, J.A., Coh, T.H.H.G., Gibson, M., Miller, S., O'Sullivan, M.C., and Ramesh, V. (1989). Corticospinal transmission excited by electromagnetic stimulation of the brain is impaired in children with spastic hemiparesis but normal in those with quadriparesis. *J. Physiol.*, **414**, 9P.

Hall, E.J., Flament, D. Fraser, C., and Lemon, R.N. (1990). Non-invasive brain stimulation reveals reorganized cortical outputs in amputees. *Neurosci. Lett.*, **116**, 379–386.

Hepp-Reymond, M.C., and Wiesendanger, M. (1972). Unilateral pyramidotomy in monkeys: effect on force and speed of a conditioned precision grip. *Exp. Brain Res.*, **36**, 117–131.

Hess, C.W., Mills, K.R., Murray, N.M.F., and Schriefer, T.N. (1987). Magnetic brain stimulation: Central motor conduction studies in multiple sclerosis. *Ann. Neurol.*, **22**, 744–752.

Lesser, R.P., Raudzens P. Lüders, H., et al. (1986). Postoperative neurological deficits may occur despite unchanged intraoperative somatosensory evoked potentials. *Ann. Neurol.*, **19**, 22–25.

Levy, W.J., Amassian, V.E., Traad, M., and Cadwell, J. (1990). Focal magnetic coil stimu-

lation reveals motor cortical system reorganized in humans after traumatic quadriplegia. *Brain Res.*, **510**, 130–134.
Macdonell, R.A.L., Donnan, G.A., and Bladin, P.F. (1989). A comparison of somatosensory evoked and motor evoked potentials in stroke. *Ann. Neurol.*, **25**, 68–73.
Merton, P.A., and Morton, H.B. (1980). Stimulation of cerebral cortex in the intact human subject. *Nature*, **285**, 227.
Muir, R. B., and Lemon, R.N. (1983). Corticospinal neurones with a special role in precision grip. *Brain Res.*, **261**, 312–316.
Rothwell, J.C., Thompson, P.D., Day, B.L., Dick, J.P.R., Kachi, T., Cowan, J.M.A., and Marsden, C.D. (1987). Motor cortex stimulation in intact man. *Brain*, **110**, 1173–1190.
Thompson, P.D., Day, B.L., Rothwell, J.C., et al. (1987a). The interpretation of electromyographic responses to electrical stimulation of the motor cortex in diseases of the upper motor neurone. *J. Neurol. Sci.*, **80**, 91–110.
Thompson, P.D., Dick, J.P.R., Asselman, P., Griffin, G.B., Day, B.L., Rothwell, J.C., Sheehy, M.P., and Marsden, C.D. (1987b). Examination of motor function in lesions of the spinal cord by stimulation of the motor cortex. *Ann. Neurol.*, **21**, 389–396.
Van der Kamp, W. Maertens de Noordhout, A., Thompson, P.D., Rothwell, J.C., Day, B.L., and Marsden, C.D. (1991). Correlation of phasic muscle strength and corticomotoneuron conduction time in multiple sclerosis. *Ann. Neurol.*, **29**, 6–12.
Zidar, J., Trontelj, J.C., and Mihelin, M. (1987). Percutaneous stimulation of human corticospinal tract: A single fibre EMG study of individual motor responses. *Brain Res.*, **422**, 196–199.

8
Motor Prostheses for Restoration of Upper Extremity Function

P. HUNTER PECKHAM AND MICHAEL W. KEITH

Clinical systems which provide upper extremity function have been developed. These systems have focused on providing control of grasp and release functions in individuals with spinal cord injury, with earlier stage development directed toward control of more proximal joints. Functional neuromuscular stimulation has also been used to provide hand opening in hemiplegic individuals. These motor protheses primarily utilize implanted electrodes, although surface stimulation systems have been used for proximal joint control. Hand control systems using implanted percutaneous electrodes have demonstrated a significant improvement in function, as compared to the user's best alternative technique. This motor prosthetic system presently is being tested in a limited multicenter clinical trail. Initial results are positive regarding the ability of the satellite centers to implement the systems and the functional capabilities achieved by the users at each of the centers. The challenge which remains is to continue to evolve the functionality of these systems by increasing their capabilities and simplifying their operation, while transferring them at the most expeditious pace into clinical utility for the enhancement of function of the disabled user.

Paralysis of the upper extremity is one of the more severely debilitating dysfunctions that humans can sustain. Without use of the upper extremity, even simple manipulative functions that are necessary for basic daily function must be replaced by alternative assistive measures. Among the more conventional means of providing increased function in the extremity treatment are orthotics and reconstructive surgery. In some injuries, specifically those which are of central nervous system (CNS) origin, the muscle may still receive innervation of the peripheral nerve, and may be

Table 8–1 Hand Configurations Used by Able-Bodied Individuals in Grasping and Holding for Use Objects Encountered in Daily Life[a]

Series	Prehension Type		
	Palmar	Tip	Lateral
Pick up	34	8	58
Hold for use	64.5	1.5	34

Source: Keller et al. (1947).
[a]Percentage frequency of three prehension patterns.

electrically excitable for indefinite periods after the CNS lesion. For individuals who have sustained these injuries, controlled movement of the limb may be induced by activation of the nerves using low levels of pulsed electrical current. This technique is known as functional electrical stimulation (FES), or functional neuromuscular stimulation (FNS). The principle focus of clinical applications of FNS in the upper extremity has been on restoration of grasp and release functions. This chapter is an overview of activities in this area of clinical research.

OBJECTIVES OF AN FNS SYSTEM IN THE UPPER EXTREMITY

The objectives of an upper extremity system must be directed clinically toward establishing independence to the user. Various etiologies and extent of injury present with different needs. The most effort in upper extremity FNS has been directed toward the individual with clinically complete spinal cord injury (SCI), meaning complete absence of motor and sensory function caudal to the lesion in the spinal cord. This description, while convenient, is generally misleading, since asymmetries in voluntary control, muscle innervation, and sensation are nearly always identified upon physical examination. In general, however, the retained function is related to the level at which the spinal cord is transected (Stauffer, 1975). Injury at the C4 results in volitional control of the scapula with lost control of the entire arm; at C5, with retained control of shoulder and elbow flexors with loss of control of the wrist and hand and lost sensation below the upper forearm; at C6, having in addition some capacity for wrist extension and sensation extending into the hand. At C7 and below, some voluntary control of the digits and sensation in the hand is retained. An international standard for categorizing the injury has been developed (McDowell et al., 1979). Approximately 13% of injuries are at C4, 17% at C5, 13% at C6, and 6% at C7 (Stover et al., 1986).

Restoration of function by FNS in the upper extremity has focused principally upon grasp-release. Consideration has been given to the type of grasp, the necessary forces to achieve, and the precision of control. Some guidance in these specifications is provided by early studies relating to prosthetics, conducted by Keller et al. (1947) and reviewed by Klopsteg and Wilson (1954). These studies related that palmar and lateral prehension accounted for approximately 90% of the hand functions in normal able-bodied individuals grasping and manipulating for use various objects encountered in daily activities. Table 8–1, abstracted from Keller (1947), relates the details. The maximal forces achieved in grasp were 103 ± 21 N in lateral prehension and

96 ± 24 N in palmar prehension. However, in grasping common objects, grasp forces were generally less than 20% of maximum. In other studies, Rohmert (1960) found that in voluntary contraction, forces of approximately 18% of maximum voluntary contraction could be sustained indefinitely (i.e., without fatigue). The resolution of force control in voluntary contraction is more difficult to assess; Klopsteg and Wilson (1954) claim values for force discrimination of 0.49 N and thickness discrimination of 0.15 cm. These measurements provide some guidelines for the specification to be obtained in restored grasp with FNS, as related to normal volitional control.

RESTORATION OF GRASP AND RELEASE MOVEMENT

Restoration of hand function has focused upon providing both lateral and palmar grasps and release, since the user should then be able to grasp and manipulate most objects they will encounter in daily living. To achieve these movements, independent control of the thumb and fingers must be achieved. For lateral prehension, finger flexion at the metacarpal-phalangeal (MP) and both interphalangeal joints, and thumb flexion and extension is required. Positioning is obtained with the finger flexors and extensors; force generation with the thenar flexors and adductor. For palmar prehension, finger flexion-extension at the MP joint and abduction of the thumb is required. Positioning is obtained with the thenar muscles for abduction; force generation by the finger flexors. In voluntary control, Hoshimiya et al. (1989) have used myoelectric recording to demonstrate the muscles which are active. Predictably, these include finger and thumb intrinsic and extrinsic muscles and wrist extrinsics, which will be active to varying levels depending upon the conditions under measurement (e.g., limb position, object weight). As demonstrated by Kilgore et al. (1990) in the hand and by Nathan (1989) at the wrist, during electrical stimulation most of the muscles generate joint torques that are not in pure flexion-extension or abduction-adduction directions, and the movements vary with the level of stimulation that is applied to the muscle. In FNS-restored grasp, a subset of these muscles generally is excited. Table 8–2 shows the muscles that generally are used for restoration of these two basic grasps. In addition, Fukamachi et al. (1987) also reported use of the intrinsic muscles of the fingers to develop isolated flexion of the MP joints of the fingers, which requires six channels of stimulation not including the lumbrical muscles. The digits are defined as either fixed or moving, indicating that the control of force generation is principally through the moving digits, while the fixed digit(s) is used to position the remaining digit(s) to provide a restraint against which the object and moving digits apply force. For lateral prehension, grasp is ideally achieved with the thumb providing force against the middle phalanx, whereas in palmar prehension grasp is ideally achieved with the index and long fingers producing force against the thumb. Figure 8–1 shows these two grasping configurations.

CANDIDATE CLINICAL ETIOLOGIES

Many factors must be considered in selection of candidates for FNS. These factors include physiological factors (e.g., muscle innervation, joint range of motion), med-

Table 8–2 Muscles Used in Restoration of Grasp in Lateral and Palmar Prehension and Release with Functional Neuromuscular Stimulation[a]

		Positioning	Force Generation
Lateral	Thumb	EPL/EPB	AdP
			FPL
			FPB
	Fingers	FDS/FDP	—
		EDC/EI	
Palmar	Thumb	AbPB	FDS/FDP
		AbPL	
	Fingers	EDC	—
		EI	

[a] The muscle groups can be separated into those which control the fixed digit(s) and those controlling the moving digit(s). EPL = extensor pollicis longus; EPB = extensor pollicis brevis; AdP = adductor pollicis; FPL = flexor pollicis longus; FPB = flexor pollicis brevis; FDS = flexor digitorum superficialis; FDP = flexor digitorum profundus; EDC = extensor digitorum communis; EI = extensor indicis; AbPB = abductor pollicis brevis; and AbPL = abductor pollicis longus.

ical factors (e.g, spasticity, autonomic stability), and psychosocial factors (e.g., family support, motivation). However, no factor is more critical than the innervation state of the muscle. Motor paralysis in the upper extremity may involve either the upper motor neurons, the lower motor neurons, or both. Functional neuromuscular stimulation utilizes relatively low-charge injection with short pulses, which is effective in exciting principally nerve rather than muscle, and thus only those muscles which have a sufficient number of motor units with retained innervation may be considered for functional restoration. In some injuries, such as nerve avulsions which may be caused by excessive stretching of the axilla, the paralysis is peripheral in origin, and the peripheral nerve will degenerate. Muscle paralysis from this type of injury is due to the denervation, and functional restoration has not been demonstrated in clinical populations. In contrast, injuries to the CNS often leave the peripheral nervous system intact and electrically excitable, without any apparent cessation of the electrical excitability for decades after the original injury. Examples of such injuries are stroke (cerebral vascular accident), cerebral palsy, and SCI. In SCI, it has only recently become appreciated that at the zone of injury, there may be damage to the anterior horn cells or spinal roots as well as the central lesion, and thus the profile of the innervation pattern to the muscle may be quite complex. This may lead to a complex neurological pattern of innervation that varies from one individual to the next. There may be varying degrees of the following conditions of paralysis in each muscle:

1. Total denervation (classical lower motor neuron lesion).
2. No central innervation, but complete peripheral innervation (classical upper motor neuron lesion).
3. Partial volitional control and partial denervation.
4. Partial denervation and partial peripheral innervation without central innervation.
5. Partial normal volitional control and partial peripherally innervated by centrally isolated motor units.

In our experience, muscles which receive their innervation just at or above the injury

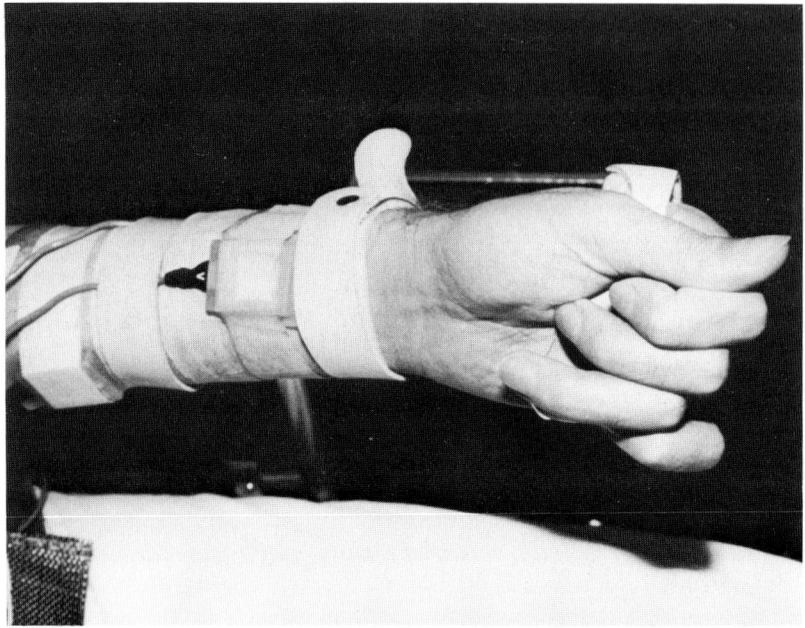

(A)

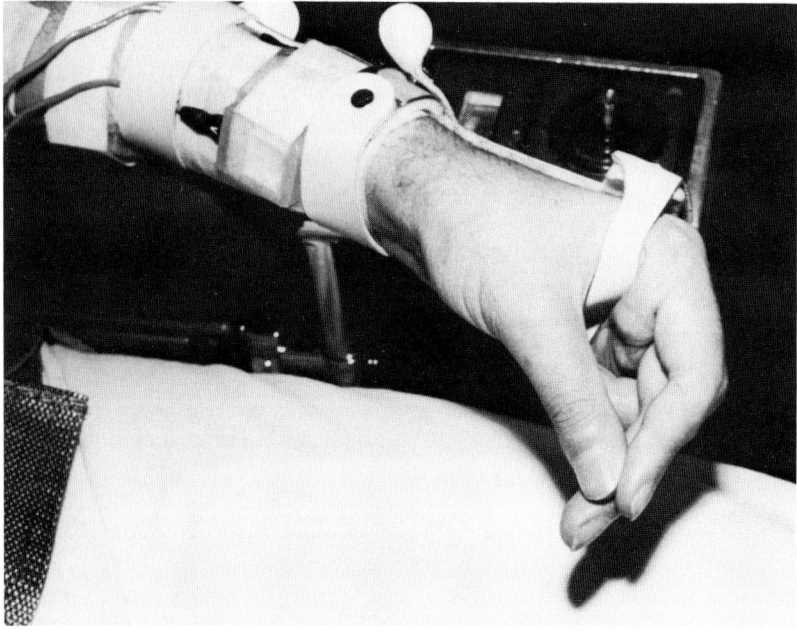

(B)

Figure 8–1 Grasp and release movements synthesized for restoring functional use in the paralyzed hand in spinal cord injury. (A) Lateral prehension is generally used for grasping small objects (e.g., fork, pen). (B) Palmar prehension is used for grasping larger objects (e.g., glass). (C) Release allows objects to be included between the thumb and fingers.

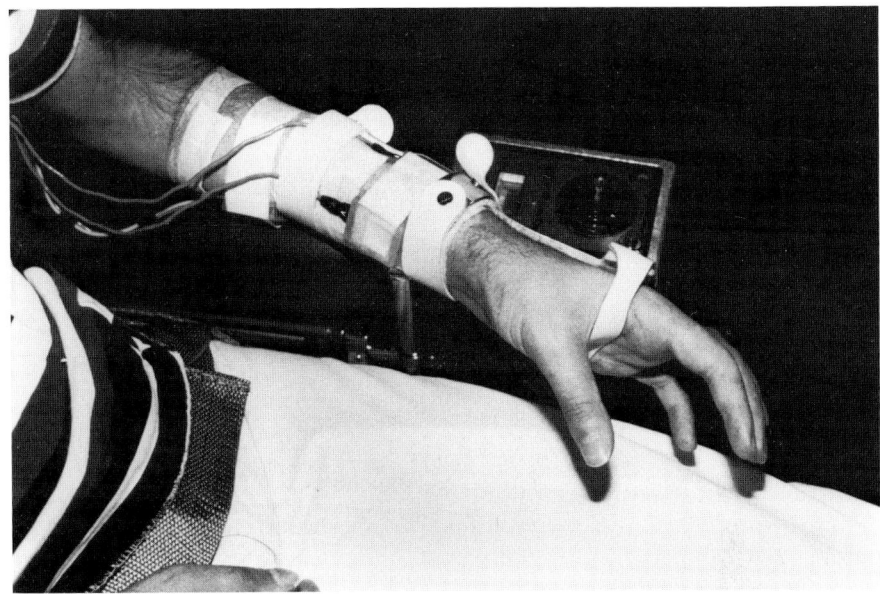

(C)
Figure 8–1 (Continued).

site present in class 3, whereas muscles which receive their innervation just at the injury level present as class 1 or 4. In clinically complete SCI, class 5 is rare. In a recent review by Gorman and Peckham (1990), researchers at Shriner's Hospital found 27% of muscles in the upper extremity to be denervated. Our studies, carried out on 32 limbs in 18 tetraplegics (8, C5; 14, C6; 10, C7), showed between 80 and 100% of muscles had innervation intact. The innervation was dependent upon the muscle group and the spinal injury level, consistent with our expectations. Surgical alternatives have been developed to substitute innervated muscles for those which are denervated, by performing tendon transfers of muscles with upper motor neuron lesions and subsequent stimulation. In planning the strategy for reconstructing hand function in the spinal cord-injured individual, this most critical determination must first be made.

SYNTHESIS OF GRASP AND RELEASE

The synthesis of movement is defined as the process of coordinating the activation of the electrically stimulated muscles to obtain the desired movements of the digits and force generation between the moving and fixed digits. In synthesis of grasp under open-loop control, the investigator must program the level of activation of the individual muscle groups to achieve the desired grasp, defined as the grasp template. In all clinical systems that have been developed to date, the objective is to enable the user of the FNS system to control their hand through a single, proportionally graded command input. This input simultaneously controls the activation of all muscles in the grasping pattern by regulation of the electrical stimuli applied to each muscle. Thus, the relationship between the stimulus input and force output of the muscle must be characterized.

It is well known that the muscle, or more precisely the number of muscle fibers activated, is controlled by the stimulus pulse width or stimulus pulse amplitude, and the level of temporal summation is governed by the rate at which stimulus pulses are applied to the muscle (Mortimer, 1981). While both recruitment and temporal summation can be employed, generally only the former has been employed in clinical systems. The stimulus frequency, which determines the level of temporal summation, is fixed at the minimum which will generate a fused response, which is approximately a stimulus period of 80 msec (i.e., a stimulus frequency of 12.5 Hz). Although higher stimulus frequencies will generate higher forces, the choice of fixing the stimulus frequency at the lowest value which produces fusion is to enable the muscle to generate force for the most extended periods, since higher frequencies of stimulation will result in more rapid decrement of the contractile force (Kugelberg and Edstrom, 1968; McNeal, 1973; Bigland-Ritchie et al., 1979), although this is not the single likely explanation (Bigland-Ritchie, 1981).

Muscle recruitment with electrical stimulation is a nonlinear relationship between the stimulus input and muscle force output. The relationship is characterized by a deadband, which is the threshold stimulus that must be delivered before excitation is achieved, and followed by an increase in force with increasing stimulus. The shape of the recruitment curve is frequently characterized by piecewise linear segments, with alternating regions of higher and lower gain (Crago et al., 1980a,b). Complete excitation of the principle "target" muscle may not be achieved before "spillover" to another muscle, depending upon many factors, such as proximity of the electrode to nerve fibers innervating those adjacent muscles. Stability of the recruitment characteristics is important in an open-loop system, since degradation of response of any one muscle will alter the characteristics of the coordinated response. The recruitment relationship is time variant, which is due to a reduction in force-generating capacity of the muscle with time. This factor is particularly critical in humans, since muscles that are paralyzed due to disuse have been demonstrated to assume an atrophied, type-II characteristic (Grimby et al., 1976). Such muscle fibers generate small amounts of force and fatigue rapidly. Considerable efforts has been directed toward using chronic electrical stimulation to investigate the plasticity of the metabolic characteristics of the muscle (Vrbova et al., 1978; Pette, 1980). To build muscle strength and fatigue resistance, chronic electrical stimulation has been used as an effective "muscle conditioning" program which reduces this factor (Peckham et al., 1973; Lieber, 1986; Ferguson et al., 1989). Other factors that may alter the stability of the muscle response include the position of the electrode relative to the nerve, which may change as a function of the magnitude of the contractile response. Various electrode types exhibit these characteristics to varying degrees.

Synthesis of grasp requires that the appropriate response be delivered by each electrode. Kilgore et al. (1989) developed a rule-based system to select electrodes, based upon the factors which are most critical for a particular muscle group (e.g., selectivity, gain, length-dependent recruitment, maximum force generation). Upon selection of the electrode, the stimulus values at threshold and spillover for each muscle are used as parameters in the grasp template to automatically generate the set of stimulus grasp parameters to be applied to each muscle group. Subsequent

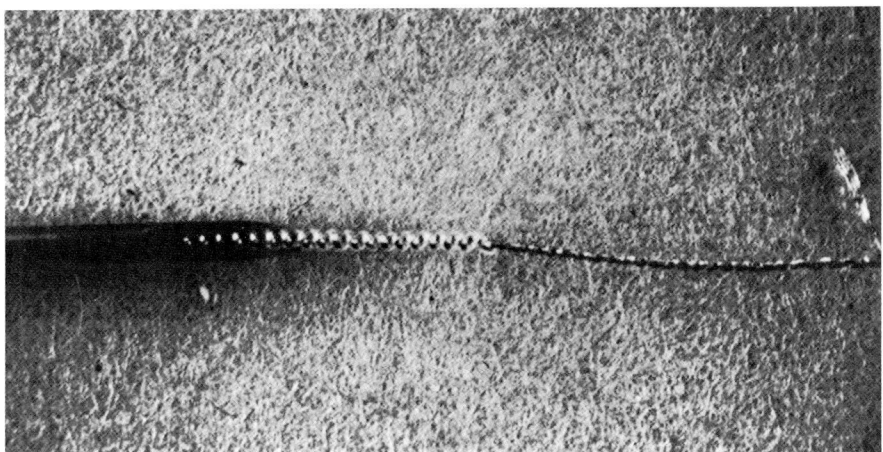

Figure 8-2 Percutaneously implanted intramuscular electrode as developed in Cleveland. The electrode is fabricated from insulated, multistand wire and formed into a helix. A hypodermic needle is used to introduce the electrode through the skin and into the muscle near the motor point.

modification of the grasp is performed empirically. In contrast, Handa et al. (1989) use the myoelectric activity of the normal muscle to perform initial estimates on the stimulus parameters.

HARDWARE FOR UPPER EXTREMITY MOTOR PROSTHESES

Both implanted and surface stimulation systems have been used for upper extremity motor prostheses. In general, the surface stimulation systems have demonstrated the ability to excite only the larger, more superficial muscles. They require that the electrode be precisely positioned and experience poor repeatability with motor-point movement as the muscle shortens during contraction (Crochetiere et al., 1967). Nathan (1989) reported efforts to overcome the positioning difficulties of surface electrodes.

Several types of implanted electrode have been used. Percutaneously implanted electrodes have been used most extensively by teams in Cleveland (Peckham et al., 1980a) and Sendai (Handa et al., 1989). Figure 8-2 illustrates a percutaneous electrode. The electrodes used are single-strand, multifilament-type 316 stainless steel wire insulated with Teflon and wound into a helical configuration. The tip of the wire is deinsulated to deliver current and a barb is formed at the tip. The electrode is inserted into a hypodermic needle, which is used as a cannula for introduction of the electrode into the muscle. Several electrodes may be inserted through the skin within a small area, and adverse tissue response is rare. In Cleveland, only 0.5% of 572 electrodes were infected, and there is a 90% probability that the electrode will be functional for 6 months and an 82% probability it will be functional for 1 year. The electrode is inserted nonsurgically using clean technique, generally without skin anesthesia. The electrode has been used in outpatient studies for over 11 years and has been an extremely effective tool for implementation of upper extremity FNS

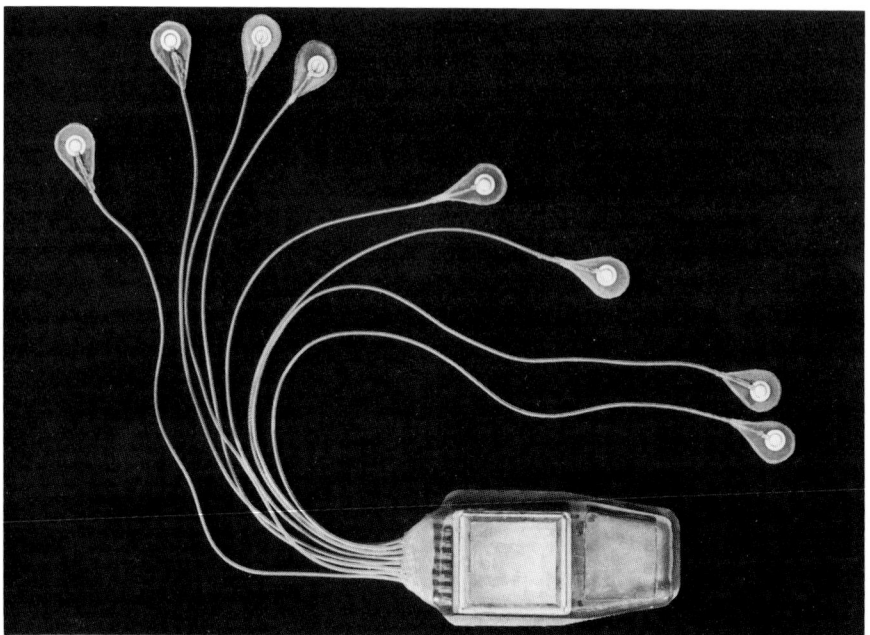

Figure 8–3 The CWRU/VA implantable receiver-stimulator showing the epimysial electrodes. The diameter of the conductive area of the disk is 3 mm.

systems. Other electrodes that have been used for upper extremity systems have been used in conjunction with an implantable stimulator. They include an epimysial electrode and a nerve cuff. The epimysial electrode is a platinum-iridium disk conductor with polymer backing for securing to the muscle epimysium. Figure 8–3 shows an epimysial electrode attached to the implantable receiver-stimulator developed in Cleveland (Smith et al., 1987). The nerve cuff is the book type (Rushton, personal communication, 1988), originally developed for the bladder neuroprosthesis (Brindley et al., 1982).

Implanted stimulator systems have been used in Konstancin, Poland (Kiwerski and Pasniczek, 1984), Cleveland (Keith et al., 1989) and London (Brindley et al., 1989). The implantable stimulator used in the first study was a single-channel device; the latter studies used multichannel radio frequency (RF) powered and controlled units. A principle advantage of using the implantable stimulator is that the reliability of the system can be improved over the percutaneous, and that the need to maintain percutaneous leads is eliminated.

The external control device is used to process the patient-generated command control signals and generate, by the preprogrammed process, the set of stimulus parameters to be used in excitation of the muscle. In the case of the implanted system, the system must generate the appropriate RF commands to communicate with the receiver. The control hardware used must be sufficiently small, reliable, and portable with self-powering, and easily programmed and maintained. Microprocessor-based systems assist in the ease of implementation and versatility of these systems. Considerable engineering effort is directed toward the development of such hardware (Buckett et al., 1988; Ignagni et al., 1980).

FACTORS AFFECTING SYNTHESIZED GRASP AND SURGICAL CONSIDERATIONS

The quality of the synthesized grasp is related to many physiological and anatomical factors. Among the most critical factors are the amount of denervation, the type of electrode and its position (which affects muscle recruitment), joint laxity, fixed contractures in the hand, and the normal biomechanical linkages of the musculoskeletal system. Denervation affects the grasp because it may eliminate a muscle from use, as described above. Muscle recruitment affects the grasp because graded output of the muscle generally is required. Muscle recruitment factors which affect the grasp quality include high gain, low force, spillover, or length-dependent recruitment (Kilgore et al., 1990). An unacceptably high gain may make control of force insufficiently graded, and thus result in objects being squeezed from the hand or crushed. Low force may result in insufficient grasping force or inability to move the hand through the entire range of motion. Stimulus parameters may have to be limited to avoid an unacceptable response (e.g., spillover), and thus limit the available force. Contractile force may change with the muscle length due to recruitment changes superimposed upon the muscle length tension properties. Joint laxity may result in insufficient transmission of force across one or more joints; joint contracture may limit the active range of motion that can be generated, thus limiting the size of objects that can be grasped. The normal biomechanical linkages which have the tendons crossing several joints may make balance and control of any joints difficult with a reduced number of actuator muscles.

Selection among available electrode types requires knowledge of the forearm muscle anatomy and some specific recruitment characteristics of available implantable electrodes. The anatomic distribution of motor points is well known from clinical experience with electromyography and, in our hands, multiple surgical explorations during tendon transfer surgery with operative subjects, intraoperative implantation, and from surface mapping with transcutaneous or percutaneous stimulation (Keith et al., 1989).

The epimysial electrode is asymmetrical, with a silastic surface which acts as an insulator on one side and the electrode on the other such that the current dispersion can be directed preferentially. Nerve fiber activation, and thus muscle fiber recruitment, will occur first on the noninsulated side bearing the conductive electrode. The surgical team can take advantage of this property in locating the electrode when motor points of two muscles are closely adjacent. The electrode should be located near the motor point such that graded recruitment of the muscle can be distributed over the available current range of the stimulator. Placement too close to the motor point causes an "all-or-none" phenomenon, with poor control of the muscle. The intramuscular electrode has a largely symmetrical current spread from the electrode tip such that it is most useful when implanted within the center of a muscle and recruits muscle force spatially.

The evolution of engineering and design of implantable electrodes has been toward greater resistance to fatigue failure of metals, including stronger leads, and better tissue incorporation and stability. Fortunately, the electrode surface area and size has not appreciably increased and remains appropriate for patient tolerance.

The electrode type selected should depend on intraoperative mapping in the patient and previous experience of the surgeon. The muscle surface must be exposed, usually over the proximal one third of the muscle belly of the facial surface. Most muscles accessible for FES are superficial in the forearm or hand with nerve branches coming from deep. The fascia should be excised in order to allow subsequent biological fixation to the muscle surface rather than the fascia. Muscle movement relative to the fascia would otherwise introduce variable length-dependent recruitment. Other factors such as recipient muscle bulk, the insulating quality of adjacent scarred or denervated muscle, and proximity to skin sensory nerve trunks may also be critical in any individual patient. These aspects are empirically determined.

Surgical intervention has been investigated as a means of mitigating the biomechanical factors identified above (Keith et al., 1989). The approach has been to use standard hand reconstruction procedures, but to apply them to the severely paralyzed hand in new ways. The procedures that have been employed are joint arthrodeses and tendon transfers. Joint arthrodesis is used to stabilize a lax joint so that moments can be generated across the joint for application to the end of the digit. This has been particularly important in the interphalangeal joint of the thumb. Tendon transfers are used in three ways. First, muscles with an intact lower neuron but no central control can be transferred to substitute for a denervated muscle group. The transferred muscle can subsequently be programmed into the grasp template as would the original muscle. Second, the tendons of muscles that insert into multiple digits can be anastomosed together to create a single muscle unit that simultaneously moves all digits. This avoids asynchrony of finger movement. Third, tendons transfers can be performed to change the biomechanical linkage, thus changing the joint moments that are produced by the stimulated muscle. Surgical intervention also allows direct access to the muscle unit, and allows precise placement of the electrode to the desired site on or in the muscle or nerve, thus avoiding muscle recruitment limitations. These procedures have been performed with 5 individuals in the Cleveland program and 1 at the satellite site in Philadelphia.

The desirable patterns of hand grasp, namely palmar prehension and lateral prehension, cannot always be obtained by stimulation of the appropriate muscles in the normal grasp. Denervation of some muscles by lower motor neuron lesion at the cord or peripheral nerve level may cause loss of critical functions and is commonly found. Typically, the finger extensors on the C6 tetraplegic or the wrist extensors in the C5 patient are affected. Restoration of these movements can be accomplished by extensive bracing or transfer of paralyzed and electrically excitable muscles employing standard surgical principles and techniques. For example, to restore finger extension, extensor carpi ulnaris may be transferred, end to side, to the extensor digitorum communis. This muscle does not have the capability of substituting for the amplitude or power of the finger extensors, but within the restricted range in these patients, it functions well. It is important to condition the muscle to be transferred prior to surgery for example by using a percutaneous electrode, in order to be able to assess flexibility and strength of the muscle during surgery. Deconditioned muscle will be stiff and its full potential uncertain. The length-tension properties may also change after transfer and thus diminish the efficiency of its new function.

All patients undergoing procedures for restoration of paralyzed limbs must accept compromises due to the lack of motors for joint motion. Accomplishing the same functions of the intact hand requires that degrees of freedom and the complexity of grasp patterns in the hand be reduced. The stabilization of joints reduces the number of muscles required to position the joint and is indicated when static positioning will suffice such as at the interphalangeal joint of the thumb. We do not recommend arthrodesis of the wrist, as a wrist orthosis is often well tolerated by the C5 patient, and we anticipate that control of the wrist by FES will be achieved in the next generation of devices. Arthrodesis of the thumb carpometacarpal (CMC) joint is often performed in tetraplegics to preposition the thumb for adduction/opposition. With the FES system, CMC motion is required as both palmar and lateral pinch are possible. Carpometacarpal arthrodesis is therefore unnecessary in FES patients.

When a single motor must replace the muscles which move several fingers simultaneously, the technique of synchronizing the tendons may be used. By creating a cross-tenodesis between the tendons and sewing the tendon transfer into the new single tendon, coordination of finger movement is possible. We recommend a different position of the fingers than is usually used in patients with peripheral nerve injuries. We recognize that patients will often develop contracture of the fingers in finger flexion due to the predominant tone of these powerful muscles when paralyzed. Unless the fingers are balanced such that the fourth and fifth fingers are less tight or flexed than the index and long, the tendency is for objects to be excluded from the hand during palmar grasp. This same tendency was noted by Hentz et al. (1988), who recommended transfer of muscles to flexor digitorum profundus of the index and long fingers but then added the flexor digitorum sublimis of the ring and fifth fingers. Pronation is a most important motion for limb position, as gravity can assist the severely impaired high-level tetraplegic patient to extend the fingers by tenodesis. To achieve pronation, we have used rotational osteotomy of the radius so that the action of the biceps brachii causes supination from full pronation to about 90°, or normal forearm position. An alternative might be the Zancolli biceps transfer (Zancolli, 1979). At this early stage of performing surgical alterations in paralyzed muscles and using stimulation for activation, the issues for concern and the success appears similar to that in tendon transfers with normal, unparalyzed hands, with particular attention to avoid adhesions.

The implantable receiver-stimulator eliminates many of the issues associated with placing external surface electrodes or maintaining a percutaneous interface. Certain surgical considerations and precautions have been learned as a result of our animal and human experience. The implantable stimulator is placed in a subcutaneous pocket created on the chest wall. Mammograms should be obtained prior to insertion in female patients. The location is similar to that used for cardiac pacemakers. The pocket is fortuitously located in sensory skin in most C6 patients with portions of the device in C5 skin. This sensibility may be important in case of infection or device malfunction, as the case of the stimulator is the anode. Stimulation of the underlying pectoralis muscle has not been noted within normal stimulation current ranges. The stimulator is connected to a lead array by in-line connectors. The connectors physically separate the lead subsystem from the implant stimulator. We expect that the array will be stabile on the muscle surfaces, and if correctly mapped will not be replaced often. The stimulator may require upgrading with design evolution and thus should be easy to replace. The leads are positioned along the neutral axis of the arm to avoid kinking and maintain a large radius of curvature. The loads are thus minimized. Redundant lead length is coiled at the connector to accommodate shoulder motion. The leads at the electrode are positioned with some redundancy, again to accommodate to elbow motion. The leads are sewn in at maximum tension with the elbow extended and the shoulder abducted. Bending is less likely than tension or traction to result in lead dislocation. The connectors and helically coiled leads are designed to tolerate tension and bending. Incorporation of the coiled leads in a silastic tube induces a light filmy encapsulation response in the subcutaneous tissue. Many forces act on the implant system in addition to the movements of the limbs. The respiratory movements, gravity, and application of external forces to the body during transfers, all may shorten the life expectancy of an implant. The overall survival rates for this device are unknown, but will surely depend on the incidence of infection, trauma, and biocompatibility in each subject. The epimysial electrodes are implanted on the muscle surface by sewing them in place over an optimum motor point. The motor point for FES applications may be different than that noted from surface stimulation. The gain (change in recruitment force per unit of current applied) and the threshold for muscle-force recruitment relative to the total current available are important parameters to optimize. Since the nerve fiber branches within a muscle are not visible from the external surface, their location can only be estimated by stimulation of the muscle surface with a trial electrode of the same surface area and current range. Improper placement of the electrode too close to the nerve branches results in a muscle that reaches full force too quickly in the control-command range and thus acts in an on/off fashion, which is hard to control. An electrode placed too far from the nerve fiber branches produces too weak a muscle response. Care must be taken that adjacent muscles are not recruited simultaneously by current spillover, as the resulting pattern may not be functional. For example, the extensor indicis proprius (EIP) is adjacent to the extensor pollicis longus (EPL) deep in the extensor musculature of the forearm. While the EPL is essential to a well-controlled hand grasp pattern, recruitment of EIP is counterproductive in the same motion. Use of a selective epimysial electrode or surgical release or transfer of the EIP may be needed if the pattern persists.

SENSORY FEEDBACK

The use of substitutional cues to provide the user of the motor prosthesis is critical to their performance with the system. The substitution can provide information of the control state (e.g., on/off, lock, grasp type) or of the input or output state. The former requires less difficult recognition, since codes are short lived, whereas the latter requires a recognition of the proportional state (e.g., how hard am I grasping?). Van Doren and Riso (1991) recently completed a review of the state of sensory feedback, which is beyond the scope of this chapter.

The Case Western Reserve University and the VA Medical Center (CWRU/VA) implanted system provides both state information and simple proportional information by electrocutaneous feedback. The epimysial electrode is used to stimulate skin afferents without exciting underlying muscle on the shoulder or chest wall by taking advantage of its asymmetrical current spread. Care must be taken not to incorporate or damage the skin sensory branches when sewing the electrode in place on the muscle fascia. Applying the electrode to the underlying moveable muscle mass is undesirable and also may cause changing sensory patterns which may be confusing to the patient. The logical commands are provided by either low- (4 Hz) or high- (40 Hz) stimulus bursts, and the magnitude of the proportional input at 20% command intervals is represented by increasing frequencies selected to be separated by at least two just noticeable differences of discrimination.

We have implanted both the intramuscular and the epimysial electrodes in research subjects for sensory feedback. The perception is that of a tapping or buzz depending on the frequency and burst length. At high current amplitude, pain may be produced. Our experience with subcutaneous stimulation has demonstrated satisfactory information transfer regarding the state of the stimulator such as on/off, grasp pattern selected, or command level. We feel this type of private sensory cues is more desirable than audible beeps and less subject to misinterpretation or accommodation than skin surface electrical or mechanical stimulation. Various paradigms, including amplitude or frequency modulation or burst encoding, have been investigated (Riso et al., 1991). A single-electrode sensory feedback system as currently configured is a compromise, because only limited information can be transferred with this simple hardware. Using a subcutaneous array is more desirable in that it provides much more information and will be incorporated into subsequent generations of stimulators.

COMMAND CONTROL OF THE MOTOR PROSTHESIS

The command interface to the motor prosthesis must provide the user with simple and complete control of their hand without interfering with their ongoing activities. The sites for command control necessarily decrease as the lesion level occurs more rostral in the cord. For the existing motor prosthesis, the command task requires that the user generate both a proportional signal for grading the strength of the grasp, and logic signals to change the state of the control function. The states that are controlled are on/off, lateral/palmar grasp, and active control/hold. The latter allows the user to override the proportional command to maintain a fixed level of command. Studies have been performed to determine the resolution of the proportional command signal. To match the resolution of the stimulus gradation, eight bits are required. To achieve dexterous manipulation, approximately 45 discrete command levels are estimated to be required (Johnson and Peckham, 1990). It may be expected that as the capacity for finer function is achieved, the requirement will increase for more precise command sources.

The sources for command control information that have been used include switches and potentiometers controlled by the opposite hand, myoelectric activity, voice control, shoulder control, and wrist position. Switches have been used to gate the command signal to increase or decrease (Mortimer and Peckham, 1973). This simple command source is basically limited by a compromise between the rate of command change and the precision in the command. Potentiometers controlled by the opposite hand provide a precise control signal. However, both the potentiometer and switches are generally undesirable because they occupy the hand which is often needed to assist in performing functional tasks, and the hand generally lacks sensation that allows the user to be certain of their command action. Furthermore, both require mounting on a stable and accessible surface, such as a wheelchair, which limits the use of the system to those sites. Myoelectric activity has been used as a switch to gate the command on and off. It has the advantage of obtaining the signal from a site which is not involved in the grasping task and allowing the "switch" to be mounted on the body (Peckham, 1980b), but has inherent limitations in the resolution of command if used as a proportional source (Vodovnik and Rebersek, 1970). Voice control has been used to control the hand, with the user providing commands to grasp and release (Handa et al., 1985). This signal source has the disadvantage that it causes attention to be drawn to the user, which may be unacceptable.

The most widely investigated signal source is the shoulder opposite to the active hand (Johnson et al., 1990). This command source provides generation of both proportional and logic signals by movement of the shoulder in one or two axes. A ball-and-socket mechanical arrangement is used with a Hall-effect sensor placed in the socket used for transduction with a magnet placed in a ball; a switch mounted near the transducer is used for on/off. The entire transducer/switch apparatus is mounted on the sternum, with a telescoping rod attached to the ball extending to the shoulder. Figure 8-4 shows subjects of the CWRU/VA program using the shoulder controller. A similar mechanism has been used at the wrist to provide command information for patients who have retained wrist extension. Wrist extension is used to generate grasp; wrist flexion for release.

CLINICAL APPLICATIONS OF FNS FOR HAND FUNCTION IN SPINAL CORD INJURY

The first application of FNS for hand control was by Long and Masciarelli (1963) in Cleveland. Surface electrodes were used to activate the finger extensors; grasp was provided by a spring on an external orthosis, which positioned the thumb and directed the fingers. Work on this orthosis was subsequently abandoned because of the physiological problems described earlier (muscle atrophy, fatigue). Efforts in Cleveland subsequently focused upon the use of chronically indwelling percutaneous electrodes for nerve stimulation (Caldwell and Reswick, 1975). Work progressed from using an external orthosis to position the wrist and thumb for palmar prehension (Mortimer and Peckham, 1973) to providing lateral prehension (Peckham et al., 1980a) and palmar prehension (Peckham et al., 1980b) with little or no orthotic support. Patients who have used this system report significant benefit from it use. They are able to perform tasks that cannot otherwise be accomplished, and often wear the system on a daily basis. Wijman et al. (1990) reported the results of a follow-up of 22 patients in the Cleveland study who were evaluated for their ability to perform various tasks of daily living with and without the motor prosthesis. The success rate of the patients in performing the activities was 89% with the motor prosthesis, but only 49% without. All patients could perform more activities with the system than without, and in only two tasks with one patient was the function less with the motor prosthesis. Stroh et al. (1991), in comparing performance with and without the motor prosthesis, showed that performance is clearly improved in 31 of 48 conditions and partially in 8 additional cases in evaluation carried out under strict testing conditions. The complete assessment of the functional outcome awaits

MOTOR PROSTHESES FOR RESTORATION OF UPPER EXTREMITY FUNCTION 177

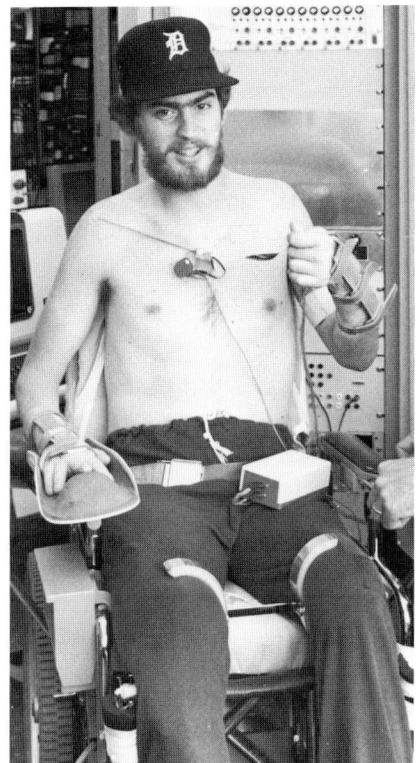

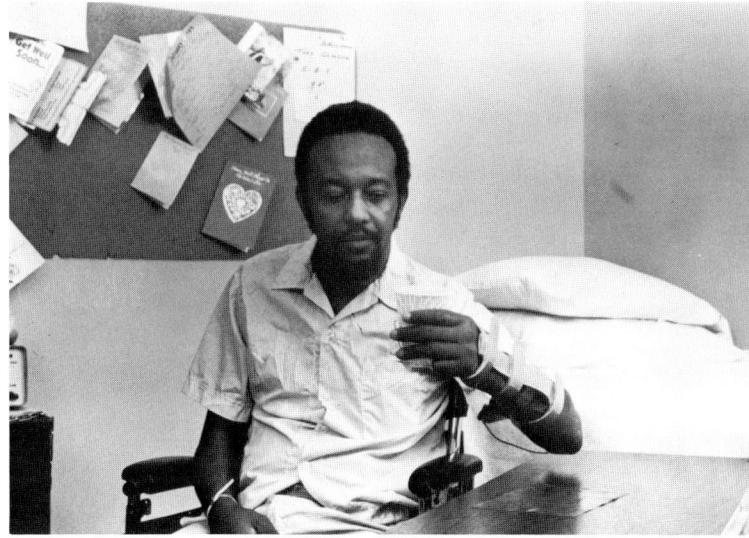

Figure 8–4 Subjects of the CWRU/VA program demonstrating functional use of the motor prosthesis with (A) apparatus uncovered, and (B) as normally worn. The external controller, described in Buckett et al. (1988) is shown on the leg of the subject in (A), but is generally mounted behind or under the wheelchair.

the completion of a multicenter study described below. Nevertheless, this result demonstrates that significant improvement can be achieved in SCI patients with FNS.

Handa and Hoshimiya and colleagues in Japan have independently developed and implemented a similar system (Handa et al., 1985; Hoshimiya et al., 1989). They have proceeded to develop innovative techniques for control, system programming, and new functional implementations, as well as electrode technology. Researchers in Poland used implanted stimulators activating the median and radial nerves to achieve grasp, with an orthosis used to stabilize the wrist, thumb, and fingers (Kiwerski et al., 1979; Weiss et al., 1981; Kiwerski and Pasniczek, 1984). Investigators led by Brindley, Donaldson, and Rushton at the MRC Neuroprosthesis Unit in London, have one patient implemented with an implanted receiver-stimulator (Brindley et al., 1989). Girbirdt (1981) reported the use of surface stimulation of finger flexor muscles for grasp.

CONTROL OF PROXIMAL JOINTS OF THE UPPER EXTREMITY IN SCI

Effort has been directed toward the control of the elbow extension in patients with C5-level injury and shoulder and elbow, as well as the hand, in patients with C4-level injury. In patients with C5 injury, the objective is to provide overhead movement using elbow extension as an active antagonist to the intact volitional control of elbow flexion (Miller and Peckham, 1989). This is achieved by stimulation of the lateral and medial heads of triceps. Control of the elbow position is determined by voluntary elbow flexion acting in opposition to the triceps. The position of the upper arm and elbow are detected by sensors on the arm. Stimulation of triceps is sufficient to cause full elbow extension; voluntary elbow flexion will enable the user to obtain a midrange elbow position. Thus, no additional command-control generation is required by the user to effect control of the elbow. This has been implemented in a laboratory, but not in a portable system in conjunction with a hand grasp system.

Control of the shoulder, elbow, and hand has been investigated in patients with C4 spinal cord injury by Nathan (1989) and Naito (1987). Each of these systems uses an ancillary orthotic support (balanced forearm orthosis) of the upper arm, since the patient presents with paresis of the shoulder girdle and upper arm muscles, as well as paralysis of the forearm and hand muscles. The extent of denervation of the muscles that are required for upper arm control has not been reported, but Nathan reported decreased force generation of wrist extensors and elbow flexors and extensors. Based upon the information presented above, it is our expectation that considerable denervation can be expected in all muscles innervated by the C5 root and some in those innervated by the C6 root in the C4 patient. To overcome this problem, Betz recently reported transfer of lattismus dorsi to biceps and electrical stimulation to provide powered elbow flexion (personnel communication). Both Nathan and Naito reported clinical success, with patients able to perform certain activities of daily living with the system.

APPLICATIONS TO THE UPPER EXTREMITY IN OTHER CNS INJURIES

Clinical applications of FNS have been introduced by Vodovnik and Rebersek (1970, 1975) to provide hand opening in individuals who have sustained cerebral vascular accidents (e.g., stroke). Surface electrodes applied to the extensor compartment of the forearm were used to excite the finger and thumb extensors to enable the patient to more easily release the flexion posture in the hand. Control of the stimulation was through the shoulder; a suspender over the shoulder pulled a linear potentiometer as the shoulder was elevated. No long-term follow-up reports are available on the efficacy or acceptance of the device.

Merletti et al. (1975) used a two- or three-channel device stimulating wrist and elbow extensors and deltoid with surface electrodes. Movement of the unaffected shoulder in two axes controlled stimulation. Five of eight patients showed improved function with the orthosis and three of the five gained a therapeutic effect. The study indicated that improved engineering for implanted stimulators and clinical training were needed. Although not implemented as a motor prosthesis, Baker et al. (1979) also noted an increase in voluntary range of motion and prevention of contractures in hemiplegic patients who were provided a program of cyclical electrical stimulation in the subacute and chronic phases.

Patients with brain injury, stroke, or brainstem injury have a different sensory nervous system than the spinal cord-injured patient. Our clinical experience has been that these patients have greater sensitivity to an improper perception of sensory-afferent electrical current and have more pain associated with electrical stimulation of muscle. The SCI patient has a more predictable sensory dermatome distribution of preserved afferents and less of the ill-defined pain. The reasons for this observation are unknown but predictable from our experience. The surgical implications are that until new methods are developed which minimize this effect, electrodes must be placed with the patient sedated but awake to avoid painful locations. In general, electrodes should be kept away from the skin surface, and intramuscular locations are preferred. We have not had sufficient experience with epimysial electrodes to determine if they will shield the skin afferents.

CLINICAL SYSTEMS FOR FUNCTIONAL USE AND TECHNOLOGY TRANSFER

Several laboratories have reported on development of systems for restoration of the upper extremity control in SCI. A inquiry was made of these investigators in January 1991, to determine the number of systems that have been implemented, the number presently being studied, and the number in regular use outside of the research laboratory, either in an extended care facility, at home, or at work, and the longest time in use outside of the laboratory. The results of this survey are given in Table 8-3.

The results of this admittedly incomplete survey suggest that a small but significant number of patients are benefitting from the regular use of FNS research systems. Studies are underway at nine centers and 21 patients are using systems on a regular basis. Our laboratory in Cleveland at Case Western Reserve University and the VA Medical Center has implemented patient-portable systems in 28 patients. All but one of these are implemented with percutaneous electrodes; the longest having been implanted for nearly 12 years. The one system which is implemented with an implanted receiver-stimulator has been in use for nearly 5 years. We have also led the

Table 8–3 Results of Survey of Investigators Performing Clinical Studies of FNS Systems

	Total Pts. Studied	No. Pts. Presently Studied	No. Pts. with Portable System	Longest at Home (months)	System Type		
					Surface	Percutaneous	Implanted
Cleveland, OH	30	5	5	155	—	4	1
London, England	1	1	1	47	—	—	1
Sendai, Japan	12	3	3	60	—	12	—
Beer Sheva, Israel	12	2	5	5	—	—	—
Cleveland Satellite Centers							
Edmonton, Alberta, Canada	3	2	2	41	—	1	—
Toronto, Ontario, Canada	2	1	1	34	—	1	—
Philadelphia, PA	6	5	5	19	—	5	
Los Angeles, CA	1	1	1	10	—	1	

clinical studies to transfer the technology to four other centers in North America, where another eight systems using percutaneous electrodes are being studied.

The system developed in Japan by Handa and Hoshimiya and colleagues is used by three patients presently in study. Brindley, Donaldson, and Rushton at the MRC Neuroprothesis Unit in London, have one patient implemented with an implanted receiver-stimulator for 47 months and in daily usage. Nathan, at Ben Gurion University in Beer Sheva, Israel, has two subjects using a surface stimulation system for control of the entire upper limb. These are considerable accomplishments, given the complexity of the systems and the absence of commercial sponsorship in supporting the technology.

The Cleveland team has been leading a study in which hand-assist systems are being implemented and tested at collaborating satellite institutions. The purpose of the study is to identify the deficiencies of the system employing percutaneous electrodes, and to test the readiness of the system for testing in more extensive clinical trials. The study is being performed in cooperation with the University of Alberta, Edmonton; Rancho Los Amigos and the Rancho Rehabilitation Engineering Center in Downey, CA; Shriners Hospital of Philadelphia; and the University of Toronto and Hugh MacMillan Center, Toronto. Several aspects are critical in order to accomplish the study and are expected to be important aspects of undertaking trials of neural prostheses for any application. These aspects are selection of centers, standardization of protocols, development and support of technology, and follow-up evaluation. The selection of clinical teams is critical to the success of the study. The teams must be of a multidisciplinary nature and consist of a therapist, medical direction and support by a physician with the active involvement of a hand surgeon, and a rehabilitation engineer. The therapist is primarily responsible for the training and evaluation of the patient; the physician is primarily responsible for selection of subjects, the medical/surgical aspects involving implantation, and long-term clinical support; the rehabilitation engineer is responsible for the technical details involving system support, and programming and troubleshooting. The teams must have an adequate commitment to the project of time and resources to fulfill support for the patients during the course of the study. Since the user who accepts the system well will come to rely on the system and therefore expect it to be functional on a daily basis and for an extended period (perhaps his lifetime) with minimal problems, this commitment to the patient is not to be underestimated.

The technology to be utilized must be at a stable stage of development, must have adequate documentation, and must be available in sufficient numbers. The technology must include not only the patient device, but also cables, controls, and peripheral devices used to program and test the units. These must be available in adequate numbers to account for replacement in the event of failure such that the patient's needs can be adequately served. Furthermore, detailed documentation on use and maintenance of the system is required. Our study has used the hardware and software fabricated entirely in our research laboratories in Cleveland, since the production of the commercially fabricated portable units has taken longer than projected. Research investigators should not underestimate the intensity required in this aspect of a project.

Each aspect of the program must be precisely documented. This involves patient selection, implementation, training, evaluation, and technical manuals on all aspects of the clinical devices. As inventors or developers of the technology, there are many small but critical steps that can be overlooked in all aspects of the program. It is critical to identify the essential aspect of "know how" that must be provided in written form and communicated to the collaborators. Detailed training on the proper implementation and use of the system is necessary. This will entail intensive training which is well planned and executed. As in any educational process, there must be ongoing follow-up once the centers start to apply the concepts to provide support and clarify ambiguities.

Follow-up with the collaborators is an ongoing and essential aspect of a technology transfer program. Follow-up enables the lead center to maintain contact on the status of each patient in the program or under consideration for participation. Follow-up also provides the opportunity to reveal deficiencies and assemble the individuals, often from several centers, to address problems at an early stage. Finally, follow-up is essential to ensure that information that is required to assess the utility of the neural prosthesis is forthcoming at regular intervals and without ambiguity.

Multicenter clinical trials are an essential step and critical element for moving neural prostheses from the clinical laboratory into clinical utilization. They require considerable planning and resources to ensure that the outcome will provide sufficient information to justify the further dissemination of the technology. Commitment from all participants, the researchers and clinicians, industry, and federal sources, is essential to ensure that the technology can be delivered to the consumer expeditiously.

COMBINED TECHNIQUES FOR RESTORING UPPER EXTREMITY FUNCTION

Functional neuromuscular stimulation is one of several techniques to be considered for restoring upper extremity control. While this chapter has focused on FNS, the use of orthotics and reconstructive surgery are the conventional procedures that are widely practiced clinically. Depending upon the specific individual, FNS provides a means of improving upon the function provided by these approaches or may be considered as an alternative to them. In many cases, the treatment of an individual may include all of these techniques. For example, an individual with C5-level SCI may be expected at present to use an orthosis to stabilize the wrist and may benefit from tendon transfers or joint arthrodeses to provide more uniform movement of the digits and force transmission in grasp. If brachioradialis has sufficient strength, it may also be considered for transfer. These scenarios must be developed for each individual candidate, since each presents a slightly different picture of voluntary muscle control, joint mobility, innervation, spasticity, and sensation. Thus the clinician can consider FNS as a technique which provides new additional "motors" to augment force and range of movement. The utilization of this technique, in conjunction with the existing conventional procedures, thus gives the clinician a new tool that has not been available previously. Its successful implementation in the rehabilitation of any single individual remains the challenge to the clinical team.

FUTURE DIRECTIONS OF UPPER EXTREMITY DEVELOPMENT

Advancements in upper extremity motor prostheses will focus on enhancements that will improve the function, user acceptance, and ease of implementation. While the quality of hand function allows for considerable utility, there are many opportunities to advance the performance of the upper extremity. The quality of movement can be improved by increasing the number of muscles that can be excited and the selectivity and repeatability of neural excitation. This will most likely entail advances in the technology of stimulation electrodes and stimulus delivery techniques, and utilization of closed-loop control of movements. Several examples of new nerve electrodes which provide selective excitation have been studied (Agnew and McCreey, 1990). Microinjectable stimulators may be used to reduce the surgical intervention required in the implementation of an FNS system (see Chapter 15). Control of additional degrees of freedom may also be expected to improve user performance and acceptance. Most current users of hand systems have limitations in their voluntary control of elbow extension, forearm pronation, and the wrist. Incorporation of control of these movements into the motor prosthesis will restore a wider work space and extend functional capabilities of the user. The challenge will be to deliver these advances in a form that does not require complexity which is too great to be clinically implementable and acceptable.

The sensors that are required to implement these systems must be easily used, and perhaps implanted, to be acceptable to the user. Access to the natural sensors through a neural interface could reduce the dependence upon artificial sensors (see Chapter 5). Advances will also come by providing the user with substitutional sensory feedback, which compensates for the absent or abnormal feeling in the hand. While relatively rudimentary sensory feedback has been provided to date, the quality of performance may be expected to increase as these techniques are introduced into the clinical system (Szeto and Riso, 1990; Van Doren and Riso, 1991).

Advances will also come through the introduction of command-control techniques which are more easily generated and are more integrated with the movement that the user is attempting to perform. Examples are to use the position of the arm in space to control elbow extension (Miller et al., 1989) and to use the voluntarily active wrist musculature to control stimulation. Eventually, the utilization of CNS control signals may be achieved, which could relieve the necessity of obtaining control through the less natural sites, as presently employed. Until these techniques evolve through the research process, more conventional control using joint position or myoelectric signals are expected to be the principle means of eliciting command signals. Enhancements will be developed by improving the efficiency of generating commands, for example, to provide a fluid means of changing the command state. Acceptance by the user is expected to be enhanced further by developing hardware for transduction of the command signal that can be fully implanted and only requires the placement of a single antenna over the implanted source to activate the system. Systems which have this capability are presently under development and may be expected to reach clinical testing within the next several years.

ACKNOWLEDGMENTS

The authors are indebted to many individuals on the faculty and staff of Case Western Reserve University, the Cleveland Veterans Affairs Medical Center, and MetroHealth Medical Center for their active participation which has made this work possible. They include Jim Buckett,

Pat Crago, Marti Gazdik, Peter Gorman, Ron Hart, Tony Ignagni, Mark Johnson, Kevin Kilgore, Tom Mortimer, Greg Naples, Brian Smith, Tom Stage, Kathy Stroh, Geoff Thrope, Clayton Van Doren, and Leon Woods. The authors acknowledge the support of the NIH Neural Prosthesis Program (Contract No. N01-NS-9-2356), the National Institute on Disability and Rehabilitation Research (Grant No. H133E80020), The Department of Veterans Affairs Rehabilitative R & D Program, and the Paralyzed Veterans of America Spinal Cord Research Foundation, for assistance in the research in Cleveland.

REFERENCES

Agnew, W.F., and McCreery, D.B. (1990). In: *Neural Prostheses: Fundamental Studies.* Englewood Cliffs, NJ: Prentice Hall.

Baker, L.L., Yeh, Ch. Wilson, D., and Waters, R.L. (1979). Electrical stimulation of wrist and fingers for hemiplegic patients. *Phys. Ther.*, **59**(12), 1495.

Bigland-Ritchie, B. (1981). EMG and fatigue of human voluntary and stimulated contractions. In: R. Porter and J. Whelan, eds., *Human Muscle Fatigue: Physiological Mechanisms*, pp. 111–156. London: Pitman Medical.

Bigland-Ritchie, B., Jones, D.A., and Woods, J.J. (1979). Excitation frequency and muscle fatigue: Electrical responses during human voluntary and stimulated contractions. *Exp. Neurol.*, **64**, 414–427.

Branstatter, M.E., and Dinsdale, S.M. (1976). Electrophysiologic studies in the assessment of spinal cord lesions. *Arch. Phys. Med. Rehab.*, **57**, 70.

Brindley, G.S., Donaldson, N., Perkins, T.A., Polkey, C.E., and Rushton, D.N. (1989). Two-stage keygrip by joystick from an 11-channel upper limb FES implant in C6 tetraplegia. *Proc. Biol. Eng. Soc.*, 41.

Brindley, G.S., Polkey, C.E., and Rushton, D.N. (1982). Sacral anterior root stimulators for bladder control in paraplegia. *Paraplegia*, **20**, 365–381.

Buckett, J.R., Peckham, P.H., Thrope, G.B., Braswell, S.D., and Keith, M.W. (1988). A flexible, portable functional neuromuscular stimulation neuroprosthetic system. *IEEE Trans. Biomed. Eng.*, **35**(11), 897–904.

Caldwell, C.W., and Reswick, J.B. (1975). A percutaneous wire electrode for chronic research use. *IEEE Trans. Biomed. Eng.*, **5**, 429–432.

Crago, P.E., Mortimer, J.T., and Peckham, P.H. (1980b). Closed-loop control of force during electrical stimulation of muscle. *IEEE Trans. Biomed. Eng.*, **27**(6), 306.

Crago, P.E., Peckham, P.H., and Thrope, G.B. (1980a). Modulation of muscle force by recruitment during intramuscular stimulation. *IEEE Trans. Biomed. Eng.*, **27**(12).

Crochetiere, W.J., Vodovnik, L., and Reswick, J.B. (1967). Electrical stimulation of skeletal muscle—a study of muscle as an actuator. *Med. Biol. Eng.*, **5**, 111–125.

Ferguson, A.S., Stone, H.E., Roessman, U., Burke, M., Tisdale, E., and Mortimer, J.T. (1989). Muscle plasticity: Comparison of the effects of a 30 Hz burst paradigm with 10 Hz continuous stimulation. *J. Appl. Physiol.*, **33**(3), 1143–1151.

Fukamachi, H., Handa, Y., Naito, A., Ichie, M., Yajima, M., Ushikoshi, K., Tuchiya, M., Matsushita, N., and Hoshimiya, N. (1987). Improvement of finger movement by intrinsic muscles stimulation of the hand. *9th IEEE EMBS Proc.*, 361–362.

Girbirdt, R. (1981). Restoration of the grasp movement of a tetraplegic with the help of functional electrical stimulation. *Proc. VII International Congress of Biomechanics*, pp. 301–306. University Park Press. Baltimore: University Press.

Gorman, P.H., and Peckham, P.H. (1990). Upper extremity functional neuromuscular stimulation. *J. Neurol. Rehab.*, in press.

Grimby, G., Broberg, C., Krotkiewska, I., and Krowieska, M. (1976). Muscle fiber composition in patients with traumatic cord lesions. *Scand. J. Rehab. Med.*, **8**, 37–42.

Handa, Y., Handa, T., Nakatsuchi, Y., Yagi, R., and Hoshimiya, M. (1985). A voice controlled functional electrical stimulation system for the paralyzed hand. *Jpn. J. Med. Electron. Biol. Eng.*, **23**, 292–298.

Handa, Y., Hoshimiya, N., Iguchi, Y., and Oda, T. (1989). Development of percutaneous intramuscular electrode for multichannel FES system. *IEEE Trans. Biomed. Eng.*, **36**(7), 705–710.

Hentz, V.R., Hamlin, C., and Keoshian, L.A. (1988). Surgical reconstruction in tetraplegia. *Hand Clin.*, **4**, 601–607.

Hoshimiya, N., Naito, A., Yajima, M., and Handa, Y. (1989). A multichannel FES system for the restoration of motor functions in high spinal cord injury. *IEEE Trans. Biomed. Eng.*, **36**(7), 754–760.

House, J.H., and Shannon, M.A. (1985). Restoration of strong grasp and lateral pinch in tetraplegia: A comparison of two methods of thumb control in each patient. *J. Hand Surg.*, **10**, 22–29.

Ignagni, A.R., Buckett, J.R., and Peckham, P.H. (1990). A programming and data retrieval system for an upper extremity FES neuroprosthesis. *12th Annual IEEE Conference*, Philadelphia, PA.

Johnson, M.W., and Peckham, P.H. (1990). Evaluation of shoulder movement as a command control source. *IEEE Trans. Biomed. Eng.*, **37**(9), 876–885.

Keith, M.W., Peckham, P.H., Thrope, G.B., Stroh, K.C., Smith, B., Buckett, J.R., Kilgore, K.L., and Jatich, J.W. (1989). Implantable functional neuromuscular stimulation in the tetraplegic hand. *J. Hand Surg.*, **14A**(3), 524–530.

Keller, A.D., Taylor, C.L., and Zahm, V. (1947). Studies to determine the functional requirements for hand and arm prosthesis. *Final Rep. Nat. Acad. Sci. Contract No. VAm-21223*.

Kilgore, K., Peckham, P.H., and Keith, M.W. (1990). Electrode characterization for functional application to upper extremity FNS. *IEEE Trans. Biomed. Eng.*, **37**(1), 12–21.

Kilgore, K.L., Peckham, P.H., Thrope, G.B., and Keith, M.W. (1989). Synthesis of hand movement using functional neuromuscular stimulation. *IEEE Trans. Biomed. Eng.*, **36**(7), 761–770.

Kiwerski, J., and Pasniczek, R. (1984). An apparatus making possible restoration of simple functions of the tetraplegic hand. *Paraplegia*, **22**, 316–319.

Kiwerski, J., Weiss, M., and Pasniczek, R. (1979). Electrostimulation of the median nerve in tetraplegics by means of implanted stimulators. *Int. J. Rehab. Res.*, **2**(1), 41–46.

Klopsteg, P.E., and Wilson, P.D. (1954). In: *Human Limbs and Their Substitutes*, New York: McGraw Hill Co. Inc.

Kugelberg, E., and Edstrom, L. (1968). Differential histochemical effects of muscle contractions on phosphorylase and glycogen in various types of fibers: Relation to fatigue. *J. Neurol. Neurosurg. Psychiat.*, **31**, 415–423.

Lieber, R.L. (1986). Skeletal muscle adaptability II: Muscle properties following spinal cord injury. *Dev. Med. Child Neurol.*, **28**, 533–542.

Long, C., and Masciarelli, V. (1963). An electrophysiologic splint for the hand. *Arch. Phys. Med.*, **44**, 499–499.

McDowell, C.L., Moberg, E.A., and Smith, A.G. (1979). Proceedings of the international conference on surgical rehabilitation of the upper limb in tetraplegia. *J. Hand Surg.*, **4**, 387.

McNeal, D. (1973). Peripheral nerve stimulation—superficial and implanted. In: W.S. Fields and L.A. Leavitt, eds., *Neural Organization and Its Relevance to Prosthetics*, pp. 77–99. New York: Intercontinental Medical Book Corp.

Merletti, R., Acimovic, R., Grobelnik, S., and Cvilak, G. (1975). Electrophysiological orthosis for the upper extremity in hemiplegia: Feasibility study. *Arch. Phys. Med. Rehabil.*, **56**, 507–513.

Miller, L.J., Peckham, P.H., and Keith, M.W. (1989). Elbow extension in the C5 quadriplegic using functional neuromuscular stimulation. *IEEE Trans. Biomed. Eng.*, **37**(7), 771–780.

Moberg, E. (1975). Surgical treatment for absent single-hand grip and elbow extension in quadriplegia. *J. Bone Joint Surg.* **57-A**, 196–206.

Moberg, E. (1978). The upper limb in tetraplegia. Stuttgart: George Thieme.

Mortimer, J.T. (1981). Motor prosthesis. In: V.B. Brooks, ed., *Handbook of Physiology, Section I: The Nervous System, Vol. 2, Part I, Chap. 5*, pp. 155–187. Bethesda, MD: American Physiological Society.

Mortimer, J.T., and Peckham, P.H. (1973). Intramuscular electrical stimulation. In: W.S. Fields and L.A. Leavitt, eds., *Neural Organization and Its Relevance to Prosthetics*, New York: Intercontinental Medical Book Corp.

Naito, A., Handa, Y., Ichie, M., Handa, T., Matsushita, N., Yajima, M., Fukamachi, H., Ushikoshi, K., Tsuchiya, M., and Hoshimiya, N. (1987). EMG analysis of elbow movements and its application to FNS. *9th IEEE Proc. EMBS*, 46–47.

Nathan, R.H. (1984a). The development of a computerized upper limb electrical stimulation system. Orthopedics, **7**(7), 1170–1180.

Nathan, R.H. (1984b). Functional electrical stimulation of the upper limb: Charting the forearm surface. *Med. Biol. Eng. Comput.*, **17**, 316–319.

Nathan, R.H. (1989). Generation of functional arm movements in C4 quadriplegics by neuromuscular stimulation. In: F.C. Rose, R. Jones, and G. Vrbova, eds., *Neuromuscular Stimulation: Basic Concepts & Clinical Implications*, pp. 273–284. New York: Demos Publications.

Peckham, P.H., Marsolais, E.B., and Mortimer, J.T. (1980a). Restoration of key grip and release in the C6 quadriplegic through functional electrical stimulation. *J. Hand Surg.*, **5**(5), 462–469.

Peckham, P.H., Mortimer, P.H., and Marsolais, E.B. (1980b). Controlled prehension and release in the C5 quadriplegic elicited by functional electrical stimulation of the paralyzed forearm musculature. *Ann. Biomed. Eng.*, **8**, 369–388.

Peckham, P.H., Mortimer, J.T., and Marsolais, E.B. (1976a). Alteration in the force and fatigability of skeletal muscle in quadriplegic humans following exercise induced by chronic electrical stimulation. *Clin. Orthop.*, **114**, 326.

Peckham, P.H., Mortimer, J.T., and Marsolais, E.B. (1976b). Upper and lower motor neuron lesions in the upper extremity muscles of tetraplegics. *Paraplegia*, **14**, 115.

Peckham, P.H., Mortimer, J.T., and Van Der Meulen, J.P. (1973). Reversal of fiber types in cat skeletal muscle following chronic electrical stimulation. *Brain Res.*, **50**, 424–429.

Pette, D., ed. (1980). *Plasticity of Muscle*, Berlin: de Gruyter.

Rebersek, S., and Vodovnik, L. (1973). Proportionally controlled functional electrical stimulation of hand. *Arch. Phys. Med. Rehabil.*, **54**, 378–382.

Riso, R.R., Ignagni, A.R., and Keith, M.W. (1991). Cognitive feedback for use with FES upper extremity neuroprostheses. *IEEE Trans. Biomed. Eng.*, **38**, 29–38.

Rohmert, W. (1960). Ermittlung von erholunspausen fur statische arbeit der menschen. *Int. Z. Agnew. Physiol.*, **18**, 123–164.

Rudel, D., Bajd, T., Kralj, A., and Benko, H. (1982). Surface functional electrical stimulation of the hand in quadriplegics. *Proc. 5th Ann. Conf. Rehab. Eng.*, Houston TX.

Smith, B., Peckham, P.H., Roscoe, D.D., and Keith, M.V. (1987). An externally powered, multichannel implantable stimulator for versatile control of paralyzed muscle. *IEEE Trans. Biomed. Eng.*, **34**(7), 499–508.

Stauffer, E.S. (1975). Diagnosis and prognosis of acute cervical spinal cord injury. *Clin. Orthop.*, **112**, 9.

Stover, S.L., Fine, P.R., Go, B.K., Lazarus, P.B., Devito, M.J., and Vaughan, D.R. (1986). *Spinal Cord Injury: The Facts and Figures*. Birmingham: University of Alabama.

Stroh, K.C., Van Doren, C.L., and Thrope, G.B. (1991). Quantitative assessment of quadriplegic patients using a hand neuroprosthesis. Submitted for publication.

Szeto, A., and Riso, R. (1990). Sensory feedback using electrical stimulation of the tactile sense. In: R.V. Smith, and J.H. Leslie, eds., *Rehabilitation Engineering*, pp. 29–78. CRC Press.

Van Doren, C.L., and Riso, R.R. (1991). Synthetic sensory feedback for motor prostheses. *J. Neurol. Rehabil.*, In press.

Vodovnik, L., and Rebersek, S. (1970). Myoelectrical and myomechanical prehension systems using functional electrical stimulation. In: P. Herberts, R. Kadefors, R. Magnussen, and I. Petersen, eds., *The Control of Upper Extremity Prostheses and Orthoses*, pp. 151–165. Charles C. Thomas.

Wijman, C.A., Stroh, K.C., Van Doren, C.L., Thrope, G.B., Peckham, P.H., and Keith, M.W. (1990). Functional evaluation of quadriplegic patients using a hand neuroprosthesis. *Arch. Phys. Med. Rehabil.*, **71**, 1053–1057.

Weiss, M., Kiwerski, J., Pasniczek, R., and Morecki, A. (1981). An electronic hybrid device for the control of hand functions by electrical stimulation methods. *Proc. VII International Congress of Biomechanics*. Baltimore: University Park Press, 397–404.

Vrbova, G., Gordon, T., and Jones, R. (1978). In: *Nerve-Muscle Interaction*. London: Chapman and Hall.

Zancolli, E.A. (1975). Surgery for the quadriplegic hand with active strong wrist extension. *Clin. Orthop.*, **112**, 101–113.

Zancolli, E.A. (1979). *Functional Restoration of the Upper Limb in Traumatic Quadriplegia*. Philadelphia: J.B. Lippincott.

III
Control of Lower Extremities

9

Simple Models of the Mechanics of Walking

R. McNEILL ALEXANDER

A concise, quantitative description of normal human gait that takes account of differences of leg length and of speed is made possible by the dynamic similarity hypothesis, which is explained. A series of simple mathematical models help to explain why we walk as we do. A model with rigid, massless legs shows that centrifugal effects set an upper limit to walking speed, and explains why walking (unlike rolling on wheels) requires positive and negative work even in the absence of friction. The synthetic wheel model shows how the inertia of the legs may also set a limit to walking speed if they are allowed to swing forward passively. Another model shows that walking gaits may have inherent stability, independent of nervous control. Finally, a model that specifies force patterns shows that walking and running may be interpreted as solutions to an optimization problem, with a bifurcation explaining the gait transition. A discussion suggests how the data and ideas presented in this chapter may help us to understand the limitations of muscle-stimulation–powered orthoses, and to suggest improvements.

The aims of this chapter are to show that normal human gait can be described very concisely by a method which takes account of differences of leg length and speed; and that simple mathematical models can help us to understand the basic principles of walking and the energy costs involved. A discussion at the end attempts to relate the data and ideas presented in the chapter to the design and evaluation of orthoses.

DESCRIPTION OF WALKING

Qualitative Descriptions

Walking is easily described in qualitative terms. It is our usual gait, but is used only at relatively low speeds; we run to go faster. Each foot is on the ground for more than half the duration of the stride so there are times when both are on the ground simultaneously. Each knee remains almost straight while its foot is on the ground. All these characteristics distinguish walking from running.

Quantitative description is complicated by the different sizes of different people. Children, from the age of about 5 years, walk much like adults, but take shorter strides at higher frequency to maintain the same speed (Grieve and Gear, 1966; Cavagna et al., 1983). They run at speeds at which adults would still be walking. However, quantitative descriptions of gait that apply to people of all sizes can be made by a method that uses the concept of dynamic similarity, which was first used in a study of dinosaurs (Alexander, 1976). This approach, which is described below, is also very convenient when actual gaits are to be compared with the predictions of the models presented in later sections.

Dynamic Similarity

Two shapes are geometrically similar if one is a scale model of the other, and so could be made identical with it by a uniform change in the scale of length. A related but less familiar concept concerns movement rather than shape: two motions are dynamically similar if they could be made identical by uniform changes in the scales of length, time, and force (e.g., two pendulums of different lengths swinging through the same angle). When gravitational forces are important (as they are in walking and in the swinging of pendulums), dynamic similarity is possible only if the motions being compared have equal Froude numbers v^2/gl: here v and l are a speed and a length characteristic of the motion and g is the gravitational acceleration.

The dynamic similarity hypothesis of walking and running (Alexander, 1976; Alexander and Jayes, 1983) predicts that similar animals or people of different sizes will move in approximately dynamically similar fashion when traveling with equal Froude numbers v^2/gl. In this context, v is defined as the mean velocity over a complete stride and l as the length of the leg (from ground to hip joint) in normal standing.

The dynamic similarity hypothesis predicts that different people will change from walking to running at the same Froude number. This prediction does not seem to have been tested by comparison between children and adults, but Alexander and Jayes (1983) found that quadrupedal mammals ranging from cats to rhinoceros all changed from walking to running at Froude numbers near 0.5. Adult humans make the change at about 2.5 m/s, at a Froude number of about 0.7 (Alexander and Maloiy, 1984).

Stride length is the distance between corresponding points on successive footprints of the same foot. In dynamically similar gaits (which are possible only at equal Froude numbers) stride length, λ, would be the same multiple of leg length, l. Thus the dynamic similarity hypothesis predicts that relative stride length λ/l will be the same function of Froude number for people of all sizes. This is found to be approximately true over the range from 4-year-old children to adults (Alexander, 1984). The relationship is quite well described by the equation

$$\lambda/l = 2.2 \, (v^2/gl)^{0.2} \qquad (1)$$

(from the data of Alexander and Maloiy, 1984, Figure 2). Thus stride length increases from about 1.4 l at a Froude number of 0.1 to 2.0 l at a Froude number of 0.7.

The duty factor β is the fraction of the duration of the stride for which each foot is on the ground. It is approximately the same function of Froude number for a wide range of mammals. Alexander and Jayes (1980) obtained the following equation for humans

$$\beta = 0.67 - 0.13 \, (v^2/gl) \qquad (2)$$

Thus, duty factor falls from about 0.66 at a Froude number of 0.1 to 0.58 at a Froude number of 0.7. It falls abruptly to about 0.35 when running starts (Alexander, 1989).

The patterns of vertical and horizontal force that the feet exert on the ground change predictably with speed. The most marked change in human walking is in the vertical component, from force records with a fairly flat plateau at speeds below 1 m/s to a markedly two-humped pattern above 2 m/s (Figure 9–1). Alexander and Jayes (1980) showed that the shapes of the force records could be described by the segment between $\omega t = -\pi/2$ and $\omega t = +\pi/2$ of the Fourier series.

$$F(t) = a_1 \cos \omega t + b_2 \sin 2\omega t + a_3 \cos 3 \omega t \ldots \qquad (3)$$

The first few terms of the series were sufficient to describe the records quite closely. They published equations relating ratios of the Fourier coefficients to Froude number, for example

$$a_3/a_1 = 0.26 - 0.69 \, (v^2/gl) \qquad (4)$$

Thus a_3/a_1 changes from -0.3 at a Froude number of 0.1 to -0.7 at a Froude number of 0.7. It rises abruptly to about $+0.1$ at the onset of running.

MODELS OF WALKING

This section shows how simple mathematical models can help us to understand the mechanics of walking.

Rigid, Massless Legs

Figure 9–2A shows the simplest model of walking that has been analyzed (Alexander, 1977). The legs have negligible mass and constant length, and remain straight while their feet are on the ground. Each foot is set down as the other is lifted, giving an unrealistically low duty factor of 0.5. The hip joint and the center of mass of the body move along a series of circular arcs of radius equal to leg length l so they rise and fall in the course of a step by $l(1 - \cos \theta)$, where θ is the angle of the legs to the vertical at the instant of changing the foot on the ground. An average walking

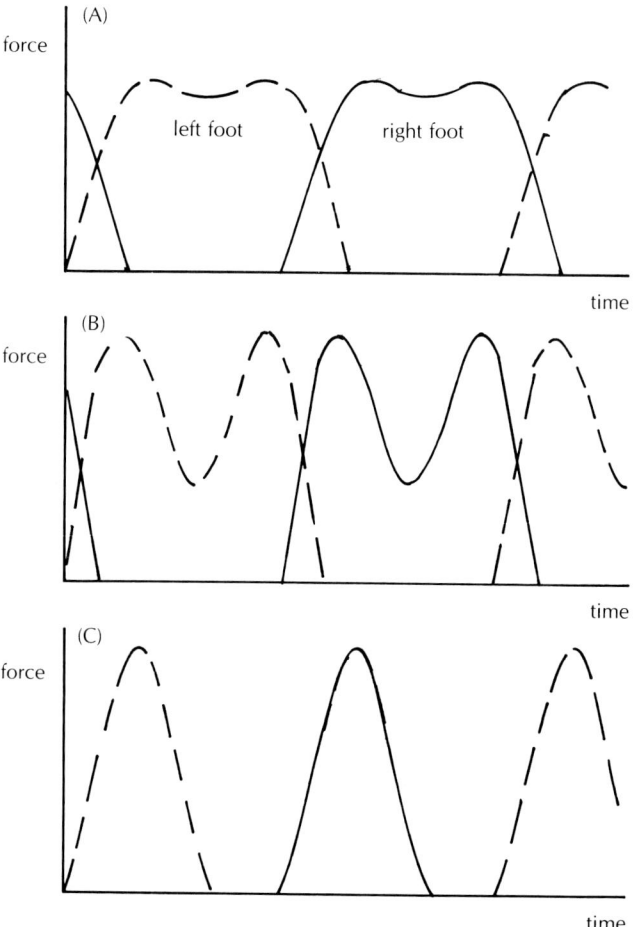

Figure 9–1 Schematic graphs of the vertical component of force exerted on the ground in walking and running. (A) Represents a slow walk; (B), a fast walk; and (C) a run. These graphs have been drawn with realistic values of the duty factor and the parameter a_3/a_1 [equation (3)], but the finer details of actual force records have not been imitated. (see Alexander and Jayes, 1980). Parameter values are: (A), duty factor = 0.65, $a_3/a_1 = -0.20$; (B), duty factor = 0.60, $a_3/a_1 = -0.55$; (C), duty factor = 0.35, $a_3/a_1 = +0.10$.

stride length of $1.7\ l$ implies $\theta = 25°$, giving a vertical excursion of almost $0.1\ l$, or 9 cm for a typical adult. Observed fluctuations of the height of the center of mass are considerably less (as indicated by the energy changes reported by Cavagna et al., 1983), largely because of the heel-and-toe action which the model does not represent.

While the body's center of mass is traveling a circular arc of radius l, at speed v, it has an acceleration towards the center of the circle equal to v^2/l. (If it did not have this acceleration it would fly off at a tangent.) The only force available to cause this acceleration is the body's weight, so it cannot be greater than g

$$v^2/l \leq g$$
$$v^2/gl \leq 1 \tag{5}$$

SIMPLE MODELS OF THE MECHANICS OF WALKING

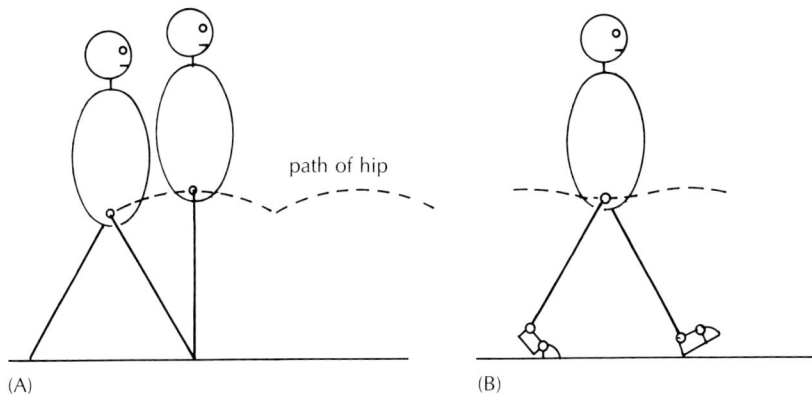

Figure 9–2 (A) A model of walking on legs that remain straight and rigid while the foot is on the ground. (B) A diagram showing how a foot with ankle and metatarsophalangeal joints can be used to eliminate the infinite accelerations in the gait of model (A).

Thus the model cannot walk with a Froude number greater than 1, which is consistent with the observation that people change to running at a Froude number of about 0.7. Higher Froude numbers are attained in the racing walk, but only by means of hip movements, which increase the radius of curvature of the path of the center of mass, reducing the vertical accelerations that are required (Cairns et al., 1986).

Force plate records show that the forces exerted on the ground in walking act fairly nearly in line with the hip (data of Alexander and Jayes, 1980). Assume that they act precisely in line with the hip of the model, whose rigid legs remain constant in length. In that case no work is done as the body moves along each circular arc, though the speed falls as the body rises, and rises as the body falls: energy is exchanged between the kinetic and potential forms. As the legs reach angles Θ with the vertical, just before the foot on the ground is changed, the body's velocity is v_θ and has a vertical component $-v_\theta \sin \Theta$. Slightly later, immediately after the change of foot, the body's vertical component of velocity is $+v_\theta \sin \Theta$. This change of velocity requires a vertical impulse supplied by forces on the feet. The foot being set down can be expected to make an inelastic impact with the ground, dissipating mechanical energy, while the foot being lifted does work as it pushes off. The body loses and regains kinetic energy $\frac{1}{2} m v_\theta^2 \sin^2 \theta$ which must be dissipated and then replaced by work. This happens after each step, in which the body of weight mg travels a distance $2\,l \sin \Theta$. Thus the positive and negative work required to move unit weight of body unit distance (the cost of transport C) is

$$C = (\sin \Theta/4)\,(v_\theta^2/gl)$$

Stride length λ is $4\,l \sin \Theta$, so this can also be written

$$C = (\lambda/16\,l)\,(v_\theta^2/gl) \qquad (6)$$

One might argue about this conclusion. A different argument in which the impact of the foot landing on the ground preceded the impulse of the other foot pushing off [as in McGeer's (1990) "rimless wheel" analysis] would have made the kinetic energy loss $\frac{1}{2} m v_\theta^2 \sin^2 2\Theta$ and given a correspondingly higher cost of transport. However, this would not alter the conclusion from equation (6). This suggests that to minimize the energy cost of walking we should take very short strides (small λ) at high frequency, which is false. Zarrugh et al. (1974) showed that oxygen consumption at any given speed of walking increases if stride frequency is made too high. The stride frequency that walkers prefer to use at a given speed is the one that minimizes oxygen consumption. The reason for the model's false prediction is that it ignores the mass of the legs: no energy is needed to make massless, frictionless legs swing backward and forward at high frequency (see Cavagna and Franzetti, 1986).

If relative stride length is proportional to (Froude number)$^{0.2}$, as it is found to be [equation (1)], equation (6) predicts that cost of transport will be proportional to (Froude number)$^{1.2}$ or (speed)$^{2.4}$. Measurements of oxygen consumption show metabolic cost of transport increasing with speed, but not in proportion to so high a power of speed. Zarrugh et al. (1974) report a quadratic relationship between rate of oxygen consumption and speed, which implies that the net cost of transport is directly proportional to speed.

The velocity used in the Froude number in equation (6) is not the mean horizontal velocity, but the peak velocity that is attained just before the foot on the ground is changed. Alexander (1977) presented a more elaborate analysis of the same model that obtained cost of transport as a function of mean velocity.

One of the unrealistic features of this model is that it requires an infinite acceleration (and so infinite force) at the instant when the foot on the ground is changed. To avoid this, the path of the center of mass must be smoothed, eliminating the cusps. This requires the legs to lengthen for part of each step, which is impossible for the simple legs shown in Figure 9–2A if the knee is already straight. It is made possible by the ankle and metatarsophalangeal joints, which are used in the heel-and-toe style of human walking (Figure 9–2B): they also make it possible for the trunk to move forward while the knees are straight and both feet are on the ground. The heel-and-toe technique is peculiar to humans, who are also peculiar in keeping the knees straight while their feet are on the ground. Chimpanzees walk on bent knees and do not use the heel-and-toe technique (Jenkins, 1972).

The Synthetic Wheel

The previous model took account of the vertical movements of the center of mass in walking, and ignored the mass of the legs. This model, presented by McGeer (1990), does the converse.

In it, each leg is represented by part of a wheel: the hub, one spoke, and a segment of rim (Figure 9–3A). The two hubs are mounted on a single axle which allows the legs to swing independently. The legs have mass that is small, however, compared to the mass of the trunk, so the trunk advances with constant velocity, unaffected by the fluctuating momentum of the swinging legs. While the left wheel-foot is on the ground it rolls, carrying the trunk forward. Meanwhile the right leg swings freely like a pendulum, having been raised slightly to enable it to clear the ground. At the instant when the point of contact with the ground reaches the "toe" of the rolling left foot, the "heel" of the swinging right foot lands on the ground and the right foot starts rolling while the left one is raised.

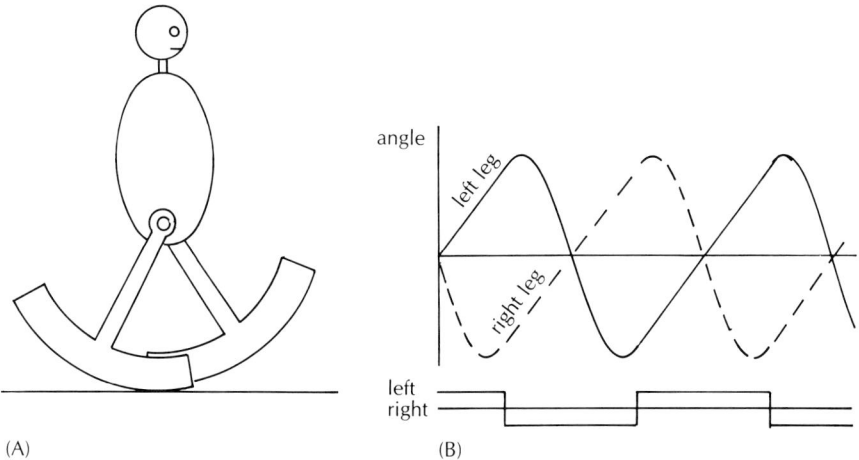

Figure 9–3 (A) The synthetic wheel model of McGeer (1990). (B) Graphs of leg angle against time for the same model. Bars below the graph show when each foot is on the ground.

Figure 9–3B is a graph of leg angles against time. During each half cycle, one leg has its foot on the ground and is rolling with constant angular velocity while the other is swinging sinusoidally as a pendulum. At the instant when the foot on the ground is changed, each leg has the appropriate angle and angular velocity for the start of the next step. McGeer (1990) shows that this implies that the duration of a complete stride is 1.29 times the period of the leg swinging as a pendulum, which for a real person would be about $5\sqrt{l/g}$ [calculated from data in Grieve and Gear (1966), assuming leg length is 0.52 times stature]. Stride duration is stride length divided by speed, λ/v. Thus

$$\lambda/v = 6.5\sqrt{l/g}$$

$$\lambda/l = 6.5\,(v^2/gl)^{0.5} \qquad (7)$$

Comparison with the observed relationship between relative stride length and Froude number [equation (1)] shows that equation (7) predicts unrealistically long strides: 2.1 l at a Froude number of 0.1 (observed stride length 1.4 l) and 5.4 l at a Froude number of 0.7 (observed 2.0 l). The latter is far beyond the bounds of possibility: even a gymnast who performed the splits in every step could not exceed a walking stride length of 4 l. This model would be incapable of fast human speeds.

The legs of the synthetic wheel swing forward passively so no energy is needed to drive them. The matching of angular velocities (Figure 9–3B) ensures that the feet are set down smoothly with no energy-dissipating impact. The trunk travels with constant potential and kinetic energy. Friction and aerodynamic drag are ignored. Once the model has been set moving on a horizontal surface it will continue indefinitely with no fresh energy input, which is, of course, unrealistic.

Despite these faults, the model is valuable in showing how legs can swing forward passively and how the time required for the swing may affect gait. Very little electrical activity can be recorded from the muscles of the leg while it is swinging forward (Basmajian and DeLuca, 1985), which indicates that the swing is largely passive.

Models with Heavy Legs

McGeer (1990) presented another model of walking with small feet, unlike the very large feet of the synthetic wheel. In this model, he allowed the legs to be a substantial fraction of body mass. The body rises and falls in each step, as in the model of Figure 9–2, and the legs swing as pendulums like those of the synthetic wheel. He built a physical model of this kind that walks downhill without any motor. (A gradient is needed, because energy is lost at each impact of a foot with the ground). The equations of motion could not be solved analytically, so the mathematical version of the model had to be investigated by numerical integration over a series of walking strides. The most interesting conclusion was that the walk was stable. For any particular gradient (above the minimum needed for walking) there was a corresponding speed and stride length into which the model settled after a few strides. If it were jostled while walking it would withstand quite substantial impulses without being knocked over and would return (over the next few strides) to the original speed and stride length.

This model, like the synthetic wheel, walks with a near-constant stride period: it travels faster down steeper slopes by taking longer strides at the same frequency. The period is shorter than for the synthetic wheel, especially if the mass of the trunk is small: most of the simulations presented by McGeer (1990) show periods between $5\sqrt{l/g}$ and $6\sqrt{l/g}$, compared to $6.5\sqrt{l/g}$ for the synthetic wheel. These periods are still unrealistically long for human walking.

A later model by McGeer (1990) has knees. It too is capable of stable passive walking down a slope, but only if the feet are asymmetrical, projecting more in front of the lower leg than behind. Human feet, or course, do just that.

Mochon and McMahon (1980) had previously presented a model of walking with knees. They allowed the angles and angular velocities of the hip and knee to be set (presumably by muscles) just before the foot left the ground, but thereafter the leg swung forward passively. The initial conditions were chosen so that the knee became straight as the foot landed on the ground again. The time taken for the forward swing might be anything from 0.55 to 0.85 of the half-period of the straight leg, swinging as a pendulum. Swing times shorter than this could not be obtained by using higher initial angular velocities, because the toe would then fail to clear the ground. Longer ones would involve unrealistic bending of the knee, to angles greater than 125°. It is difficult to compare the results from this model with those from the others because the simulations cover only the part of the stride when one foot was off the ground and ignore the part when both were grounded, but the range of calculated swing times agree well with ranges observed for children and adults by Grieve and Gear (1966).

Force Patterns

The last model to be considered differs from the others in specifying the patterns of force that the feet exert, rather than the form of the legs (Alexander, 1980). In the bipedal version of the model the body was treated as a point mass. The force pattern was used to calculate its velocity fluctuations throughout the stride. At a time when its horizontal and vertical components of velocity were dx/dt, dy/dt, a leg exerting components of force F_x, F_y on the ground was doing work at a rate $F_x.dx/dt + F_y.dy/dt$. Equal positive and negative work was done over a complete stride (because frictional losses were ignored), but they were summed separately. Different force patterns were tried, to find the one that minimized total positive work.

Two variables were used to specify the vertical component of force: the duty factor, and the ratio a_3/a_1 [equation (3)] which can describe force-time graphs of a range of shapes with either one or two peaks (Figure 9–1). The horizontal component of force was then defined by keeping the resultant force aligned with a point in the trunk, above the hip. The combination of duty factor and a_3/a_1 that minimized work was found, for each of a range of Froude numbers.

For Froude numbers corresponding to walking speeds, the predicted optima closely resembled observed gaits: their duty factors were high, and a_3/a_1 became increasingly negative as Froude number increased. At high Froude numbers, the model predicted that the duty factor should be as small as possible and a_3/a_1 positive, as in running (Figure 9–1). The optimum moved suddenly from a walking to a running gait at a bifurcation which, however, occurred at a higher Froude number than the one at which people make the change. This bifurcation could have been shifted to a lower, more realistic Froude number by incorporating elastic elements in the model that would have stored strain energy as the force on a foot increased, and returned it in a subsequent recoil. The Achilles tendon and the ligaments of the arch of the foot play such a role in running, greatly reducing the positive and negative work that the muscles have to do (Ker et al., 1987).

This model was notably successful in predicting the patterns of force that the feet should exert on the ground, but we must nevertheless question its assumption that work should be minimized. The metabolic energy consumption of muscles is a function not only of the rate at which they are doing work, but also of the force that they are exerting (Heglund and Cavagna, 1987). We do not yet know enough to assess the relative importance of the costs of performing work and of exerting force (to do that we will need more information about the physiological properties of muscles and the rates at which they contract in locomotion), but it is possible to argue fairly convincingly that the cost of force may be dominant (see Alexander, 1989). This view has been greatly strengthened by a paper by Kram and Taylor (1990), which explains the scaling of metabolic costs of running with body size in mammals, solely in terms of the costs of exerting force. The walking gaits used by humans require little work, but they also require smaller forces in muscles than if we walked on bent legs: the straightness of our legs keeps the moments acting about leg joints small. It is possible that minimization of muscle force has been more important than minimization of work in the evolution of our gait.

DISCUSSION

The frequent remarks in this chapter, that this or that feature of a model is unrealistic, may seem disheartening, but these simple models are nevertheless very important to our understanding of walking. Also, they may help us to evaluate orthoses and to understand their limitations.

The models tend to support the suggestion that the movements of normal walking are adapted to minimize energy costs. For this reason, an early stage in the evaluation of an orthosis might be to compare the gaits performed in it to normal human gait. How do stride length, duty factor, and force patterns compare to those observed *at the same Froude number* in normal walking? Orthoses that allowed near-normal gaits would probably be more economical of metabolic energy than existing orthoses, as well as being cosmetically preferable.

Muscles have to do work and metabolic energy is used whenever kinetic energy is lost and has to be replaced. In normal walking, most of the body's kinetic energy is carried forward from one step to the next, and metabolic energy costs are low. The model illustrated in Figure 9–2A indicated that the kinetic energy lost at each footfall need be no more than $\frac{1}{2} m v_\theta^2 \sin^2 \theta$ (or $\frac{1}{2} m v_\theta^2 \sin^2 2\theta$, depending on the assumptions made). In slow walking, θ would be 20° or even less, and these kinetic energies would be much less than the total kinetic energy of the body, $\frac{1}{2} m v_\theta^2$. If a patient using an orthosis stops between each step and the next, the metabolic energy cost of walking will be abnormally high. This helps to explain why walking with a long leg brace is more expensive of energy than normal walking, but fails to explain the even higher energy costs measured by Marsolais and Edwards (1988) for walking with functional neural stimulation: they report that with FNS "it was possible to make the gait more dynamically continuous without stopping and starting with each stride."

The model shown in Figure 9–3 emphasizes that the economy of walking depends on allowing the legs to swing forward more or less passively: more metabolic energy may be needed when muscles are stimulated to make the leg swing forward.

Finally, McGeer's (1990) conclusion that bipedal walking is not inherently unstable seems to raise the hope of developing orthoses that will enable paraplegics to walk without the need for support from a walking frame.

REFERENCES

Alexander, R.McN. (1976). Estimates of speeds of dinosaurs. *Nature*, **261**, 129–130.

Alexander, R.McN. (1977). Mechanics and scaling of terrestrial locomotion. In: T.J. Pedley, ed., *Scale Effects in Animal Locomotion*, pp. 93–110. London: Academic Press.

Alexander, R.McN. (1980). Optimum walking techniques for quadrupeds and bipeds. *J. Zool.*, **192**, 97–117.

Alexander, R.McN. (1984). Stride length and speed for adults, children, and fossil hominids. *Am. J. Phys. Anthropol.*, **63**, 23–27.

Alexander, R.McN. (1989). Optimization and gaits in the locomotion of vertebrates. *Physiol. Rev.*, **69**, 1199–1227.

Alexander, R.McN., and Jayes, A.S. (1980). Fourier analysis of forces exerted in walking and running. *J. Biomech.*, **13**, 383–390.

Alexander, R.McN., and Jayes, A.S. (1983). A dynamic similarity hypothesis for the gaits of quadrupedal mammals. *J. Zool.*, **201**, 135–152.

Alexander, R.McN., and Maloiy, G.M.O. (1984). Stride lengths and stride frequencies of primates. *J. Zool.*, **202**, 577–582.

Basmajian, J.V., and DeLuca, C.J. (1985). In: *Muscles Alive*, 5th ed. Baltimore: Williams & Wilkins.

Cairns, M.A., Burdett, R.G., Pisciotta, J.C., and Simon, S.R. (1986). A biomechanical analysis of racewalking gait. *Med. Sci. Sports Exerc.*, **18**, 446–453.

Cavagna, G.A., and Franzetti, P. (1986). The determinants of the step frequency in walking in humans. *J. Physiol.*, **373**, 235–242.

Cavagna, G.A., Franzetti, P., and Fuchimoto, T. (1983). The mechanics of walking in children. *J. Physiol.*, **343**, 323–339.

Grieve, D.W., and Gear, R.J. (1966). The relationships between length of stride, step frequency, time of swing and speed of walking for children and adults. *Ergonomics*, **5**, 379–399.

Heglund, N.C., and Cavagna, G.A. (1987). Mechanical work, oxygen consumption and efficiency in isolated frog and rat striated muscle. *Am. J. Physiol.*, **253**, C22–C29.

Jenkins, F.A. (1972). Chimpanzee bipedalism: Cineradiographic analysis and implications for the evolution of gait. *Science*, **178**, 877–879.

Ker, R.F., Bennett, M.B., Bibby, S.R., Kester, R.C., and Alexander, R.McN. (1987). The spring in the arch of the human foot. *Nature*, **325**, 147–149.

Kram, R., and Taylor, C.R. (1990). Energetics of running: A new perspective. *Nature*, **346**, 265–267.

Marsolais, E.B., and Edwards, B.G. (1988). Energy costs of walking and standing with functional neuromuscular stimulation and long leg braces. *Arch. Phys. Med. Rehabil.*, **69**, 243–249.

McGeer, T. (1990). Passive dynamic walking. *Int. J. Robotics Res.*, **9**, 62–82.

Mochon, S., and McMahon, T.A. (1980). Ballistic walking: An improved model. *Math. Biosci.*, **52**, 241–260.

Zarrugh, M.Y., Todd, F.N., and Ralston, H.J. (1974). Optimization of energy expenditure during level walking. *Eur. J. Appl. Physiol.*, **33**, 293–306.

10

Biomechanics and Physiology of a Practical Functional Neuromuscular Stimulation Powered Walking Orthosis for Paraplegics

MOSHE SOLOMONOW

The elementary biomechanical and physiological processes necessary for simple locomotion are determined and used to derive the design specifications for a FES powered mechanical orthosis which can allow thoracic paraplegics simple, efficient and practical means of locomotion. The mechanical orthosis—the LSU Reciprocating Gait Orthosis (RGO)—was utilized to provide anti-gravity support and standing balance while surface electrical stimulation of the hip flexor and extensor muscles provided the necessary power for simultaneously executed swing phase and contralateral push-off. The efficiency of the FES powered RGO was assessed from a group of paraplegics with injury levels ranging from T-1 to T-10. It was shown that such a hybrid orthosis allows paraplegics to ambulate with greater efficiency than that observed in patients using only FES or only mechanical orthosis. Additional discussion recounts some practical aspects associated with the use of this orthosis including training requirements, patient selection criteria, cost, reliability and function.

Spinal cord injury (SCI) patients classified as paraplegics are confined to a wheelchair for prolonged periods of time, and use it as their sole way of transportation. Prolonged sitting, however, results in compounded medical, physiological, social, and psychological problems, which severely compromise the patient's health and quality of life. Pressure sores, deteriorating bone density in the legs (and exposure to fractures), bowel and bladder stagnation, and increased incidences of urinary tract infection, deteriorating cardiopulmonary and circulatory conditions, and spasticity and joint contractures are the most common problems in wheelchair-bound paraplegics. Spasticity, in particular, is a most debilitating problem, since it requires muscle relaxants for suppression. Muscle relaxants also cause general depression of the patient, reduced ambition and ability to negotiate with the challenges of daily living such as employment, family relationships, personal needs, self-image, environmental barriers, and so on. The patient is left drowsy in the wheelchair, enhancing the development of pressure sores, stagnant bladder, and deteriorating cardiopulmonary and circulatory conditions, which ultimately result in his detachment from society. The overall quality of life of such individuals is clearly substandard, with very little hope for improvement, and the burden to family members and society is simultaneously increased.

Providing SCI patients with some practical means to walk independently, therefore, satisfies the most elementary requirement (locomotion), as well as the overall rehabilitation objectives if one considers the secondary, but very important, effects of walking on the medical problems described above. At present, there is no *practical* orthosis or method which allows paraplegics to stand-up and walk independently for periods of time considered as functional or useful in daily routines, or even as an exercise modality.

Routine attempts to provide paraplegics with limited walking functions consist of fitting them with long leg braces (LLB) or its various versions. This is a rigid knee-ankle-foot orthosis, (KAFO) which requires significant amounts of metabolic energy consumption to elicit ambulation. Reports of long-term evaluation (Chantraine et al., 1984; Rosman and Spira, 1974) point out that this orthosis is abandoned by most patients, with only a few using it for exercise purposes.

In the 1970s, work was initiated in Ljubljana, Yugoslavia for developing an electrical stimulation system to elicit locomotion in paraplegics (Kralj et al., 1983; Kralj and Bajd, 1989). The system used the flexion reflex as the activator to induce simultaneous hip and knee flexion for the swing phase of gait, yet did not gain wide acceptance by patients or rehabilitation personnel. Review reports (Dimitrijevic and Nathan, 1970, 1971) have shown that the flexion reflex is highly unpredictable. It changes in responsiveness not only from day to day, but often within the same day. The reflex gradually weakens over 15 to 20 repetitions due to accommodation, and requires alternating the electrode location (Dimitrijevic and Nathan, 1971; Nicol et al., 1989; Lee and Johnston, 1976; Popovic et al., 1989), which severely limits the practicality of the system. We have tested a large number of patients within the first 6 weeks postinjury at the LSU Medical Center and have found that more than 75% did not exhibit a flexion reflex. Of the remaining 25%, half had it in one leg, but not in the other. The patients who had it in both legs demonstrated accommodation after 6 to 15 repetitions. We therefore did not consider the flexion reflex as either a practical or reliable approach to provide useful and safe locomotion as a standard, general rehabilitation tool in paraplegia. The flexion reflex technique was adapted by Graupe et al. (1983), Popovic et al., (1989), and Andrews and Baxendale (1988) with modifications. This has not yet resulted in any practical application.

Recently, Marsolais (Marsolais and Edwards, 1988) has developed an electrical stimulation system for ambulation consisting of 14 to 52 implanted wire electrodes in various leg and spine muscles. Although locomotion was obtained, limitations prevent this system from acceptance at the present time. The most important limitation is the relatively fast onset of fatigue, which limits the duration of its use to several minutes. Second, recent comparative studies (Marsolais and Edwards, 1988) show that the energy cost of locomotion in that system exceeds that of the LLB at slow to moderate walking speeds. Hopefully, with additional long-term development the limitations may be overcome successfully.

In Oswestry, England, the ORLAU group has developed the hip guidance orthosis (HGO), also known as the ORLAU Parawalker (Rose, 1979). This is a hip, knee, ankle, foot orthosis with free hip joints. It allows locomotion to paraplegics, and a recent version is offered as a hybrid, incorporating electrical stimulation of the gluteal muscles for hip extension. An evaluation by the Oxford Biomechanics Unit in England (British Health Authority Report, 1989), the HGO and the Louisiana State University-reciprocating gait orthosis (LSU-RGO) were applied to a group of 19 paraplegics. After using each orthosis for 6 months, three out of every four patients selected the LSU-RGO as the orthosis of choice for home use.

The RGO was developed at LSU in the 1970s. The RGO was first applied to pediatric patients with severe musculoskeletal disabilities of the lower extremities which prevented them from walking independently (e.g., spina bifida, muscular dystrophy, sacral agenesis, osteogenesis imperfecta, and limited cases of cerebral palsy). In the late 1970s and through the 1980s, successful applications were made to SCI cases, mostly paraplegics, although some quadriplegics with residual upper extremity function benefited as well. Since 1983, it is estimated that 5000 RGO units were made and applied in the United States, Canada, Great Britain, The Netherlands, France, Israel, Australia, and South Africa.[1] At present, the RGO is fully covered by Medicare/Medicaid, private insurers, and by the health authorities of the various countries.

Although encouraged initially with the application of the RGO to SCI cases, it became apparent that several limitations exist, the major one being a still relatively high energy cost during ambulation when compared to the gait of healthy subjects or to wheelchair transportation. To reduce the energy cost to our patients, in 1983 we developed a simple but effective and practical electrical muscle stimulation unit to power the RGO during the walking cycle.

The following sections will describe the biomechanical and physiological foundation of the design of the functional neuromuscular stimulation (FES)-powered RGO with the objectives of providing SCI patients with a practical walking orthosis to be used independently.

BIOMECHANICS OF SIMPLE LOCOMOTION

Four distinct biomechanical factors are involved in the most simple human locomotion (Solomonow et al., 1985):

1. Upright posture.
2. Execution of the swing phase of one leg.
3. Execution of simultaneous push-off with the contralateral leg.
4. Maintaining balance and stability during upright posture and locomotion.

In humans, it is obvious that the prerequisite for walking is the assumption of the upright position. This posture should be fully supported by weight bearing on the lower extremities, and not by the arms. It is also important that during standing upright, balance and stability are available to maintain such posture for prolonged

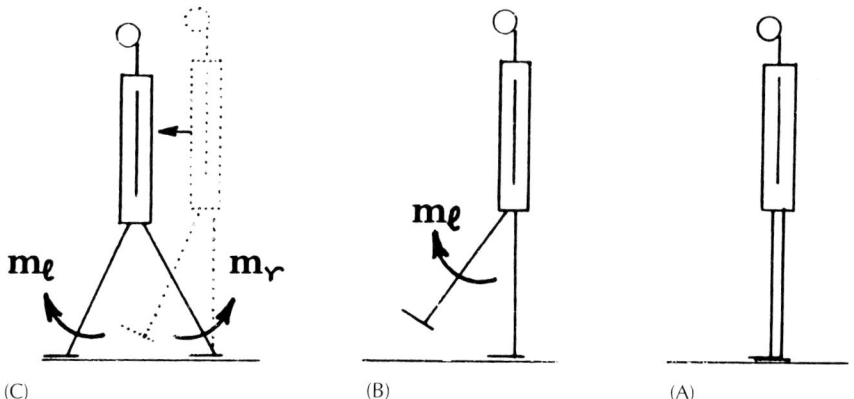

Figure 10–1 The simplest "stiff-knee" locomotion requires (A) upright posture, (B) hip flexion of one leg, and (C) simultaneous contralateral hip extension. Note that in order to create forward progression such as in (C), it is necessary to provide contralateral hip extension simultaneously with hip flexion.

periods of time at minimal metabolic energy cost which is, at least, near that measured in healthy persons.

The swing phase of one leg is a relatively complex function requiring activation of the hip, knee, and ankle in the flexion mode. For the most elementary swing phase, however, hip flexion is the minimal prerequisite for the "stiff-leg" walk (i.e., extended knee and rigid ankle). This type of stiff-leg locomotion, however, requires some lateral sway and elevation of the trunk so that the foot will clear the floor as the leg trajectory from the posterior (toe-off) to the anterior (heel-strike) positions take place.

Contralateral push-off function is accomplished by hip extension of that leg accompanied by knee extension and ankle plantar-flexion. Considering the elementary "stiff-knee" gait, only hip extension is required. Isolated swing of one leg without contralateral push-off, however, will result in zero forward progression (known as wheel spinning), underscoring the importance of hip extension. Figure 10–1 illustrates this concept graphically.

The issue of balance and its stability requires that the trunk's center of gravity is positioned within a prescribed region between the feet. The estimated region, as shown in Figure 10–2, allows certain amounts of anterior-posterior and lateral sway,

Figure 10–2 The projection of the body's center of gravity must lie within the area bounded by the two feet in order for the patient to maintain balance and stability.

while still preserving balance. Shifting the projection of the trunk's center of gravity across the boundaries of that region will upset the balance and may cause an ultimate fall if not corrected fast enough.

PHYSIOLOGY OF SIMPLE LOCOMOTION

Upright Posture

Physiologically, upright posture requires that muscles maintain extension of the hip and knee joints simultaneously with fixing the ankle in the neutral position (i.e., halfway between dorsiflexion and plantar flexion) so that antigravity support is provided to prevent the joints from flexing. At the hip, the muscles responsible for extension are primarily the gluteus, and secondarily, the hamstrings.

Knee extension is accomplished by the quadriceps, with the vasti muscles dedicating their full force for extension, while the rectus femoris, being a biarticular muscle, provides secondary hip flexion function in addition to knee extension.

Muscles crossing the ankle joint and capable of causing its motion are the triceps surae (soleus, medial and lateral gastrocnemius, and plantaris), the tibialis anterior and posterior, and the peroneous muscles.

Balance and subsequent stability during upright posture are also maintained by minor adjustments in the forces of the muscles crossing the lower extremity joints, and to a significant degree by adjusting the sway in the trunk's center of gravity so that it will stay between both legs in the lateral and anterior-posterior directions. The role of the spinal-abdominal muscles and upper limb muscles in providing this balance and stability is accomplished by swaying the trunk's weight into the stable position.

Locomotion

The swing phase of one leg, as mentioned in the previous section, is a complex function of the hip, knee, and ankle joints, not to mention the trunk. For hip flexion (considering stiff-leg gait), the primary muscles are the illiacus and psoas muscles, while the secondary flexor is the rectus femoris.

Contralateral hip extension is necessary to generate the push-off of the leg if we are using a simple stiff-leg gait. Hip extension is generated by the gluteus as the primary muscle, with the hamstrings serving in a secondary role.

BIOMECHANICAL AND PHYSIOLOGICAL ANALYSIS IN THE DESIGN OF A PRACTICAL WALKING ORTHOSIS

With an understanding of the biomechanical factors and their physiological correlates involved in simple locomotion, it is now possible to analyze the options available in the design of a walking orthosis for paraplegics.

Preferably, one would like to use a stimulation system that will simulate, as close as possible, the lost motor control of the various muscle groups. This approach, however, has at present significant limitations. First, we do not know how to efficiently stimulate muscles without imposing undue fatigue on the muscles. Fast-setting fatigue renders such an approach functionally impractical. Second, many muscles are biarticular, crossing two joints. In order to direct their force to act on the desired joint, it is necessary to coactivate the antagonist muscle of the other joint to create zero net torque. At present, our knowledge of the coactivation patterns of antagonist muscles is largely incomplete or unknown, with some data becoming available only recently (Solomonow et al., 1986, 1988; Baratta et al., 1988; Hagood et al., 1990). Therefore, trial-and-error stimulation of antagonist coactivation results in large amounts of unnecessary metabolic energy consumption due to the many activated muscles, requiring additional research to solve this problem.

An attractive alternative is to use a sophisticated mechanical orthosis to provide antigravity control to the leg muscles for the upright posture and balance functions. With a properly designed orthosis, the SCI patient may remain standing for prolonged periods of time at minimal or no metabolic energy cost, since the leg muscles are not stimulated, while the joints are held in an appropriate position by the rigid frame of the brace.

The combination of the LSU-RGO with FES is very appropriate for such an approach, because the FES can be used to initiate the swing phase and contralateral push-off (i.e., brief phasic activities) at minimal energy cost.

It is necessary, however, to determine what muscles to stimulate in order to achieve the swing phase simultaneously with contralateral push-off.

As mentioned previously, hip flexion is primarily accomplished by the illiopsoas muscles. These muscles are, however, deep and not accessible by surface electrical stimulation, since they originate in the spine or illiac crest and cross the floor of the abdomen to terminate on the proximal femur underneath many superficial muscles (Solomonow et al., 1985). In fact, even the use of implantable nerve cuff electrodes is difficult, since the nerve supply to this muscle emerges from the lower spinal roots and immediately terminates in the muscle's motor point with many branches. The nerve to this muscle, therefore, is short and requires a separate electrode for each branch. In addition, implantation of electrodes requires surgery, and most SCI patients are reluctant to have any additional surgical intervention.

Marsolais et al., (1988) and Prochazka, (Stein et al., 1990) have developed a technique by which a percutaneous wire could be inserted into close proximity to the nerves supplying the illiopsoas, and thereby circumventing the need for surgical implantation of electrodes. Marsolais' experience shows that electrode movement and breakage are major problems in attaining functionally stable hip flexion. They also pointed out that optimal placement and unwanted stimulation are additional problems associated with this approach. Surface stimulation at this stage is therefore the preferred approach.

The logical alternative is to stimulate the rectus femoris as the sole hip flexor. It is superficial and easily accessible by surface stimulation. It is also a large muscle which can generate sufficient force to bring a stiff leg into the hip flexion position. The fact that this muscle also crosses the knee creates a limitation if simultaneous hip and knee flexion are contemplated, but has no adverse action in a stiff-leg gait, where the knee is always extended.

Hip extension during push-off requires stimulation of the gluteal muscles. These muscles are large and covered by a thick layer of adipose tissue which creates serious obstacles to surface stimulation. The position of the motor point relative to the skin shifts significantly from the standing to seated or lying prone position, adding to the problem. Furthermore, it is a difficult area to reach for electrode placement by the patient and there is a risk of compressing the electrode and the gel if the patient sits. Another limitation of this muscle is that it produces hip abduction as a component of hip extension, requiring correction by coactivation of other muscles. Experience with stimulating this muscle shows that it also produces a reflex contraction of the abdominal muscles and the consequent trunk flexion, and accidental voiding, both of which are highly undesirable artifacts (personal communication, Dr. A. Nene, Oswestry). The preference then is to avoid using the gluteal muscles if there are other options.

The hamstrings, secondary hip extensors, are easily stimulated by surface electrodes and can provide sufficient force for hip extension. Since the hamstrings also cross the knee joint and can cause simultaneous knee flexion, they would create a significant complication for the push-off function with knee flexion. Since the knee is kept in full extension by a rigid brace, the hamstrings present a superior option for purposes of generating hip extension.

In summary, the swing phase of one leg with simultaneous push-off of the contralateral leg can be accomplished by surface stimulation of the quadriceps and hamstrings, respectively.

DESIGN RATIONALE FOR FES POWER

In our experience over the last 10 years, it is clear that most patients can achieve reasonable locomotion with the LSU-RGO alone (without FES). Why then employ FES power to complicate the system?

It is well known that isolated upper body work consumes much more metabolic energy per kg body mass of active tissue when compared to combined work of upper and lower body (Aastrand and Rodal, 1977; Hirokawa et al., 1990). With this fundamental concept of work physiology in mind, it is clear that during locomotion with the LSU-RGO alone (without FES), the trunk and arm muscles are active (the legs being paralyzed). This, of course, results in excessive energy cost and stress on the arms. By using FES to power the LSU-RGO we can produce strong enough contractions of the large thigh muscles to provide the swing/push-off functions while simultaneously creating combined upper and lower body work and thereby reducing the overall energy cost of locomotion. An additional advantage gained is the reduction of work and stress of the spinal and arm muscles which produced the swing/push-off in the absence of FES. This issue is very important to note as a design concept, as will become obvious later when the system evaluation is presented.

The rationale for designing a practical hybrid locomotion system is, therefore, based on biomechanical, physiological, ergonomic, surgical/medical, and realistic factors. The design itself should further allow for several other important factors, which are the foundation of orthotics/prosthetics practice; that is, function, ease of donning-doffing the device, safety, reliability, independence of assistance in operation, cost, and cosmesis. These factors are addressed in the following sections.

THE LSU-RGO

The LSU-RGO is a passive mechanical orthosis generally categorized as an HKAFO (hip, knee, ankle, foot orthosis). It consists of a polypropylene AFO splint which is custom made to the size of the patient and worn inside the shoe. Its function is to give stability to the ankle joint, keeping it rigidly in the neutral position to allow balanced upright posture. From each AFO, two aluminum uprights extend on the lateral and medial sides, terminating in bilateral knee joints. Two additional uprights extend from each knee joint, the lateral one terminating in a hip joint, while the medial upright extends only two thirds of the way along the thigh. A polypropylene posterior cuff connects the medial and lateral thigh uprights, while anterior Velcro straps insure that the thigh stays in position. An additional upright extends from each hip joint along the lateral aspects of the trunk to just below the axilla. Two Velcro straps, one posterior and one anterior, connect the proximal ends of the uprights to ensure proper placement of the trunk.

The knee joint was specifically redesigned for applications in SCI patients. Our experience shows that nearly all paraplegics suffer from significant hamstring contractures. Attempts to stand from a seated position with the aid of FES or with arm strength alone does not result in full knee extension. In order to allow the patient to remain upright, preventing his collapse into the wheelchair, we incorporated a ratchet knee joint which would freely move into extension, but will not return into knee flexion. This important feature allowed the patient to remain upright, even if a 10- to 25°-knee flexion still exists. Once the patient takes the first step, the shear force developed at the knee with heel strike fully extends the knee and locks the joint in position for the desired duration of locomotion. When the patient wishes to be seated, specially designed posterior bales are engaged by the edge of the chair, which unlocks the ratchet mechanism and allows the knee to flex freely. The bales are spring loaded, which cause the ratchet mechanism to be engaged as soon as they are removed from the edge of the chair. The patient does not have to use his arms for locking or unlocking the knee joint.

The hip joints of the RGO are connected to each other with two stainless steel cables guided inside a low-friction conduit. The cables function to satisfy two objectives, the first of which is to prevent simultaneous hip flexion of both hips and the consequent collapse of the patient. This feature allows the patient to remain upright without using his upper extremities for support for prolonged periods of time with minimal energy cost.

The second objective of the cables is force transmission from one hip to the contralateral one such that reciprocal movement of the legs is possible. If one hip goes into flexion, force is transmitted via the cables to create contralateral hip extension—a reciprocal motion identical to the swing of one leg simultaneously with contralateral push-off.

The reciprocal mechanism may be disengaged to allow simultaneous flexion of both hips for purposes of sitting down. This is accomplished by the patient pressing on a small pin which disengages the reciprocal mechanism. The pin, however, is spring loaded, and will engage the cables automatically if the patient stands and extends his hips sufficiently. This pin is also equipped with two locking positions: one at full hip extension and the second at 20° hip flexion. The position of 20° hip flexion gives the patient the option to walk up a handicapped ramp while his center of gravity is shifted forward sufficiently to prevent the loss of balance to a backward fall (Solomonow et al., 1989). This position of partial hip flexion also allows patients with some hip flexion contracture, which is common after prolonged sitting, to stand up in two stages. Standing or hip extension may easily lock in the 20° position, relieving the patient's upper extremities from providing antigravity support. The patient, then, can at his convenience attempt to extend his hip further into the fully extended position.

A photo of the RGO is shown in Figure 10–3.

Principle of Operation

The RGO allows the patient stable upright balance without using his arm against the walker, at minimal metabolic energy cost. As the patient decides to initiate locomotion, several physical functions are taken in sequence which are best explained with the aid of Figure 10–4.

Step 1 (Figure 10–4A): The patient shifts his weight over one leg (normally the stance leg which will consequently execute the push-off function). This is accomplished by executing elbow extension with the contralateral arm, tilting the trunk toward the leg. This results in slight elevation of one leg, allowing it to clear the floor as the swing phase is initiated next.

Step 2 (Figure 10–4B): The patient exagerates his lordosis, applying force against the posterior thoracic strap of the RGO. This force, acting upon the lateral thoracic uprights of the RGO, creates a moment about the hip joint, forcing the stance leg to undergo hip extension.

Step 3 (Figure 10–4C): The dual cable mechanism linking the two hip joints transmits part of the torque created about the hip of the stance leg to the contralateral hip in a reciprocal manner, initiating hip flexion. This results in the execution of the swing phase simultaneously with contralateral push-off.

Needless to say, the above sequential steps require some coordination, which are easily learned by the patient with the appropriate guidance and instruction of a well-trained physical therapist and by several hours of supervised practice.

THE STIMULATION SYSTEM

As was noted in a previous section, the objective of the muscle stimulation is twofold. The first is to initiate the swing of one leg simultaneously with contralateral push-off and thereby provide the power for locomotion, releasing the upper extremities and spinal muscles from that task. Second, because both the upper and lower extremities are active, it reduces the energy cost per kg of body mass.

In order to stimulate the rectus femoris of one leg simultaneously with the hamstring of the contralateral leg, two channels are necessary. Furthermore, to initiate the next step, the cycle is reversed, requiring stimulation of the hamstrings of one leg with simultaneous activation of the contralateral rectus femoris. Overall, four stimulation channels are required, with each pair active simultaneously.

The stimulation is accomplished with monophasic, charge-balanced pulses of 0.5 msec duration at a rate which varies from 18 to 26 pulses per second, according to the individual patient. The objective of the rate adjustment is to generate a contraction of a strength near 50 to 70% of the maximal tetanic force without inducing fatigue. Lower rates are well known to accomplish such an objective (Solomonow, 1984a, 1984b). Individual adjustments were made to accommodate the fiber composition of each patient, and the changes due to the FES therapy administered to reverse muscle atrophy.

The current pulses are applied to the patient via the conventional carbon impregnated rubber electrodes covered with karaya solid gel, (Uni-Patch, Inc., Wabash, MN).

We strongly advise against the use of liquid/paste gel due to the potential difficulties or unsafe conditions experienced in our earlier phase of this work.

> Paste gel tends to liquify after prolonged contact with the skin due to body temperature. The gel will then run down the skin, stimulate undesired muscles, and create unpredictable and unwanted motion which compromises safety. Eventually, running gel can short circuit the active/passive electrodes and damage the stimulator, battery, or wires.
>
> Moderate pressure on electrodes due to Velcro straps, not to mention the additional pressure from body weight when the patient sits and squeezes the paste gel out, results in similar deficiencies as described above.
>
> Finally, if the gel is not applied uniformly, leaving the exposed electrode surface to the skin (air bubbles), serious skin burns may result.

The use of elastic stockinettes with gel pockets should also be avoided for the above reasons.

Karaya gel is a solid and prevents the possibility of melting/running even after many hours in contact with the skin. It is also resistant to deformation under pressure even when the patient is seated over the electrodes. It does not soil clothing, is not messy to handle, and a single sheet covering one electrode can last 4 to 7 days before it has to be replaced.

Severe formidable human-factor problems emerge if one requires patients to apply four sets of electrodes (two per muscle or eight electrodes altogether) over the same location every day.

> Most patients are not familiar with polarity, wiring, and other aspects or electricity.
>
> Duplicating the location of placement from day to day about the motor point with reasonable accuracy is difficult.
>
> Placing an electrode over the hamstrings is difficult due to indirect field of vision.
>
> Connecting the correct wires to the appropriate electrode from the eight possible is too much to be expected from all patients.
>
> How to keep the electrodes fairly snug to the skin and without irritating it.

We designed a flexible copolymer electrode cuff, custom made for each patient. The electrodes are placed in the cuff properly predistanced about the motor point. All electrode wires are passed between the outer shell and the internal foam cover (excluding electrodes surface) and emerge from the cuff in a single cable with a plug connector. The connector is inserted into the stimulator only in one way—the correct

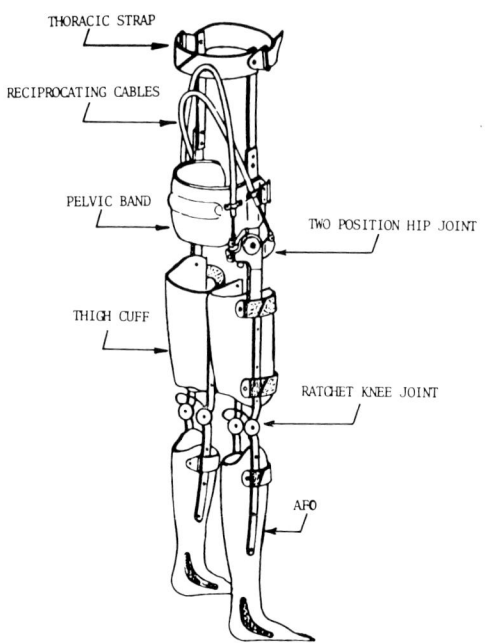

(A)

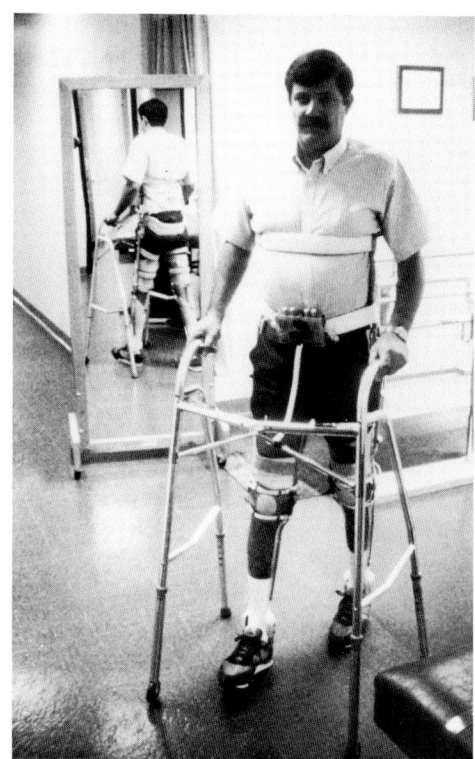

Figure 10–3 Showing the schematic of the LSU-RGO in (A), and a patient walking with the LSU-RGO powered with FES in (B). Note that (B) gives also the rear view of the patient as reflected in the mirror. In (C) an enlarged view of the hip joint and the associated reciprocating cable assembly is shown.

(B)

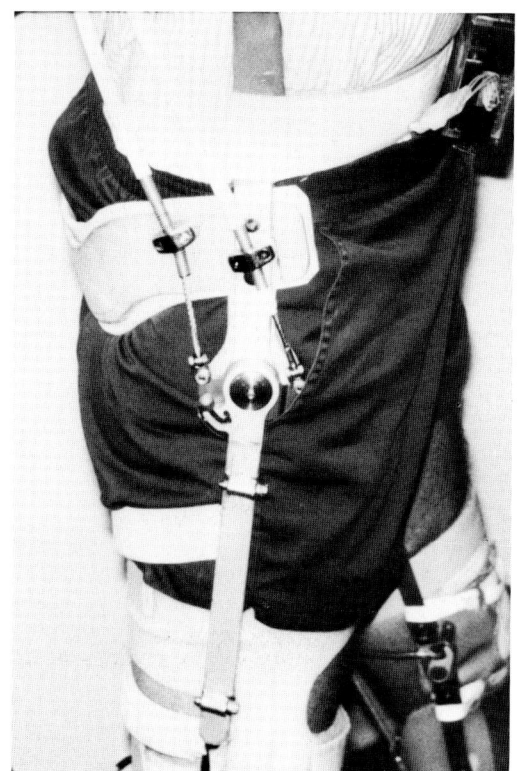

Figure 10–3 (Continued). (C)

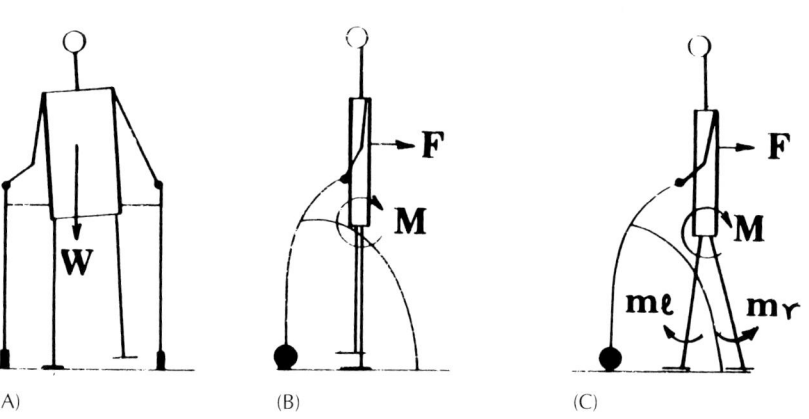

Figure 10–4 The operation of the LSU-RGO when used without electrical stimulation is shown. (A) Step 1 requires shifting of the weight towards one leg by extending the contralateral arm and thrusting with the shoulder such that the foot is raised slightly above the floor. (B) The patient then exaggerates his lordosis applying force, F, on the posterior thoracic strap of the RGO, which results in the moment, M, about the hip joint. (C) The moment about the hip is decomposed into moments m_l and m_r about the left and right hip joints by the reciprocating cables to create hip flexion simultaneously with contralateral hip extension.

way. The inside foam cover can be peeled off for washing or for replacing the karaya gel over the electrodes as necessary. It also allows for ventilation of the skin, preventing temperature build-up and absorption of sweat while providing comfort.

Velcro straps fasten the cuffs snugly about the thigh as shown in Figure 10–5.

The stimulator is in the "off" mode at all times except when the patient decides to initiate walking. By triggering a miniswitch mounted on each handlebar of his rolling walker, the patient applies activation to the rectus femoris on the same side of the switch while stimulating the hamstrings on the contralateral side. The trigger signal from the switch is transmitted to the belt-worn stimulator via a spiral cable emerging from the walker. The complete stimulation system is shown in Figure 10–6.

REHABILITATION PROGRAM

Evaluation

Clear, universally accepted guidelines for acceptance of SCI patients to a rehabilitation program including locomotion with an orthosis or FES-powered orthosis do not exist. Current criteria as pointed out by Kralj et al., (1983, 1989) are an initial attempt. Our aggressive research-oriented experience with applying the RGO to a variety of patients with musculoskeletal diseases yielded additional important knowledge. Once the patient was cleared by the physician as having a stable spine and in general good condition, we found that the major factor was *motivation*. Once the patient demonstrated motivation by requesting to join the program and attending some preliminary sessions, we proceeded with the evaluation.

To date, patients who completed the training or are in training include:

Injury level: C5–6 incomplete to T11.
Age: 18 to 62 years.
Time since injury: 11 months to 22 years.
Spasms: none to severe.
Contractures: none to severe (but not ossified joints).
Weight: normal to very overweight.
Pressure sores: none to some.

The reason for such liberal acceptance criteria is based on experience and the need to experiment. We found that even severe spasticity is significantly diminished or even disappears with the application of FES or with locomotion in the RGO with or without FES. This could be due mostly to muscle stretching, range-of-motion exercise, or to the FES alone as was reported before (Kralj et al., 1983). It should be noted that the FES by itself was an important factor in reducing or eliminating spasticity, and consequently, the antispastic medication. The effect of FES on spasticity, however, had only a short-term carryover, with a gradual return of spasticity after 3 to 4 days of the last FES application.

Similarly, contractures of the hip, knee, and ankle joints were initially regarded as contraindications. After some experimentation with such patients, we found that as long as the joints are not ossified, application of FES and/or locomotion with the

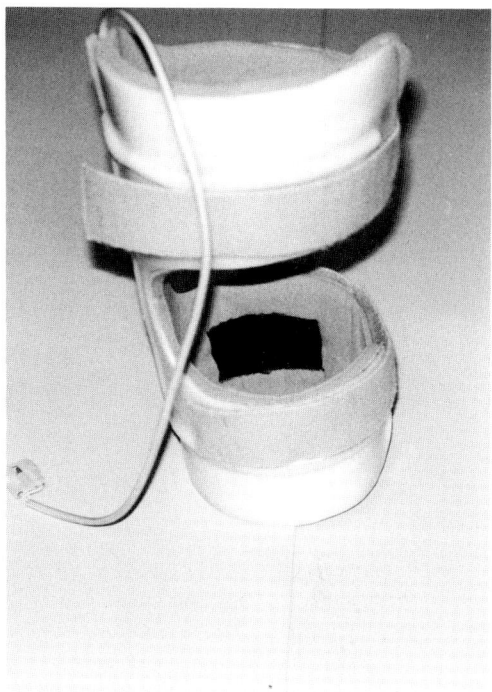

(A)

Figure 10–5 The electrode cuff with the single cable and connector is shown in (A). In (B), the soft foam cover and the location of the electrodes is shown, as well as the flexibility of the cuff which allows its easy application on the thigh.

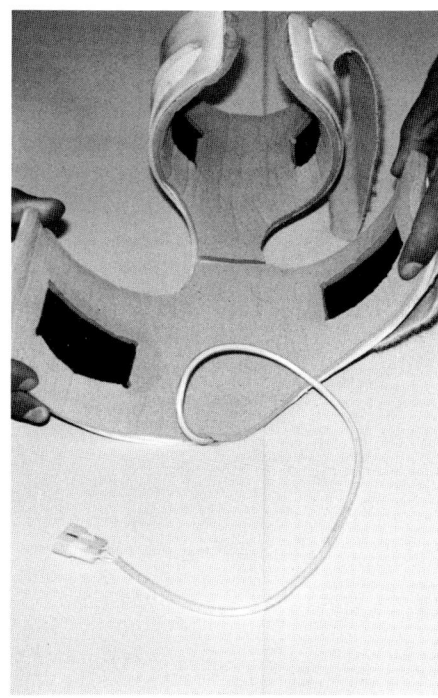

(B)

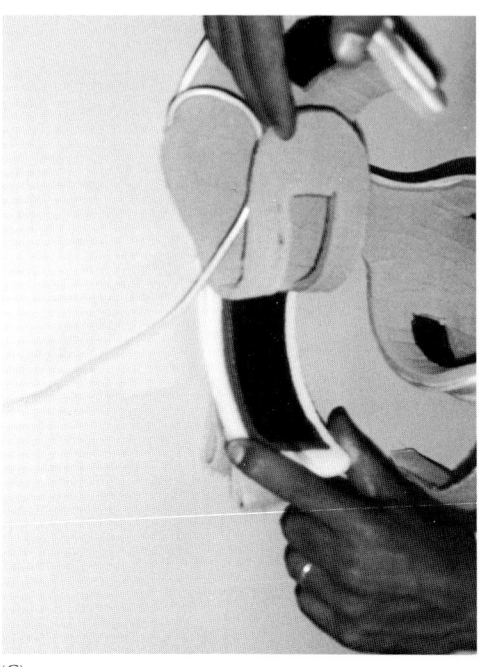

Figure 10–5 (Continued). The interior foam cover could be easily peeled as shown in (C) to expose the electrodes, giving direct access to replace the karaya gel sheet or for periodic washing of the foam.

(C)

RGO significantly decreased the contracture and increased the joints' range of motion. Continuation of locomotion with the RGO powered by FES assured the consolidation of such gains, which were quickly lost if the patients did not ambulate for 2 to 3 weeks.

Long periods of sitting in the wheelchair accelerate gain in weight. We accepted overweight patients with motivation and realized that rapid loss of weight was possible as soon as locomotion began. This could not be attributed to the FES alone, but rather to the locomotion function and the high rate of metabolic energy consumption associated with it. These patients were eventually good walkers despite the initial hardship.

Patients with relatively short duration since injury demonstrated rapid reversal of muscle atrophy, although other patients at 10, 17, and 22 years postinjury demonstrated equal improvements, but required longer periods of FES therapy. The latter patients had some initial hardship to overcome when locomotion training began due to deficiency of the cardiopulmonary system encumbered over the many inactive years.

Patients with injury level of T1 to T11 were relatively easy to rehabilitate, although we accepted patients with lesions above and below that range. One patient, for example, had complete lack of sensorimotor function below T1 and incomplete damage up to the C5-6 level. After several weeks of arm-hand strengthening exercise, he was accepted to the program and is now, 3 years later, one of the best users. High lesions which completely affect the arms and hand, however, are contraindications.

Patients with lesions below T11 have partial or complete damage to the lower

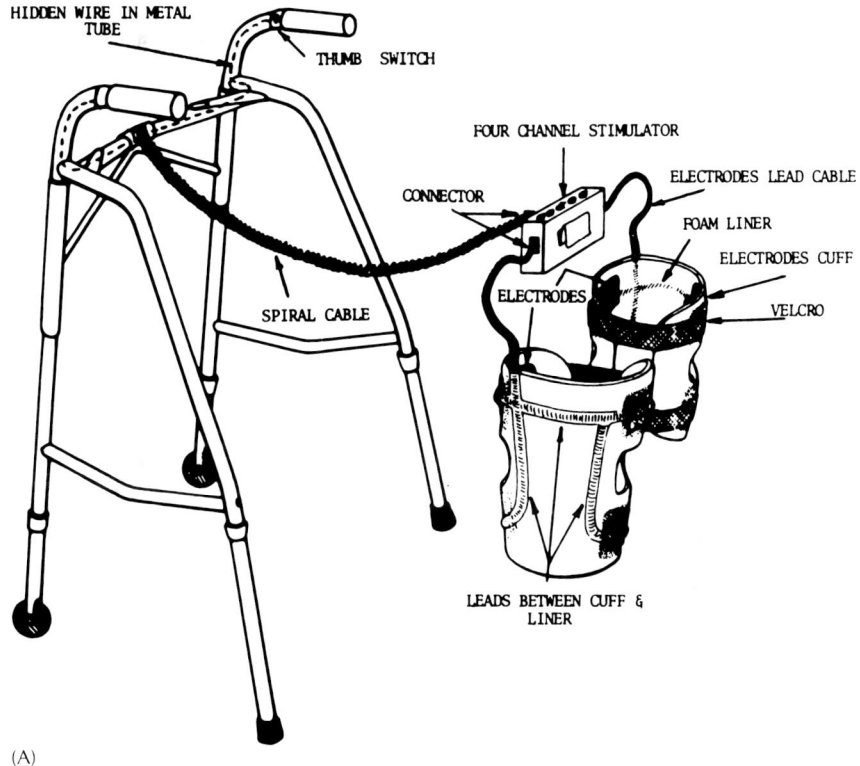

Figure 10–6 (A) shows a schematic of the stimulation system, while (B) shows the real components. (*Continued*)

motor neurons, and therefore do not respond to FES. Such patients are, as a rule, better walkers with the RGO alone, especially if some hip flexion is available.

The preexistence of pressure sores or some skin lacerations show a rapid healing once FES and locomotion are initiated. We suspect that the improvement in circulation in the lower extremities due to FES, muscle hypertrophy, revascularization, and general increase in metabolism are responsible.

In summary, experience shows that acceptability to the program should not be limited to a certain group, but open for the general paraplegic population. It is obvious that additional hardship and perseverance are required to bring to a successful conclusion some patients with severe deficiencies, but it is possible and should be done. It is also obvious that a systematic study should be conducted to determine evaluation guidelines based on sound medical experience as it is acquired.

RGO Fitting and Training

Each patient underwent a preambulatory training which consisted of 3 to 4 weeks (3 1-hour sessions per week) of arm and shoulder girdle muscle strengthening, back extensor, and abdominal muscles strengthening and trunk balance. The objective of this preambulatory training is to reduce contractures, maximize the strength and

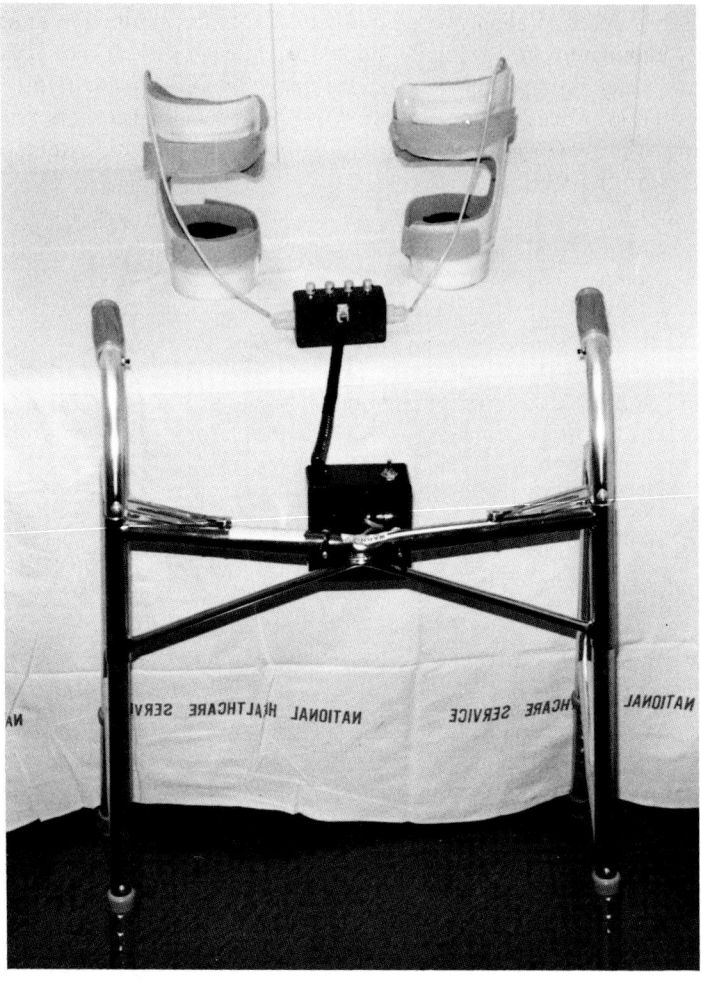

Figure 10–6 (Continued).

control of any innervated muscles, increase the strength of the arms and shoulders (which is essential for ambulation in the RGO), and retrain the patient to control the trunk's center of gravity (a function which is limited and gradually lost after prolonged sitting in the wheelchair). Another objective is to improve the patients general physical conditioning (i.e., cardiopulmonary condition and endurance).

The significance of this preambulatory training is underscored, since in our experience, patients who successfully completed it became good users of the RGO in relatively short time, whereas patients who did not participate in it exhibited low acceptance rate, even after prolonged ambulatory training.

Patients are fitted with a custom-made RGO by a certified orthotist with prior experience with this orthosis. Care is employed to properly calibrate the RGO uprights and cables so that the patient can stand fully balanced and stable without holding on to any object with their hands for at least one continuous minute. Additional care is taken to align the leg uprights so that circumduction or scissoring is completely eliminated. Following the initial fitting, each patient receives 6 weeks of training consisting of three 1-hour session per week in donning and doffing the RGO, walking on level surfaces, sitting and standing up, and making corners and full turns. All training is provided by a registered physical therapist with extensive previous experience with the RGO.

Patients with injury to the T1 spine and/or incomplete damage to the low cervical level receive an additional 3 weeks of arm-strengthening therapy prior to initiating the RGO training.

It should be also emphasized that the proper fitting and calibration of the RGO by a qualified and experienced orthotist is essential for its successful performance. Alignment of leg members, symmetry, proper tension in cables, adjustment of thoracic straps, and other features of the unit . . ., makes unimaginable differences in the ability of the patient to perform, and consequently, in his acceptance of the orthosis.

FES Therapy

Each patient receives 6 weeks of FES therapy to the quadriceps and hamstrings muscles. The therapy consisted of three sessions per week lasting from 2 to 40 minutes each. The objective of the therapy is to reverse thigh muscle atrophy and increase strength. A pair of carbon-impregnated surface electrodes are placed over the hamstrings and another pair over the quadriceps of each leg. The patient is raised with a specially designed hydraulic lift while sitting on a narrow, bicycle-like seat with free space around his legs as shown in Figure 10–7. A specially designed four-channel electrical stimulator delivers 0.5 msec rectangular pulses at a rate of 20 pulses per second to one quadriceps and the contralateral hamstrings resulting in a hip flexion and contralateral hip extension and knee flexion, respectively, simulating swing and push-off phases of the gait cycle. Then the stimuli are switched off and applied to the contralateral quadriceps and hamstrings.

Initially, the stimuli are applied for a 1-minute duration at a rate of 0.3 steps/sec (i.e., a swing and contralateral push-off were held for 3 seconds before reversing the stimuli to the muscles of each leg). A 10-minute rest is given to the patient following another minute of "walking-like" session.

The duration of the FES therapy is increased by 2 minutes each session as the muscles became conditioned. In the final 2 weeks of FES therapy, the patients are given 2 20-minute sessions spaced by a 10-minute rest period. A 25-N weight is also wrapped around the ankles to load the movement and improve strength and fatigue resistance of the thigh muscles. Furthermore, during the last 2 weeks, the stimuli cycle rate is increased to 1 step/sec (i.e., the patient performed swing and contralateral push-off 60 times in each minute).

Care is taken to monitor the heart rate during the therapy with an earlobe sensor to avoid undue stress and exertion of the patients. Some patients demonstrate rapid increase in heart rate during the first week of FES therapy. As a routine, if the heart rate increases over 140 beats per minute, the patient is lowered to the supine position and closely monitored for 20 to 25 minutes until his condition returns to normal. Occasionally, additional preconditioning is prescribed on the tilt table to allow the

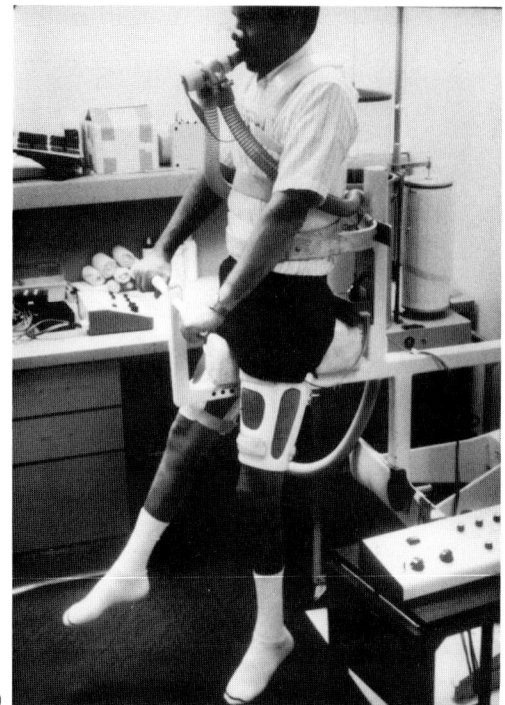
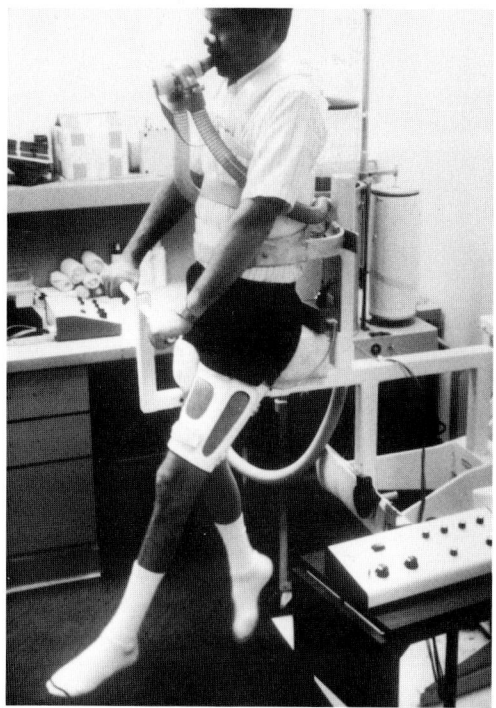

Figure 10–7 Showing a patient during the FES therapy. The patient is seated on the hydraulic lift and the table top stimulator is shown on the lower right. Note the electrode cuffs on the patient's thighs. In this picture, the oxygen consumption of the patient was also measured (with the spirometer in the background) to calculate the energy cost of the muscles stimulated.

cardiovascular system exposure to compensate for upright posture that the patient was lacking for prolonged durations.

Gait Training with FES-Powered RGO

Once a patient completes the 6 weeks of gait training with the RGO and the FES therapy, which is administered simultaneously, an additional 6 weeks (three 1-hour sessions, 3 times a week) of gait training with the FES-powered RGO (FES & RGO) is administered to develop and improve skill and performance in level walking when using FES for the thigh muscles.

ENERGY CONSUMPTION

Protocol

Patients are instrumented with a nose clip and a mouthpiece from which two flexible tubes are connected to a volume spirometer containing oxygen mounted on a rolling cart which is pushed behind them during locomotion as shown in Figure 10–8. The tubes are mounted on a lightweight plastic shoulder harness to allow the patient to freely move his head during locomotion. Expired, excess oxygen is filtered back to the spirometers reservoir so that net oxygen consumption during each breath and overall oxygen consumption are recorded.

Initially, the patient stands quietly for 5 minutes to establish basal heart rate and energy consumption during rest. The patient is then instructed to walk a level, straight 30-meter track at a speed set to him by a metronome. At the end of the 30-meter track, measurements are made of final heart rate and total oxygen consumed. Following a 20-minute rest, the metronome speed is changed and the procedure is repeated for another walking speed. Walking speeds are set at random to prevent biased errors. Care is also taken to insure that the patient's heart rate at the end of each trial returns to within ±3 beats/min of the original resting heart rate before the next trial is initiated.

Patients were instructed to avoid food consumption 3 to 4 hours before coming to the clinic and another 1.5 hours without food elapses in the clinic before initiating the trials.

Each patient was also instructed to walk a 30-meter distance at a speed he feels is the most comfortable for his circumstances (e.g., injury level, training period, height, weight, and other physical factors). Two such trials are performed by each patient, and are included in calculating the average preferred walking speed of all the patients. The preferred walking speed of a group of six patients with T1 to T10 injuries is 0.2 m/s.

RESULTS

Discussion of energy cost data associated with a new orthotic device is meaningful only if a comparison is made to a well-known device such as the LLB, or other

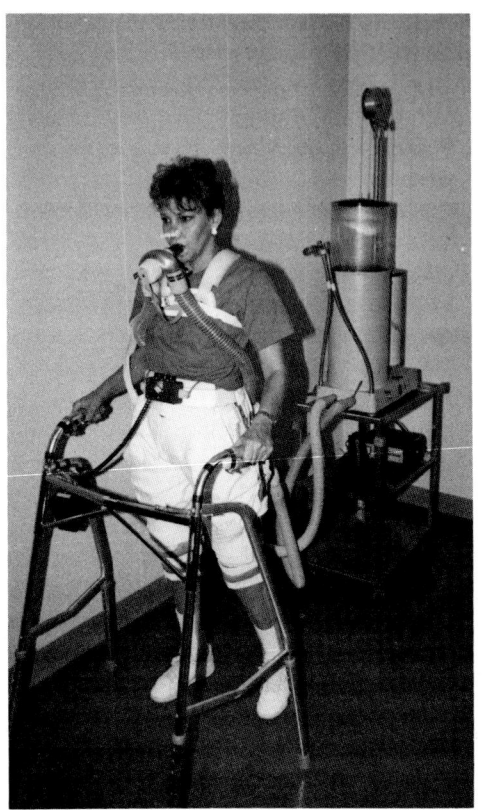

Figure 10–8 Showing a patient during the assessment of the energy cost associated with ambulation with the RGO powered by electrical stimulation of the thigh muscles.

devices available as an option for the same patient category. This data is presented with a comparative analysis among the RGO, RGO & FES, HGO (Nene and Patrick, 1989), LLB, and the FES system of Marsolais (Marsolais and Edwards, 1988).

Figure 10–9 depicts the energy expenditure in Kcal/kg/min versus walking speed for the LLB, HGO, RGO, RGO & FES, and the Marsolais FES. The lowest energy cost associated with the FES-powered RGO at walking speeds from 0 to 0.27 m/s is immediately evident. Ranking second in energy expenditure per minute is the RGO, which displays a nearly parallel curve to the RGO & FES, but spaced 0.01 Kcal/kg/min upward. The energy expenditure associated with the LLB displays a fast rate of increase as walking speed increases and is ranked third for walking speeds ranging from 0 to 0.1 m/s. The HGO demonstrates a rapid decline in energy cost at low speeds, becoming lower than the LLB at 0.1 m/s, and even lower than the RGO and RGO & FES at 0.2 and 0.27 m/s, respectively. At a walking speed of 0.28 m/s the energy expenditure required for walking with the LLB exceeds that of the Marsonlais FES and continues to rise as a function of speed. Conversely, the Marsolais FES requires the highest energy expenditure at low to moderate walking speeds in

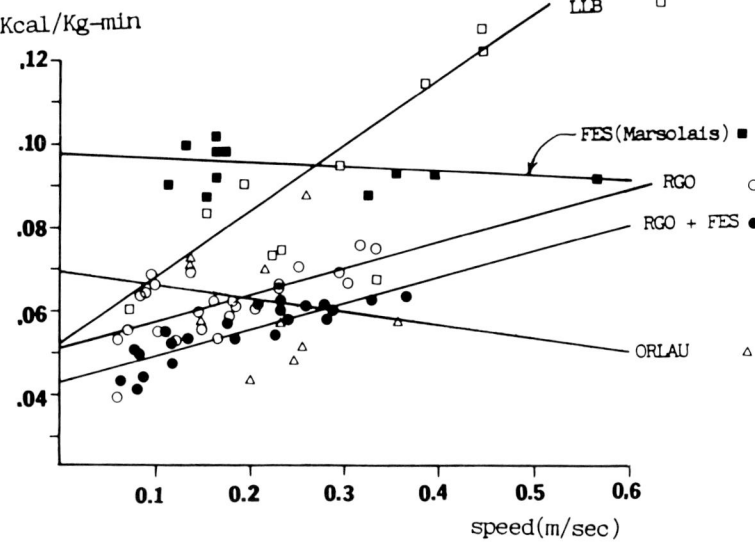

Figure 10–9 The energy cost in Kcal/Kg/min versus walking speed for the RGO, RGO & FES, the ORLAU orthosis, the LLB, and the FES system developed by Marsolais.

the range of 0 to 0.25 m/s, and then improves its ranking to fourth place as the walking speed increases further.

Considering again 0.2 m/s as the preferred walking speed which will be utilized in daily living activities, the ranking of the five types of walking aides show that the RGO & FES is first, having the lowest energy cost, with the RGO and HGO second, LLB third, and the Marsolais FES fourth, with the highest energy cost.

Figure 10–10 displays the energy expenditure per meter versus walking speeds for the RGO, RGO & FES, HGO, LLB, and the Marsolais FES system. The Marsolais FES system was the least efficient, requiring the highest energy expenditure throughout the full range of walking speeds, and especially in the preferred mean speed of 0.2 m/s. The LLB and the HGO rank second and third, respectively, although the HGO became highly efficient at 0.25 m/s only, equalizing the RGO & FES as the most efficient. At low walking speeds the LLB and RGO have nearly the same energy cost, but the RGO requires lower energy cost as the speeds increase. At high speeds the difference between the LLB and the Marsolais FES diminishes, indicating the inefficiency of the LLB relative to the FES-based walking aide for brisk locomotion. The RGO & FES demonstrates the highest efficiency relative to the other four devices almost throughout the full range of walking speed. Only at speeds exceeding 0.35 m/s did the energy cost associated with the RGO & FES equal that of the RGO, indicating that at high walking speeds the RGO & FES is as efficient as the RGO. The fact that the HGO had high energy cost throughout the range of walking speeds except at 0.25 m/s, where it equaled the cost of the RGO & FES, is supported by the finding that patients using this orthosis preferred 0.25 m/s as the most comfortable walking speed (British Health Authority Report, 1989). This fact emphasizes the importance and implications of energy cost on the per-

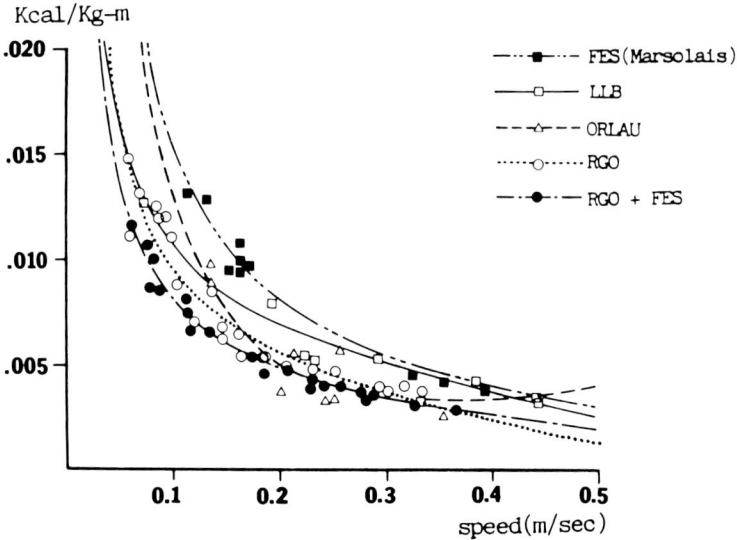

Figure 10–10 The energy cost in Kcal/Kg/m versus walking speeds for the RGO, RGO & FES, ORLAU orthosis, LLB, and the Marsolais FES system.

formance of the patients, who intuitively select the walking speed associated with minimum energy cost.

Heart Rate

Figure 10–11 displays the mean and standard deviation of the pooled pretrial and posttrial heart rate (HR) for the RGO and RGO & FES along with heart rate data for the LLB and the Marsolais FES as obtained from the literature (Marsolais and Edwards, 1988). Heart rate data for the HGO is not available in the literature.

The mean pretrial heart rate for patients using the RGO & FES was 88 beats/min (standing quiet) and the posttrial HR was 119 beats/min, representing a 35.2% increase. For the RGO, the HR rose from 86 beats/min at rest (standing), to 131 beats/min posttrial, a 52.3% increase. The mean HR of patients using the LLB rose from 80 beats/min (seated) at rest to 150 beats/min postwalking, an 87.5% increase. For patients using the Marsolais FES system, the mean HR increased from 80 beats/min (seated) at rest to 161 beats/min posttrial, representing a 101.25% increase.

The addition of FES power to the RGO resulted in 12 beats/min lower HR at the end of at least a 30-meter walk as compared to the HR of the same patients using the RGO alone. It was 31 beats/min less than the HR of patients using the LLB and 42 beats/min less than the HR of patients using the Marsolais FES system. The lower HR resulting from walking in the RGO & FES reflects the low stress associated with the use of this device as compared to the RGO, LLB, and FES alone, further confirming the advantages of a walking aid in which a passive mechanical orthosis is coupled with FES of the leg muscles.

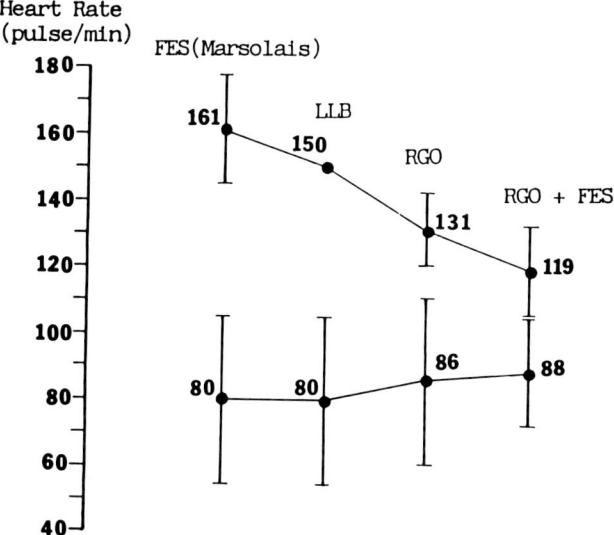

Figure 10–11 The initial and final heart rate after walking 30 meters in the RGO, RGO & FES, the LLB, and the Marsolais FES system.

GENERAL DISCUSSION

The lowest energy expenditure in Kcal/kg/min (at low to moderate walking speed) and Kcal/kg/m was evident for the RGO & FES throughout this study, was expected, and is due to several important factors.

A mechanical orthosis such as the LLB provides energy-free antigravity support to the knee and ankle. Hip stability during quiet standing is also possible by teaching and training the patient to hyperextend this joint, but such training is often neglected. The patient, therefore, is required to prevent his hip joints from yielding to gravity by excessive exertion of force with his arms, shoulders, and any voluntary controlled spinal muscles. This high level of force required by the upper extremity and trunk muscles has to be exerted continuously even for purposes of quiet standing. Furthermore, the LLB is a passive orthosis and requires the paraplegic patient to exert additional forces by the arms and trunk muscles in order to provide forward progression—or walking. Such a high level of forces generated by the arm and trunk muscles result in high energy expenditure which increases with walking speed.

The RGO is also a passive mechanical orthosis providing energy-free antigravity support to the hip joints in addition to the knees and ankles. The uprights extending from the hip joints to the midthoracic region provide additional support, and when properly aligned, the patient can assume a fully balanced and stable upright posture with minimal manipulation of trunk muscles. No support is required from the upper extremities. Balanced upright posture, therefore, is nearly free from any energy expenditure. This hip stability, provided by hip joints and associated cable mechanism, is the major advantage of the RGO over the LLB and the HGO during standing and over the range of increasing walking speeds. Upon initiation of locomotion, relatively high forces are required from the arm and shoulder muscles to lift the swing leg off the ground, while the spinal muscles are required to contract to provide the required lordosis which triggers the swing phase of one leg and the contralateral push-off. The net effect still results in high energy expenditure to propagate the paralyzed legs—a passive weight—into the appropriate movements. The reduction in the energy cost of the RGO relative to the LLB, then, is due to the fact that the RGO provides antigravity support to the hip joints and nearly energy-free balance and stability which requires less effort and less energy expenditure from the arms and trunk.

The HGO is a HKAFO orthosis of similar construction to the RGO. Its functional properties are, however, widely different. The RGO includes two cables connecting the hip joints and preventing their flexion in response to gravity. This in essence allows energy-free standing. The HGO, however, allows free motion of the hip joint over a limited range of flexion and extension, requiring the patient to prevent the gravitational forces acting on the hip joints by strong opposition with the arms against the walker. This fact is manifested in the relatively high energy cost during standing as well as during slow walking speeds. As the walking speed increases, the double-stance phase of the gait cycle becomes shorter, requiring less upper extremity energy to prevent hip collapse. It is also self explanatory why patients selected a somewhat higher preferred walking speed with the HGO than that of the RGO. Although the study by Marsolais and Edwards (1988) did not include the determination of the preferred walking speed for their FES system in their study, it is conceivable that their patients select higher walking speed, about 0.3 m/s, to benefit from the slight reduction in energy cost evident in using the FES system at increased speeds.

The highest energy expenditure was associated with the Marsolais FES system. Many of the stimulated muscles are biarticular (two-joint muscles) and therefore exert forces on both joints upon contraction. To direct the force into the necessary joint, antagonist muscles had to be stimulated to increase the joint stiffness. The large number of concurrently stimulated muscles resulted in high levels of energy expenditure.

Furthermore, initiation of hip flexion to generate the swing phase of one leg tends to force the trunk forward as well and causes the patient to lose balance. To prevent a fall, the patient exerts undue force with his arm and shoulder muscles against the rolling walker, consuming large amounts of energy.

Another important factor for the high energy cost associated with the Marsolais FES system is that upright posture alone requires active tension in many muscles to provide antigravity support, while the RGO requires nearly none. The high energy expenditure required just for quiet standing was evident in the curve depicting the high value of Kcal/kg/min at zero speed and the slight decrease as walking speeds increased. The LLB, HGO, RGO, and RGO & FES required less than half the energy expended by the Marsolais FES system at zero and slow walking speeds. It is important to note that the Marsolais FES system requires slightly less energy as the walking speeds increase because the patient is not required to maintain continuous upright posture with his arms, demonstrating the exceptionally high energy cost associated with quiet standing. This phenomena should be emphasized, since the energy cost associated with the other three walking orthosis increases as the speed increases, while the Marsolais FES system required slightly less energy as walking speed increases. It is conceivable that when more basic knowledge is gained on how biarticular muscles function, and how cocontraction patterns of agonist-antagonist muscles affects joint dynamics (Solomonow et al., 1986, 1988; Baratta et al., 1988) optimal patterns of FES could be devised to reduce the energy cost of locomotion with such orthoses based on FES alone.

The low energy cost of locomotion with the RGO & FES was expected, since the system was designed with that purpose in mind. The design criteria for this hybrid system combined the advantages of the mechanical orthosis, RGO, with the advantages of FES of two muscle groups. As indicated above, the RGO allows the patient antigravity support, balance, and stability at low energy cost. The FES of the quadriceps and contralateral thigh muscles was applied to generate the gait cycle, substantially reducing the need to do so by the arm and spinal muscles. The only involvement of the upper extremity required was to push the walker forward while depressing one arm on the walker to elevate the swing leg, allowing it to clear the floor. Overall, the gross reductions in activity of the arm and trunk muscles to maintain balanced antigravity standing and initiation of motion is manifested by the low energy expenditure of this system, which is primarily due to the simultaneous contraction of the quadriceps and contralateral hamstrings. Additional minor energy is expanded by one arm/shoulder muscle to raise and clear the swing leg over the floor. It should be noted that the powerful contraction of the spinal muscles into exaggerated lordosis was no longer required for triggering the swing phase, since that was provided by the stimulated thigh muscles. It should be also noted that the moderate simultaneous activity of the upper and lower extremity imposes less stress on the patient than strenuous activity of the arms alone. This was clearly manifested by the 12 beats/min reduction in HR when patients used the RGO & FES as compared to the RGO alone.

COST

One of the important factors among the many others that influence the acceptance of an orthotic device by patients and health professionals is its cost. It is, therefore, necessary to contain such a factor to a level which is not inhibitory for its utilization.

The RGO has been available commercially since the mid 1970s from Durr-Fillauer Orthopedics, Inc., of Chattanooga, TN. At present, its cost, including the hardware shipped from the manufacturer, assembly by a local orthotist, and custom fitting (casting, alignments, calibration, and so on) is $4200. The cost of the rolling walker necessary for ambulation is $155 and the custom built stimulator is $1200. The total cost of the hardware, therefore, is $5555.

The success of an orthosis measured by its acceptance by patients also depends to a large extent on the quality of training in its use. In this case, the training proved to be a most important element in acceptance. Well-trained patients became routine users, whereas poorly trained patients (primarily out-of-towners who had limited duration of stay as outpatients) were not frequent users. The training requires at least 6 weeks of supervised and guided ambulation by a physical therapist at the rate of three sessions per week. The cost of this gait training averages $1200, although it varies from patient to patient depending on age, weight, sex, level of injury, duration of disability, and aggressiveness. Some patients needed only 2 to 3 weeks of gait training, whereas in difficult cases, up to 15 weeks were required. The latter cases consisted of patients with joint contractures, high level of injury, high level of spasticity, overweight, and relative advanced age (oldest patient was 62 years old at the time of rehabilitation).

An additional cost was the reversal of muscle atrophy therapy. The FES sessions last on the average 6 weeks for three sessions per week at an average cost of $2500.

The overall average cost of the rehabilitation, therefore, is $9255. Compared to other orthotic or prosthetic devices, the cost is realistic and acceptable. The cost of a below-knee prosthesis, for example, ranges from $1800 to $4000, while an above-knee prosthesis ranges from $3200 to $10000, excluding the gait training. On a comparative basis, an overall cost of $9255 for hardware and training for the FES-powered RGO is very reasonable.

RELIABILITY AND MAINTENANCE

The RGO has evolved through the years with improvement in its reliability and a significant reduction in the frequency of service and repairs. At present, based on experience with a large number of patients, the RGO requires about two service visits per year for a patient who is a daily user. Less frequent users require an average of one service visit every 2 years. This service/repair frequency is equivalent to that of other prosthetic devices which are routinely applied, such as above- and below-knee prosthetics, and are accepted by patients as reasonable. Repairs, if any, normally occur during the gait-training period when the brace is new and undergoes calibration to optimize its performance to the patient. Repairs generally consist of a broken cable or a fractured AFO, and are usually secondary to the patients' weight. The above components are immediately replaced with heavy duty components which can last satisfactorily for many years.

CONCLUSIONS

The use of the reciprocating gait orthosis powered with brief electrical stimulation of the thigh muscles to initiate the gait cycle of thoracic paraplegics results in substantial reduction of energy expenditure when compared with other currently available options including the mechanical or the FES orthosis. The advantages of such a properly fitted hybrid orthosis combined with the appropriate training can provide selected paraplegics with an attractive alternative to wheelchair transportation, with the added benefits of preventing osteoporosis and pressure sores, improving cardiopulmonary, kidney, bladder, and circulatory functions (Rosman and Spira, 1974), as well as improved attitude and daily living functions.

To date, we have fitted 700 patients with the RGO and over 27 patients with the FES-powered RGO and followed them up to nearly 3 years. We had two failures, namely patients who abandoned the program before training was completed. Both patients were subject to social problems which hindered their successful completion of the program. The remaining patients pointed out that they are regular users, daily or at least three times a week. Patients who use the orthosis daily employ it at the workplace, in daily exercise walks in their neighborhood, or as a means for home ambulation for over 40 hours weekly. Other weekly users employ the system for special occasions (i.e., going to church, family barbeques, social gatherings) for at least 12 to 15 hours weekly.

Patients are trained to don and doff the orthosis either in bed or when seated. This procedure normally takes 15 to 20 minutes when performed without help. Although this did not bother patients, they expressed dismay that the brace has to be taken off when performing personal toilet functions in the bathroom. The source was the inability to perform hip abduction. Lack of this function was also a limitation for patients when transporting themselves in and out from cars, beds, and so on. We have designed, and are now testing, a newly developed hip abduction joint that will eliminate this limitation.

Although rehabilitation of many functions are provided to patients who use the RGO powered by electrical stimulation of the thigh muscles, many limitations still exist. Inability to safely walk up stairs or on uneven surfaces (e.g., dirt, grass, gravel), and the need to abduct the hips during transportation from chairs to cars or from bed to its edge, as well as for purposes of toilet and self-cleaning functions, are primary limitations. Current work directly addresses such limitations and demonstrates that significant improvements in function could be possible along with an increase in the acceptance of the orthosis as a routinely worn accessory.

It is difficult to conclude this type of an article without putting its content in perspective. Obviously, research and development focusing on rehabilitation of locomotion was initiated several decades ago. Over the years there were successes and failures which provided researchers with invaluable lessons. The work presented in this chapter utilized the lessons learned in the development of a reasonably practical walking orthosis with seemingly good potential for acceptance by patients. We consider it practical, since it could be used by patients without assistance in the home, work place, school, and other environments. It is commercially available, has a reasonable cost, and was found useful by many outside of our group. This is the first time an orthosis with such features has been available. In retrospect, such development marks an important milestone in this field. Yet when comparing the function and quality of gait provided by the LSU-RGO powered by FES with that of healthy persons, it reminds us how primitive this orthosis is. This should not, however, be a source of frustration, but a motivating force to aggressively tackle the problem. Based on recent development in our laboratory, we have seen the potential for significant advancement in the future. We have developed a technique which is capable of orderly stimulation of motor units according to their size with simultaneous changes of their firing rate (Baratta et al., 1989). This will allow control of muscles in a mode similar to that known to be used by the motor system under voluntary contraction. We have also initiated and made good progress on obtaining basic information on how agonist and antagonist muscles coactivate or cocontract about a joint (Solomonow et al., 1986; Solomonow et al., 1988; Hagood et al., 1990; Baratta et al., 1988) and what the dynamic properties of the muscle are (Baratta et al., 1989; Baratta and Solomonow 1990). We are also studying the feasibility of using EMG as a force feedback in a closed-loop FES control scheme (Solomonow et al., 1986, 1987, 1990a, 1990b). It is obvious that completing this research and development will require a good number of years, yet the expected results are well worth the wait. Looking into the future, we anticipate an orthosis with a significant improvement in function and acceptance by patients, but for the present, a reasonable and practical orthosis is available as a contemporary alternative for the wheelchair.

ACKNOWLEDGMENTS

This work was supported by a LSU Board of Regents Grant (LEQSF) and in part by the NSF Grants EET 8613807 and EET 8820772. The original research was conducted in collaboration with R.V. Barrata, R. D'Ambrosia, M. Harris, P. Beaudette, N. Rightor, and W. Walker, whose contributions are gratefully acknowledged.

NOTES

1. Source: Durr-Fillaver, Inc., RGO manufacturer.

REFERENCES

Andrews, B., and Baxendale, R. (1988). A hybrid orthosis incorporating artificial reflexes for spinal cord damaged patients. *J. Physiol.*, **198**, 380.

Aastrand P., and Rodal, K. (1977). In: *Textbook of Work Physiology: Physiological Basis of Exercise*, 2nd ed., New York: McGraw-Hill.

Baratta, R.V., Ichie, M., Sung, K., and Solomonow, M. (1989). Orderly stimulation of motor units with tripolar nerve cuff electrode. *IEEE Trans. Biomed. Eng.*, **36**, 836–843.

Baratta, R.V., and Solomonow, M. (1990). The dynamic response model of nine different muscles. *IEEE Trans. Biomed. Eng.*, **37**, 243–251.

Baratta, R.V., Solomonow, M., Zhou, B., Letson, R., Chuinard, R., and D'Ambrosia, R. (1988). Muscular coactivation: The role of the antagonist musculature in maintaining knee stability. *Am. J. Sports Med.*, **16**, 113–122.

Baratta, R.V., Zhou, B., and Solomonow, M. (1989). Frequency response model of skeletal muscle: Effect of perturbation level and control strategy. *Med. Biol. Eng. Comput.*, **27**, 337–345.

British Health Authority Report. (1989). *A Comparative Evaluation of the HGO and the RGO*. National Health Service of England, Health Equipment Information, #192.

Chantraine, A., Crielaard, J., Onkelinx, A., and Pirmay, F. (1984). Energy expenditure of ambulation in paraplegics: Effects of long term use of bracing. *Paraplegia*, **22**, 173–181.

Dimitrijevic, M., and Nathan, P. (1970). Study of spasticity in man: Changes in flexion reflex with repetitive stimulation in spinal man. *Brain*, **93**, 743–768.

Dimitrijevic, M., and Nathan, P. (1971). Dishabitation of the flexion reflex in spinal man. *Brain*, **94**, 77–90.

Graupe, D., Kohn, K., Kralj, A., and Basseas, E. (1983). EMG controlled electrical stimulation via EMG signature discrimination for providing certain paraplegics with primitive walking. *J. Biomed. Eng.*, **5**, 220.

Hagood, S., Solomonow, M. Baratta, R.V., Zhou, B., and D'Ambrosia, R. (1990). The effect of joint velocity on the contribution of the antagonist musculature to knee stiffness and laxity. *Am. J. Sports Med.*, **18**, 182–187.

Hirokawa, S., Grimm, M., Le, T., Solomonow, M., Baratta, R.V., Shoji, H., and D'Ambrosia, R. (1990). Energy consumption of paraplegics ambulating with the reciprocating gait orthosis powered by electrical stimulation of the thigh muscles. *Arch. Phys. Med. Rehabil.*, **71**, 687–694.

Kralj, A., and Bajd, T. (1989). In: Functional Electrical Stimulation for Standing and Walking. Boca Raton, FL: CRC Press.

Kralj, A., Bajd, T., Turk, R., Krajnik, J., and Benko, H. (1983). Gait restoration in paraplegic patients: A feasibility demonstration using multi channel surface electrode FES. *J. Rehabil. Res. Dev.*, **20**, 3–20.

Lee, K., and Johnston, R. (1976). Electrically induced flexion reflex in gait training of hemiplegic patients: Induction of the reflex. Arch. Phys. Med. Rehabil., **57**, 311–314.

Marsolais, B., and Edwards, B. (1988). Energy cost of walking and standing with functional neuromuscular stimulation and long leg braces. *Arch. Phys. Med. Rehabil.*, **69**, 243–249.

Marsolais, B., Kobetic, R., and Komp, M. (1988). Illiopsoas stimulation for hip flexion in paralyzed individuals. *Proc. ORS*, 432.

Nene, A., and Patrick, J. (1989). Energy cost of paraplegics locomotion with the ORLAU Parawalker. *Paraplegia*, **27**, 5–18.

Nicol, D., Granat, M., Andrews, B., and Baxendale, R. (1989). Characterization of the flexion withdrawal reflex. *3rd Vienna Workshop on Functional Electrostimulation*, 303–306.

Popovic, D., Tomovic, R., and Schwirtlich, L. (1989). Hybrid assistive system—the motor neuroprosthesis. *IEEE Trans. Biomed. Eng.*, **36**, 729–737.

Rose, G. (1979). The principles and practice of the hip guidance orthosis. *Prosthet. Orthot. Int.*, **3**, 37–43.

Rosman, N., and Spira, E. (1974). Paraplegic use of walking braces: Survey. *Arch. Phys. Med. Rehabil.*, **55**, 306–314.

Solomonow, M. (1984a). External control of the neuromuscular system. *IEEE Trans. Biomed. Eng.*, **31**, 752–763.

Solomonow, M. (1984b). Restoration of movement with electrical stimulation: A contemporary view of the basic problems. *Orthopedics*, 7, 245–250.

Solomonow, M., Baratta, R.V., Hirokawa, S., et al. (1989). The RGO generation II: Muscle stimulation powered orthosis as a practical walking system for paraplegics. *Orthopedics*, **12**, 1309–1315.

Solomonow, M., Baratta, R.V., Shoji, H., and D'Ambrosia, R. (1986). The myoelectric signal of electrically stimulated muscle during recruitment. *IEEE Trans. Biomed. Eng.*, **33**, 735–745.

Solomonow, M., Baratta, R.V., Shoji, H., and D'Ambrosia, R. (1990a). The EMG-force relations of skeletal muscle: Dependence on contraction rate. *EMG Clin. Neurophysiol.*, **30**, 141–152.

Solomonow, M., Baratta, R.V., Zhou, B., and D'Ambrosia, R. (1988). Electromyogram coactivation pattern of the elbow antagonist muscles during slow isokinetic movement. *Exp. Neurol.*, **100**, 470–477.

Solomonow, M., Baratta, R.V., Zhou, B., Shoji, H., and D'Ambrosia, R. (1987). The EMG-force model of electrically stimulated muscle. *IEEE Trans. Biomed. Eng.*, **34**, 692–703.

Solomonow, M., Baten, C., Smit, J., Baratta, R.V., Hermens, H., D'Ambrosia, R., and Shoji, H. (1990b). EMG power spectra frequencies associated with motor units recruitment strategies. *J. Appl. Physiol.*, **68**, 1177–1185.

Solomonow, M., Guzzi, A., Baratta, R.V., Shoji, H., and D'Ambrosia, R. (1986). EMG-force model of the elbow antagonistic muscle pair: Effect of joint position, gravity and recruitment. Am. J. Phys. Med., **65**, 223–244.

Solomonow, M., Shoji, H., D'Ambrosia, R., and Douglas, R. (1985). Electromechanical walking system for paraplegics. *Proc. 7th Ann. Conf. IEEE-EMBS*, 4–7.

Stein, R., Prochazka, A., Popovic, D., Edamura, M., Llewellyn, M., and Davis, L.A. (1990). *Technology Transfer and Development for Walking Using FES in Advances on External Control of Human Extremities*, pp. 161–175. Belgrade: Nauka.

11

Functional Electrical Stimulation for Lower Extremities

DEJAN B. POPOVIĆ

This chapter describes trends in the use of patterned electrical stimulation for restoration of functional movements of lower extremities. In addition to effective applications of Functional Electrical Stimulation (FES) for lower extremities, attention is given to major limitations and difficulties in existing systems and possible future developments. Potential improvement of locomotor function by combining a powered mechanical brace and an FES system, called a Hybrid Assistive System (HAS), is described. The aim is to explain how different techniques can cope with complex problems in a man-machine system. These considerations are classified in three groups: 1) Neuro-musculo-skeletal questions; 2) Technical and technological aspects and 3) Control problems. A broad list of references, helpful for better understanding of FES systems for lower extremities, is included.

A human spinal cord injury (SCI) can cut off the transmission of neural information between the central nervous system (CNS) above the lesion and the CNS and peripheral nerves below the lesion. Such an injury results in muscular paralysis and lack of proprioceptive and exteroceptive sensations. Functional electrical stimulation (FES) can help in regaining limited locomotor activities in numerous humans with paralysis. However, there are many unsolved questions relating to how and when to use FES for locomotion restoration, and what the real benefits of this technique are.

Neuromusculoskeletal questions arise from muscle fatigue, reduced joint torques generated through FES in comparison to CNS-activated torques in healthy subjects, modified reflex activities, spasticity, functional and joint contractures, and osteoporosis and stress fractures. Recent FES systems stimulate motor units (synchronously) with stimulation frequencies above usual physiological values in normal subjects, affecting the duration of FES use because of muscle fatigue (Bigland-Ritchie et al., 1979; Bigland-Ritchie and Woods, 1984; Kralj and Bajd, 1989; McNeal et al., 1989; Solomonow et al., 1983). From animal and human experiments it is evident that low-frequency chronic electrical stimulation is effective in increasing fatigue resistance. This proves that muscle fatigue associated with low-frequency electrical stimulation is of peripheral origin, and that the loss of force is probably due to fatigue of fast-contracting glycolytic fatiguable type-II motor fibers, and is not caused by failure of neuromuscular transmission or conduction of the peripheral nerve (Kralj and Bajd, 1989).

It is impossible to control redundant muscle groups in the same way that the CNS does this, so joint torques are smaller in comparison with healthy subjects. A CNS injury results in modified reflexes (Stein and Capaday, 1988), so numerous unexpected situations may occur, resulting in inappropriate antagonist contractions. In addition, these CNS changes are responsible for the reorganization in tonic and phasic properties of different muscle groups (i.e., spasticity) (Stefanovska et al., 1989). In some applications it may be very difficult to create functional movement because of these changes.

In our own research, these changes sometimes result in an inability to functionally ambulate because of so-called "functional contractures." The term functional contracture relates to lack of performance caused by one joint movement restricting the movement of the neighboring joint. This is probably caused by shortening of the two-joint muscle-tendon systems. Clinical measurements of the joint range of motion usually do not include the testing of this behavior. Joint contractures reduce the range of motion and thus compromise the FES-activated functional movements (Perry, 1981).

Osteoporosis (Lukert, 1982), normally found in SCI patients, may compromise the use of legs for support and may lead to stress fractures (Rafil et al., 1982) if used inappropriately. In the literature there are some speculations that patterned electrical therapy can decrease osteoporosis (Phillips et al., 1984), but recent results with chronic patients have been negative (Leeds et al., 1990). It might still be possible to prevent osteoporosis with chronic stimulation, if applied immediately after the onset of injury. Our recent findings in chronic stimulation indicate that the decrease in bone density may be reduced. These findings are preliminary, because there are no data on bone density in normal humans and we don't have results from a control group.

Technical and technological problems relate to the FES-neuromuscular interface, as well as to biocompatibility and practicality of the FES system. The FES-neuromuscular interface is realized with electrodes. Currently, several different types of electrodes are in use or under development. The least invasive is transcutaneous electrical stimulation with surface electrodes, while other techniques use percutaneous or implanted electrodes. Percutaneous or implanted electrodes are applied to muscles, close to the motor point, or to the nerve directly. The use of other types of electrodes is in its early developmental phase. The use of implanted electrodes and implanted stimulators in totally implanted systems requires the use of biocompatible materials and safe packaging of the device. The important aspect is the pattern of stimulation which will prevent tissue damage and any contamination due to changes on electrodes.

Computer-controlled stimulators are being developed in addition to hand-controlled stimulators. Some stimulators use isolated output stages, requiring two electrodes per channel, while others use one common anode and several cathodes. The trend in the development of stimulators is to use constant-current, monophasic, charge-compensated pulses.

The use of closed-loop control systems requires sensory feedback. Sensory feedback uses artificial sensors (see Chapter 4) or natural sensors. The use of natural sensors is based on recording of neural and muscular activity (see Chapter 5 and Hoffer, 1988).

Practicality of the system relates to the ease of donning and doffing, safety, and reliability. These elements determine how much the system will be used and what is the improvement of the quality of life of the handicapped human.

The difficulties in interfacing artificial and natural control is the third group of questions to be solved for effective and practical FES systems. We should emphasize that basic research results in neurophysiology indicate that computer-oriented analytic control algorithms, like the one used in industrial robots, are not found naturally in animals, including humans. In biological control, the simplest behavioral acts are reflexes (Carew, 1985), machine-like responses that are elicited by particular types of sensory stimuli. The motor system of humans is arranged in hierarchical fashion (Stein and Oguztoreli, 1984). Spinal reflexes modify the most peripheral elements (i.e., the muscles). The spinal cord can also produce some of the basic patterns such as those required for locomotion. Finally, higher centers such as the motor cortex have executive control of the whole motor system. Although such general ideas are widely accepted, the details and specific roles remain obscure. For example, even the simplest spinal pathway, the monosynaptic reflex, varies in a task-specific way during movement (see Chapter 13).

A non-numerical method based on symbolic representation of motion in animals and humans, called artificial reflex control, was proposed (Tomovic, 1984). The term "symbolic" refers here to representation of the motion in the form of discrete events. A discrete event is recognized as a specific sensory pattern occurring during a particular motor activity. The current state of the system and a sensory input define the corresponding functional movement to be executed (Tomovic, 1984; Tomovic et al., 1987). Different variants of such a control system (Andrews et al., 1987, 1988; Joonkers and Schoute, 1990; Mulder et al., 1991; Veltink et al., 1990) are currently under development.

In principle, closed-loop systems offer substantial increases in input-output linearity and repeatability, along with a substantial decrease in the sensitivity of the system to parameter variations (internal disturbances) and load changes (external disturbances). Recently, digital closed-loop methods using proportional (P) and proportional plus integral (PI) controllers were studied for both recruitment and fatigue of muscles. The increase of the loop gain in these controllers improved compensation for variation in muscle properties, but brought the system closer to instability. The effects of the simultaneous control of interpulse interval and pulse width was investigated, and promising results were obtained (Bernotas et al., 1987; Chizeck et al., 1988; Wilhere et al., 1985).

MEDICAL INDICATION AND LEVEL OF IMPAIRMENT WHERE FES CAN BE USED

Our own research indicates that the usual classification of CNS lesions is applicable as a guideline, but is not convenient as a selection criterion for FES candidates. Functional neuromuscular stimulation users and an appropriate FES system should be selected through a functional diagnosis. The term "functional diagnosis" is used to express that the functional status after the injury determines the type of treatment.

General statements about FES systems indicate that it is suitable for subjects with preserved peripheral neuromuscular structures, moderate spasticity, without joint contractures, and with limited osteoporosis. Subjects should be able to control their balance and upper body posture using the upper extremities for assistance (e.g., parallel bar, walker, crutches). Subjects with pathologies affecting the heart, lung, or circulation should be treated with extreme care, and often should not be included in an FES walking program. A satisfactory mental and emotional condition is extremely important, since an FES treatment requires a certain degree of intelligence and understanding of the technical side of the system. High motivation and good cooperation with medical staff is a significant aspect for the efficacy of the FES. Surface stimulation may be applied only in subjects with limited sensation, because it activates pain receptors. Subjects suitable for FES can be found within head and spinal cord injuries, cerebral paralysis, multiple sclerosis, various types of myelitis, and others. Many of these subjects may benefit from other bracing technique regarding their mobility, but there are numerous other benefits for the overall health.

Recently, within the group of paralyzed subjects, the number of functionally incomplete quadriplegics is rising compared to earlier times. This is connected with numerous improvements of emergency and other aspects of medical care. There are individuals within this population (SCI at the cervical level) considered for the FES program. Some of these individuals succeed to perform ambulation and standing.

The application of FES to the restoration of gait was first investigated systematically in Ljubljana, Yugoslavia (Bajd et al., 1982; Gracanin et al., 1967; Kralj et al., 1980, 1987; Vodovnik et al., 1965, 1967). Currently, FES for gait rehabilitation is used in a clinical setting in several rehabilitation centers (Andrews et al., 1988; Brindley et al., 1978; Hermens et al., 1986; Jaeger et al., 1989; Kralj and Bajd, 1989; Marsolais and Kobetic, 1983; Mizrahi et al., 1985; Petrofsky and Phillips, 1983; Solomonow et al., 1989; Stein et al., 1990; Thoma et al., 1987; Vossius et al., 1987; Waters, 1977) and there is a growing trend for the design of devices for home use.

FES SYSTEMS WITH SURFACE ELECTRODES

Current FES systems use various numbers of stimulation channels. The simplest one, from a technical point, is a surface single-channel stimulation system. This system is only suitable for stroke patients and a limited group of incomplete spinal-cord-injured patients. These individuals can perform some ambulation with assistance of the upper extremities without an FES system, although this ambulation may be both modified or impaired or both. The FES in these systems is used to activate a single muscle group. The first demonstrated application of this technique was in stroke patients (Gracanin et al., 1967). The stimulation is applied to ankle dorsiflexors so the "footdrop" can be eliminated. The stimulating electrode is generally placed so that many sensory fibers from the common peroneal nerve are stimulated, in addition to descending motor fibers innervating ankle dorsiflexors. Sensory stimulation can lead to a flexor reflex. In many stroke patients sensation is normal, so the surface stimulation, strong enough to elicit a reflex, is painful. This was the original reason for using a fully implanted system (Waters et al., 1985). In spinal-cord-injured patients, sensation is often absent or reduced, and flexor reflexes can be elicited without causing pain or skin problems.

A multichannel system with a minimum of four channels of FES is required for ambulation of a patient with a complete motor lesion of lower extremities and preserved balance and upper body motor control (Kralj and Bajd, 1989; Petrofsky and Phillips, 1986). Appropriate bilateral stimulation of the quadriceps muscles locks the knees during standing. Stimulating the common peroneal nerve on the ipsilateral side, while switching off the quadriceps stimulation on that side, produces a flexion of the leg. This flexion, combined with adequate movement of the upper body and use of the upper extremities for support, allows ground clearance and is considered as the swing phase of the gait cycle. Hand or foot switches can provide the flexion-extension alternation needed for a slow forward or backward progression. Sufficient arm strength must be available to provide balance in parallel bars (clinical application), and with a rolling walker or crutches (daily use of FES). Interesting research with computer-controlled electrical stimulation was proposed by Petrofsky and his colleagues (Phillips, 1989). The magnitude of electrical pulses was controlled according to sensory feedback from forces and position transducers. This research found application in the development of exercise bicycles and exercise procedures (Petrofsky et al., 1985). The possibility to use biological signals as a trigger signal in an FES system was proposed by Graupe and his collaborators (Graupe and Kohn, 1988). The advantage of Graupe's method was the control of stimulation sequences through an electromyogram (EMG) recorded above the lesion. The recorded EMG was from voluntary contraction of erector spinae and lower back muscles. Four different signals were identified and used in experimental work in a microprocessor FES system. These signals allowed stand-up, sit-down, and left and right leg-up commands (initiation of the swing phase).

ELECTRODES FOR FES

The systems described rely on the use of surface electrodes. A large variety of surface electrodes are now available (Bajd et al., 1982; Bowman and Baker, 1985; McNeal and Baker, 1988). These electrodes are relatively easy to apply and replace, are noninvasive, and in some cases are designed to stay attached for days and even weeks. However, they suffer from the following drawbacks: (1) activation of skin pain receptors underlying an electrode, (2) difficulties of positioning, (3) poor selectivity, (4) insecure fixation on moving limbs, (5) skin irritation, and (6) cosmetics.

These drawbacks of surface electrodes have made it desirable to develop implantable electrodes which are biocompatible and have satisfactory mechanical and electrical properties (Mortimer, 1981, 1987). The implantable electrodes currently in use are: intramuscular, epimysial, nerve cuffs, and intraneural electrodes. Wire intramuscular electrodes are the most commonly used, and are generally inserted through a cannula (Marsolais and Kobetic, 1983, 1987; Handa et al., 1989; Mortimer, 1983, 1987). Positioning and anchoring of the wires are still very uncertain procedures, and incorrect placement, pull-out, corrosion, and encapsulation have frequently led to malfunction of entire FES systems in patients. Epimysial stimulating electrodes sutured to the muscle fascia were recently developed (Grandjean and Mortimer, 1986) and require a full surgical procedure for implantation. Various types of nerve cuff electrodes have been developed (Juch and Minkels, 1989; Naples et al., 1988; Stein et al., 1977; Sweeney and Mortimer, 1986). Open surgery is required for the implantation of nerve cuff electrodes, and after some time they may cause damage to and block conduction in the nerves they enclose. Intraneural electrodes for intrafascicular stimulation and spinal nerve-root stimulation (Bowman and Erickson, 1985; Hoffer and Loeb, 1980; Nannini and Horsh, 1990) are new techniques still in the developmental stage. However, various technical problems associated with the insertion and stability of intraneural electrodes have yet to be overcome.

FES SYSTEMS WITH PERCUTANEOUS ELECTRODES

Multichannel percutaneous systems for gait restoration, with many channels, were suggested by Brindley et al. (1978) and Marsolais and Kobetic (1983, 1987). The main advantage of these systems is the possibility to activate many different muscle groups. A preprogrammed stimulation pattern very similar to the one in a healthy human is delivered to ankle, knee, and hip joints, as well as to paraspinal muscles. The experience of the Cleveland research team suggests that 48 channels are required for a complete SCI walking system to achieve a reasonable walking pattern. Fine-wire intramuscular electrodes (cathodes) are positioned close to the motor point within selected muscles. Knee extensors (rectus femoris, vastus medialis, vastus lateralis, vastus intermedius), hip flexors (sartorius, tensor fasciae latae, gracilis, iliopsoas), hip extensors (semimembranosus, gluteus maximus), hip abductors (gluteus medius), ankle dorsiflexors (tibialis anterior, peroneus longus), ankle plantar flexors (gastrocnemius lateralis and medialis, plantaris, and soleus), and paraspinal muscles are selected for activation. A surface electrode is used as a common anode. Interleaved pulses are delivered with a multichannel, battery-operated, portable stimulator. The hand controller allows the selection of gait activity. These systems are limited to the hospital environment. The application was investigated in complete spinal cord lesions and in stroke patients (Marsolais et al., 1990). The same strategy and selection criteria for implantation were used for both stroke and SCI patients. An eight-channel system was sufficient for stroke patients. An interesting phenomenon of motor control improvement, or "short-term carryover," was demonstrated by some stroke patients and not usually demonstrated by the SCI patient. Short-term carryover refers to changes in neuromuscular activities of impaired structures for a period after the electrical stimulation is discontinued. It is possible to observe improved function for a day or more without the FES device. The repetition of the proper pattern can result in permanent change in the stroke subject.

TOTALLY IMPLANTED FES SYSTEMS

A multichannel totally implanted FES system (Thoma et al., 1983, 1987) was proposed and tested in few subjects. This system uses a 16-channel implantable stimulator and is attached to the epineurium electrodes. Femoral and gluteal nerves were stimulated for hip and knee extension. The so-called "roundabout" stimulation was applied in which four electrodes were located around the nerve and stimulated intermittently. This stimulation method reduces muscle fatigue.

Another interesting approach to multichannel stimulation was suggested recently. Practical artificial control of lower limb muscles for standing and walking in paraplegia requires patterned electrical stimulation of motor axons at some site between the anterior horn cell and the motor endplate. One difficulty has been to devise an adequate, reliable, simple-to-use system which minimizes excessive muscle fatigue. The possibility of using long-term connections to many spinal roots for electrical stimulation for useful leg movements was suggested by Rushton (1990), using intradural electrode arrays to trap up to 12 roots at a time. However, there seem to be several disadvantages to the method. Whole roots gave rather complex movements, while splitting motor roots reduced their viability. There are now over 300 patients with this design of implant for bladder control, which has proved to be safe and reliable (Rushton, 1990). The question is whether a pattern of root stimulation can be found which adequately mimics the normal gait sequence. The sequence of torques and angles is required for the basic components of a synthetic dynamic gait. The EMG recording from the more accessible muscles of the lower limb (not including hip flexors), as well as hip, knee, and ankle angle and floor loading during normal gait was done. This allowed derivation of hip, knee, and ankle torques in the sagittal plane. These diagrams were used to build a sequence of torques, attempting to use single-joint and double-joint muscles appropriately, and using synergists which have the same root value as much as possible. It appears that through the gait-cycle from toe-off to toe-off the sequence of activation of ipsilateral roots is L2-L3-L4-L5-S1-S2-L2-.. (with some overlap). This method is in its pioneering stage.

POWERED HYBRID ASSISTIVE SYSTEMS

At this stage, FES systems are not sufficiently safe and reliable for daily use. A specific approach of integration of two assistive systems (FES and an external mechanical orthosis) was proposed. These systems are called hybrid assistive systems (HAS) or hybrid orthotic systems (HOS) (see Chapter 10). A few possibilities for HAS design have been suggested, combining relatively simple rigid mechanical structures for passive stabilization of lower limbs during stance phase and FES systems. These systems combine use of reciprocal gait orthosis with multichannel stimulation (see Chapter 10), the use of an ankle-foot orthosis or an extended ankle-foot orthosis with a knee cage (Andrews et al., 1987), or the use of a self-fitting modular orthosis (Schwirtlich and Popovic, 1984). A few more sophisticated laboratory systems were demonstrated by Phillips (1989) and Andrews et al. (1989). Each trend in the design of HAS implies different applications as well as specific hardware and control problems. On the basis of accumulated experience, the following features can serve as criteria for a closer description of various HAS designs (Tomovic et al., 1990): (1) partial mechanical support, (2) parallel operation of the biological and mechanical system, and (3) sequential operation of the biological and the mechanical system. The partial mechanical support refers to the use of braces to assist FES only at specific events within a walking cycle (Andrews et al., 1989). Parallel use of two systems assumes permanent exchange of power and control between the biological and mechanical system during a complete gait cycle. Parallel operation of the biological and the mechanical system requires complete dynamical modeling and stored reference joint trajectories of lower limbs and mechanical orthosis segments in the controller. The reason for the use of HAS is, however, compensating for the inadequacy of FES-provoked muscle responses by external supply of power and control to match the desired gait performance. The sequential operation of the biological and the mechanical system, in its pure form, consists of two contiguous phases: (1) a gait segment driven by biological actuators only, and (2) a gait segment driven by mechanical actuators only. Phase (1) is, clearly, under FES control with participation of internal sensorimotor control, if available; phase (2) is supported by the active brace. An overlapping interval must be provided to assure efficient and smooth transfer between these two actions.

We will present a case study to explain reasons for the use of powered HAS.

> Patient B.T., male, 43 years old, suffered a spinal cord injury. He was treated surgically, and since then he has a complete motor paralysis below the level T6. Upper extremities are well developed; the grasp force is limited because of previous fractures of both wrists (during the accident). Paraspinal and back muscles are well preserved above the lesion and minimal activity of the upper part of abdominal muscles exists. Balance in the sitting position, as well as in the standing position is good. Spasticity is moderate and the patient does not use any antispastic drugs. The x-ray and CT scans show no stress fractures or other deformities, and limited osteoporosis. We considered him as a good candidate for the FES system. The multichannel FES treatment pointed to a lower motor neuron lesion, which prevented functional movements. This fact imposed inclusion of the powered external brace to compensate for FES inadequacy. The powered HAS (PHAS) integrated: (1) multichannel electronic stimulator with surface electrodes, (2) powered external brace, (3) microcontroller, (4) sensors.
>
> At the point of admittance to the Rehabilitation Institute his muscles were very weak, spasticity was moderate, and no contractures were registered. Using a slightly modified four-channel FES procedure (Kralj and Bajd, 1989) he was prepared to start standing and walking. Simultaneously, B.T. was included in the program for standing and walking with callipers in parallel bars. Initially, we carefully checked the bone and joint status. Once B.T. learned to perform a swing-through gait in parallel bars we switched him to a nonpowered, self-fitting, modular orthosis (SFMO) (Popovic, 1986). He was taught to don and doff the SFMO on his own, to transfer with it from the bed to the wheelchair, and to stand up from the wheelchair into the parallel bars. Functional improvement was not achieved because of the lower motor neuron injury. We added the powered hip joint, and the electrically controlled locking device at the knee joint of the SFMO (Popovic et al., 1989; Schwirtlich and Popovic, 1984). The control method for this brace was suggested by Tomovic et al. (1990).

FUNCTIONAL ELECTRICAL STIMULATION FOR LOWER EXTREMITIES

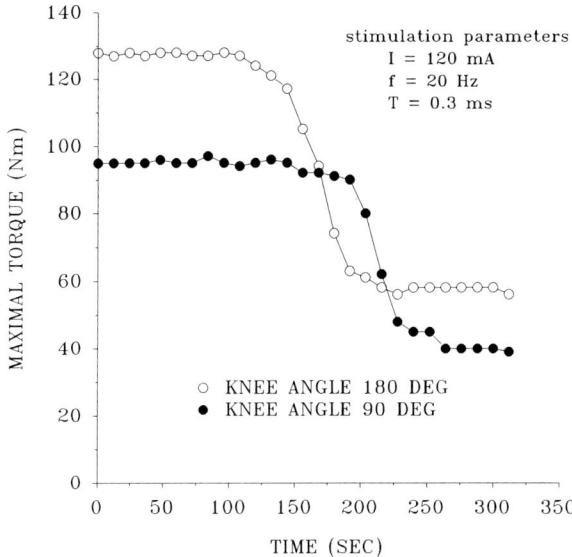

Figure 11–1 Maximal knee-joint torque when quadriceps muscle, was stimulated with two large surface electrodes. The contractile force started to decrease from its maximal value (M_{max} = 127 Nm) after about 2 minutes, for measurements done in flexed position (90°). The contractile force decreased from its maximal value (M_{max} = 95 Nm) after 204 seconds in the extended position. The torque was reduced to 50% of its initial value after 192 seconds in the flexed position, and after 264 seconds in the fully extended position. Stimulus parameters were fixed during stimulation (I = 120 mA, IPI = 50 msec, T = 300 μsec). (From Popovic et al., 1990, with permission.)

Results with the Four-Channel FES System

Maximal torque generated in the knee joint (Figure 11–1) when quadriceps muscle was stimulated with two large surface electrodes reached a maximal value of 127 Nm and started decreasing after 132 seconds when measured in a flexed position (90°). The lower trace, when the knee is extended (180°) starts to decrease from its maximal value of 95 Nm after 204 seconds. The torque was reduced to 50% of its initial value after 192 seconds in a flexed position, and after 264 seconds in the fully extended position. Stimulus parameters were fixed during stimulation (I = 120 mA, IPI = 50 msec, T = 300 μsec).

Figure 11–2 presents the duration of full extension of the knee joint, with a loaded thigh (resistive torque 12 Nm obtained with sand bags at the ankle joint). The left leg was slightly less fatigable, flexing by more than 20° at just about 4 minutes, compared to 3 minutes and 40 seconds for the right leg.

An important movement, although rather difficult to measure, is stimulated hip flexion and extension. We measured these movements while the subject was standing. Hip flexion obtained through a withdrawal reflex involved a painful and uncontrollable dorsiflexion, external rotation and eversion of the foot, and knee flexion. This was completely inadequate for the swing phase. The stimulation strength was selected for the desired knee and ankle movement. Maximal recorded hip flexion for such a movement was less than 35°. Our computer simulation indicates that reasonable gait

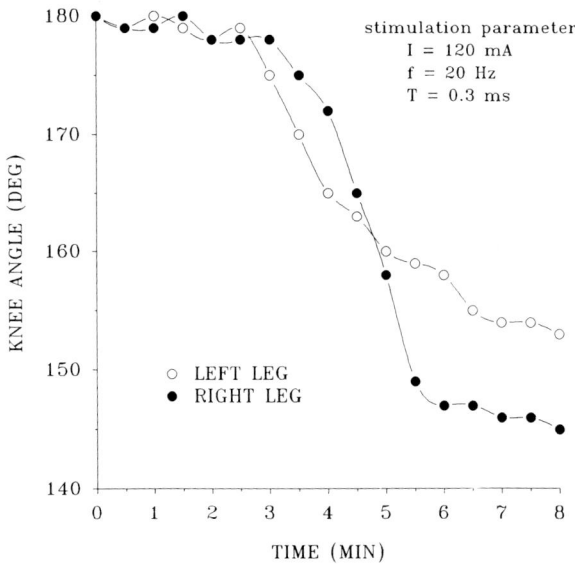

Figure 11–2 The uninterrupted stimulation of quadriceps muscle with constant-current monophasic compensated pulses (I = 120 mA, IPI = 50 msec, T = 300 μsec). The shank of the leg was horizontal, and it was loaded with a sand bag (m = 4 kg) at 30 cm from the knee axis. As expected, asymmetry between the legs was found, and the maximal duration was limited to less than 4 minutes. (From Popovic et al., 1990, with permission.)

speed requires a hip flexion angle of at least 50°. The average angular speed measured at the hip joint was less than 0.5 radian/s, which is also unacceptable for the gait speed required (Figure 11–3).

The maximal recorded gait speed was 0.28 m/s, the maximal distance was limited to six lengths of parallel bars (30 m), including turning around at both ends of the parallel bars, and the maximal standing period was less than 5 minutes. The patient was able to stand up from sitting position and to maintain upright posture in parallel bars more than four times, in series, standing every time for at least 3 minutes, while resting for 5 minutes between standing periods.

Results with the Use of PHAS

There is no need to measure the muscle fatigue because of the presence of the brace mechanism in the knee joint and a fully controllable hip joint. The brace limits the ankle movement and acts partially as a foot reaction orthosis. Our main concern was how much we could increase hip function with the powered external brace. With the motor selected we succeeded in increasing the maximal hip flexion to 50° and in increasing the angular speed to 1.2 radian/s, which is still much less than in normal individuals. The angular velocity was limited because of the need to design a portable, battery-operated system, and to maintain the safety of the patient skin, tissue, and bones. Maximal standing was prolonged to at least 30 minutes, and it depended only on overall patient fitness. The maximal distance of gait was prolonged to 100 m. The maximal measured speed in parallel bars was 0.7 m/s, while with the walker was still rather low, v = 0.47 m/s.

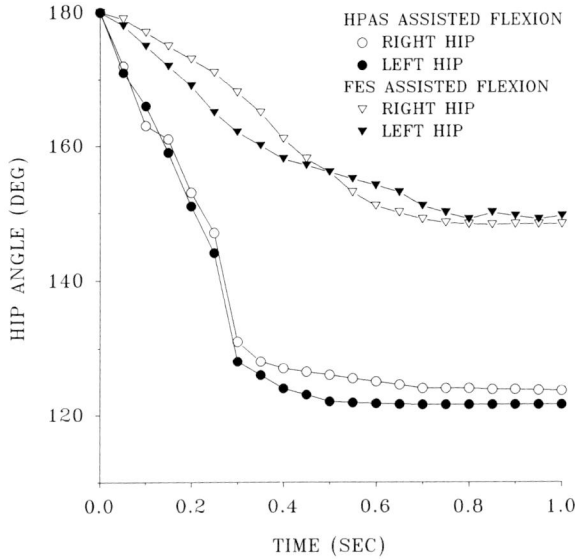

Figure 11-3 The angular changes in the hip joint while standing in a fully erect position. Lower traces are for the FES-generated movement in the left and right legs, and upper traces for the PHAS-generated movements in both legs. The use of PHAS, as expected, provided bigger hip flexion and corresponding angular velocity. The criterion for the set-up of the stimulation strength was the knee angle and ankle movement during the elicited movement. (From Popovic et al., 1990, with permission.)

One of the most interesting results is presented in Figure 11-4, which shows the angular changes in the gait cycle with the four-channel FES system and PHAS. The greater stride length, the higher cycle rate, and greater hip flexion all indicate the value for the use of the PHAS.

These results are included to describe how a powered brace can improve functioning of the assistive system. The results show that a powered and controlled external mechanical brace can replace FES during static phases of the locomotion activities (e.g., standing) and that it can produce functional movements when FES is not effective. In this way a powered mechanical brace used sequentially with FES increases the assistance of the system. However, the increased functional value is compromised at this stage of development because of the system's complexity. Often, the use of the FES and powered mechanical brace surpasses the so-called "gadget tolerance" of the patient.

CONTROL METHODS FOR STANDING AND GAIT

Many control FES algorithms for lower extremities have been developed in the last decade. The first control algorithms applied to FES systems for gait restoration were of the open-loop type. Open-loop control assumes a complete knowledge of the system and its behavior in different environmental conditions. Only a simplified "hand switch" control and preprogrammed automatic control mechanisms have been applied so far. Available data on gait performance of paralyzed individuals are often

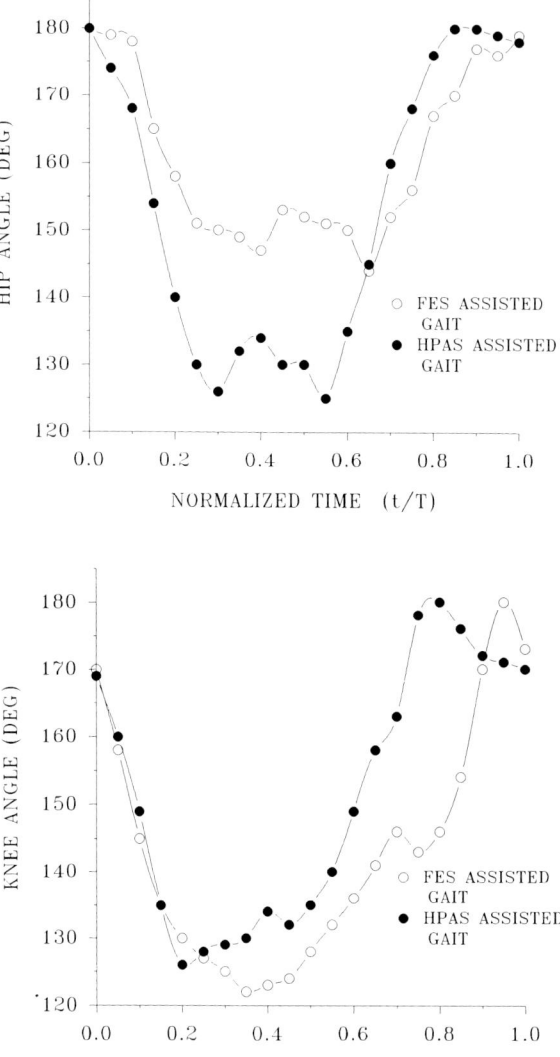

Figure 11–4 The knee and hip angles during a normalized gait cycle. The gait cycle with FES was $T = 2.06$ sec, while with PHAS it was shorter, $T = 1.29$ sec. The average record from 50 steps is presented. The step length was 0.64 m with FES, and 0.88 m with PHAS. Knee movements were very similar, but the difference occurred in hip movements. Bigger flexion and faster movement were obtained when applying PHAS, so a faster gait was achieved. The speed was $v_{PHAS} = 0.682$ m/s, $v_{FES} = 0.31$ m/s. (From Popovic et al., 1990, with permission.)

inadequate, which makes the application of the open-loop controllers in rehabilitation very difficult. In addition to the difficulties mentioned above, individual properties such as muscle fatigue, spasticity, joint contractures, and muscle denervation must be modeled quantitatively for the synthesis of an open-loop controller. Most of control systems adopted the principle of memorized and triggered FES sequences. These sequences are based on recorded average EMG patterns in normal individuals

(Marsolais and Kobetic, 1983; Thoma et al., 1983). Direct, computer-controlled electrical stimulation was proposed by the Cleveland group (Chizeck et al., 1988), emphasizing muscular properties and a discrete event model with control goals for restoring locomotion functions.

Some investigators have introduced formal modeling to solve global issues such as standing stability, control strategies, feedback design (Khang and Zajac, 1989), or synthesis of rhythmic joint trajectories for gait (Hemami et al., 1989). Kralj et al. (1990) proposed the synthesis of FES sequences on an execution level after the required joint torques were determined. It is important to mention that the open-loop control relates to activation of the FES system, but the upper part of the body, including the hands and arms over the parallel bars, walker, or crutches, actually works as a correction mechanism and provides feedback control. The preserved voluntary motor control above the lesion allows the use of open-loop control, because the compensatory forces and movements can be accomplished. A certain programming (feed-forward) control is required for fast movements and it is very convenient for cyclic motions. However, the environmental changes in addition to muscle fatigue decrease the efficacy of the feed-forward control.

CLOSED-LOOP CONTROL SYSTEMS

The second approach, which has been suggested and is used for some present FES systems, involves closed-loop control, which relies on the use of feedback. When introducing feedback, questions arise about the nature and quality of sensors and their applicability in real time. Two different feedback approaches exist. One is based on natural sensors (e.g., myoelectric activity) as a source of control signals (Graupe and Kohn, 1988; see also Chapter 5, this volume). The second analytic closed-loop control method uses artificial sensory feedback (Crago et al., 1986). What actually matters is not just the output of sensors, but their overall properties. Man-machine systems are in great need of distributed matrix-type sensory systems with high resolution. Several strategies were tested for FES systems. At Wright State University, computer-controlled walking incorporating feedback principles was proposed (Petrofsky et al., 1984).

Tomovic (1984) proposed a closed-loop, non-numerical, control method, called artificial reflex control (ARC). Artificial reflex control refers to a skill-based expert using rules that have an *If-Then* structure (Popovic et al., 1991). The cyclic locomotor activity is presented as a sequence of discrete events. Each of these discrete events is associated with a unique sensory pattern. A sensory pattern occurring during particular motor activity is recognized with the use of artificial and/or natural sensors. The specific discrete event is called the "state of the system," by analogy to the state of a finite-state automata. A recognized sensory pattern during a specified state of the system initiates corresponding functional movement (Tomovic, 1984; Tomovic et al., 1987). This skill-based expert system is of the *On-Off* type and does not consider explicitly the system dynamics. The ARC method belongs to a group of so-called "rule-based" control methods.

A rule-based control system has a hierarchical structure. The highest level is under volitional control of the user. Automatic adaptation to environmental changes and modes of gait is realized using artificial reflex control. The execution of the artificial reflex has to be tuned for smooth functional movements. Digital closed-loop methods using proportional (P) and proportional plus integral (PI) controllers should be used at the lowest actuator level of control (Chizeck et al., 1988).

Advantages of this hierarchical control method are: (1) adaptivity, (2) modularity, (3) ease of application, and (4) possibility of integration into a man-machine system. The latter is of greatest interest. Man-machine integration implies that numerous functions are volitionally controlled by the intact part of the SCI patient, depending, for example, on his current training, ability, skill, and environment. These volitionally started movements will be recognized by a controller and included in the machine part of the control. Volitionally initiated movements occur also in paralyzed extremities due to gravitational and inertial forces, as well as to the modified reflex activities mentioned above.

Rule-based control was tested in hybrid assistive systems (Andrews et al., 1989; Popovic and Schwirtlich, 1987; Popovic et al., 1990; Tomovic et al., 1990). Phillips (1989) proposed an interactive principle for controlling a hybrid gait system. Different variants of rule-based control can be found in the recent literature (Andrews et al., 1987, 1988; Joonkers and Schoute, 1990; Mulder et al., 1991; Phillips, 1990; Veltink et al., 1990).

This brief review of control principles proposed and applied for control of gait raises the question: "Why have so many different control systems not solved the problem adequately?" Regardless of the technology or control principle utilized, it can be concluded that the achievements (including practicality, gait quality, endurance, and efficiency) in complete SCI patients, are very similar. The simplest control mode in which the patient himself is controlling the FES timing (Kralj and Bajd, 1989) provides comparable results to the rather complicated computerized systems. The basic difference between available systems is the gait speed and distance of locomotion.

Advances in control theory and computer sciences give new hope that important breakthroughs into the understanding of life phenomena may be accomplished. However, the basic issues relating man and machine interface have remained unsolved. No evidence has been produced that control theory, relying on analytical and computer tools, can replace motor control or the performance of the nervous system. The complexity of biological entities is beyond the reach of the mathematical control theory in its present form. Dynamical systems, whose variables are linked by a fixed functional relation, have the great advantage that their past and future behavior may be determined analytically or by computer procedures, once the mapping operator is known. However, man-machine systems do not belong to this class, since they contain many stochastic time-varying elements. Thus, mathematical modeling produces the best results only when applied to limited periods and structures. The advent of the computer was helpful in establishing new directions in the study of man-machine relations. Great progress in the understanding of similarities and differences between the machine and the biological systems were made possible when ways to transfer knowledge from the man to the machine were developed. Symbol processing has been used in artificial intelligence (AI) to extend computer power in the cognitive direction, while neural networks (NN) simulate the functions of the nervous system by connectivism. The term "symbol processing" is used to express that the behavior of the dynamical system is modeled using symbols, rather than numerical values. Opinions about the computer's capabilities to reproduce activities of the nervous system are currently quite divided. Both optimistic and pessimistic forecasts are found in the scientific community. Such discussions are to a large extent arbitrary, unless a fuller understanding of the skeletoneuromuscular system exists.

PROSPECTIVE

The aim of this chapter was to review methods of patterned electrical stimulation for restoration of locomotor functions. This type of patterned electrical stimulation is meant to allow paralyzed humans to perform limited bipedal activities. Therapeutic effects of electrical stimulation should improve overall health conditions, and functional effects should improve the quality of life of paralyzed humans.

Handicapped humans need practical, portable, reliable systems. The system should be easy to don and doff and to use daily at home. Available FES systems meet many of these requirements, but still suffer from several drawbacks. The small number of FES system users (on a daily basis) is a significant indicator that these systems are not perfect. Recent neurophysiological findings on muscle properties and strengthening techniques, in addition to improved percutaneous or implantable stimulators, will increase the applicability of FES systems. Major limitations in daily use are connected with insufficiently adaptive and robust control methodologies for FES systems. The complexity of CNS control and the interface between voluntary control and external artificial control are still challenging, unsolved questions. Closed-loop control methods, combining symbolic models at the highest level and analytic models at lower levels, give hope for further progress.

The controller should allow the user to ambulate while concentrating on his normal daily activities, not on controlling the system. Sensory feedback is essential for effective closed-loop control. In addition to artificial sensors, hopes are directed toward the use of natural sensors and the development of an "intelligent" movement controller. There will be further and better applications of FES systems, but some patients will still require a certain degree of external mechanical bracing. The major reason for the use of HAS is safety. Some of the handicapped may improve and extend their locomotion activities with the use of HAS. The bulk of an external mechanical brace, poor cosmesis, increased power consumption, and gadget tolerance are limiting factors for the hybrid assistive system.

There are limitations for the effective use of FES systems. These limitations are connected with peripheral lesions, skin and tissue sensitivity, severe spasticity, poor vision and hearing, obesity, pressure sores, and deficit in the autonomic system, among others. Finally, we would like to mention that FES and HAS are techniques under development and that several research and development centers throughout the world will no doubt present interesting and important results on their clinical and daily use in the near future.

REFERENCES

Andrews, B.J., Baxendale, R.M., Barnett, R.W., Phillips, G.F., Paul, J.P., and Freeman, P.A. (1987). A hybrid orthosis for paraplegics incorporating feedback control. In: D.

Popovic, ed., *Advances in External Control of Human Extremities IX*, pp. 297–311. Belgrade: ETAN.

Andrews, B.J., Baxendale, R.H., Barnett, R., Phillips, G.F., Yamazaki, T., Paul, J.P., and Freeman, P. (1988). Hybrid FES orthosis incorporating closed loop control and sensory feedback. *J. Biomed. Eng.*, **10**, 189–195.

Andrews, B.J., Barnett, R.W., Phillips, G.F., Kirkwood, C.A., Donaldson, N., Rushton, D.N., and Perkins, T.A. (1989). Rule-based control of a hybrid FES orthosis for assisting paraplegic locomotion. *Automedica*, **11**, 175–199.

Bajd, T., Kralj, A., and Turk, R. (1982). Standing-up of a healthy subject and a paraplegic patient, *J. Biomech.*, **15**, 1–10.

Bernotas, L., Crago, P.E., and Chizeck, H.J. (1987). Adaptive control of electrically stimulated muscle. *IEEE Trans. Biomed. Eng.*, **34**, 140–147.

Bigland-Ritchie, B., Jones, D.A., and Woods, J.J. (1979). Excitation frequency and muscle fatigue: Electrical responses during human voluntary and stimulated contractions. *Exp. Neurol.*, **64**, 414.

Bigland-Ritchie, B., and Woods, J.J. (1984). Changes in muscle contractile properties and neural control during human muscular fatigue. *Muscle Nerve*, **7**, 691.

Bowman, B., and Baker, L. (1985). Effects of waveform parameters on comfort during transcutaneous neuromuscular electrical stimulation. *Ann. Biomed. Eng.*, **13**, 59–74.

Bowman, R.B., and Erickson, R.C. (1985). Acute and chronic implantation of coiled wire intraneural electrodes during cyclical electrical stimulation. *Ann. Biomed. Eng.*, **13**, 75–93.

Brindley, G.S., Polkey, C.E., and Rushton, D.N. (1978). Electrical splinting of the knee in paraplegia. *Paraplegia*, **16**, 428–435.

Carew, T.J. (1985). The control of reflex action. In: E. Kandel and J. Schwartz, eds., *Principles of Neural Science*, 2nd edition, pp. 457–468. New York: Elsevier.

Chizeck, H.J., Kobetic, R., Marsolais, E.B., Abbas, J.J., Donner, I.H., and Simon, E. (1988). Control of functional neuromuscular stimulation system for standing and locomotion in paraplegics. *Proc. IEEE*, **76**, 1155–1165.

Crago, P.E., Chizeck, H.J., Neuman, M.R., and Hambrecht, F.T. (1986). Sensors for use with functional neuromuscular stimulation. *IEEE Trans. Biomed. Eng.*, **33**, 256–268.

Gracanin, F., Prevec, T., and Trontelj, J. (1967). Evaluation of use of functional electronic peroneal brace in hemiparetic patients. In: *Advances in External Control of Human Extremities III*, pp. 198–210. Dubrovnik.

Grandjean, P.A., and Mortimer, J.T. (1986). Recruitment properties of monopolar and bipolar epimysial electrodes. *Ann. Biomed. Eng.*, **14**, 53–66.

Graupe, D., and Kohn, K. (1988). A critical review of EMG-controlled electrical stimulation in paraplegics. *CRC Crit. Rev. Biomed. Eng.*, **15**, 187–210.

Handa, Y., Hoshimiya, H., Iguchi, Y., and Oda, T. (1989). Development of percutaneous intramuscular electrode for multichannel FES system. *IEEE Trans. Biomed. Eng.*, **36**, 705–710.

Hemami, H., Baj, J.S., and Evans, J.B. (1989). A preliminary study of rhythmic movement. *Automedica*, **11**, 71–89.

Hermens, H.J., Mulder, A.K., Tijhaar, W.H., Heijden, G.V.D., and Zilvold, G. (1986). Research on electrical stimulation with surface electrodes. *Proc. of the 2nd Vienna Int. Workshop on Functional Electrostimulation*, pp. 321–324. Vienna.

Hoffer, J.A., and Loeb, G.E. (1980). Implantable electrical and mechanical interfaces with nerve and muscle. *Ann. Biomed. Eng.*, **8**, 351–360.

Hoffer, J.A. (1988). Closed loop, implant sensor, functional electrical stimulation system for partial restoration of motor functions. United States Patent [19], *Patent Number 4,750,499*, June 14.

Jaeger, R., Yarkony, G.Y., and Smith, R. (1989). Standing the spinal cord injured patient by electrical stimulation: Refinement of a protocol for clinical use. *IEEE Trans. Biomed. Eng.*, **36**, 720–728.

Joonkers, H., and Schoute, A.L. (1990). High-level control of FES-assisted walking using path expressions. In: D. Popovic, ed., *Advances in External Control of Human Extremities X*, pp. 21–38. Belgrade: Nauka.

Juch, P.J.W., and Minkels, R.F. (1989). The strap-electrode: A stimulating and recording electrode for small nerves. *Brain Res. Bull.*, **22**, 917–918.

Khang, G., and Zajac, F.E. (1989). Paraplegic standing controlled by functional neuromuscular stimulation: Part I—computer model and control system design. *IEEE Trans. Biomed. Eng.*, **36**, 873–894.

Kralj, A., Bajd, T., and Turk, R. (1980). Electrical stimulation providing functional use of paraplegic patient muscles. *Med. Prog. Technol.*, **7**, 3–9.

Kralj, A., Bajd, T., Turk, R., and Benko, H. (1987). Results of FES application to 71 SCI patients. In: *Proc. of RESNA 10th Annual Conference on Rehabilitation Technology*, pp. 645–647. San Jose, CA.

Kralj, A., Bajd, T., Turk, R., and Munih, M. (1987). Mathematical synthesis of FES sequences. In: D. Popovic, ed., *Advances in External Control of Human Extremities IX*, pp. 249–260. Belgrade: ETAN.

Kralj, A., and Bajd, T. (1989). *Functional Electrical Stimulation, Standing and Walking after Spinal Cord Injury*. Boca Raton, FL: CRC Press.

Kralj, A., Bajd, T., and Munih, M. (1990). Model based FES control utilizing formal and natural like synthesis of muscle activation. In: D. Popovic, ed., *Advances in External Control of Human Extremities X*, pp. 55–66. Belgrade: Nauka.

Leeds, E.M., Klose, K.J., Gang, W., Serafini, A., and Green, B. (1990). Bone mineral density after bicycle ergometry training. *Arch. Phys. Med. Rehabil.*, **71**, 207–209.

Lukert, B. (1982). Osteoporosis—a review and update. *Arch. Phys. Med. Rehabil.*, **63**, 480–484.

Marsolais, E.B., and Kobetic, R. (1983). Functional walking in paralyzed patients by means of electrical stimulation. *Clin. Orthop.*, **175**, 30–36.

Marsolais, E.B., and Kobetic, R. (1987). Implantation techniques and experience with percutaneous intramuscular electrode in the lower extremities. *J. Rehabil. Res.*, **23**, 1–8.

Marsolais, E.B., Kobetic, R., and Jacobs, J. (1990). Comparison of FES treatment in the stroke and spinal cord injury patient. In: D. Popovic, ed., *Advances in External Control of Human Extremities X*, pp. 213–218. Belgrade: Nauka.

McNeal, D.R., and Baker, L. (1988). Effects of joint angle, electrodes and waveform on electrical stimulation of the quadriceps and hamstrings. *Ann. Biomed. Eng.*, **16**, 299–310.

McNeal, D.R., Nakai, R.J., Meadows, P., and Tu, W. (1989). Open-loop control of the freely-swinging paralyzed leg. *IEEE Trans. Biomed. Eng.*, **36**, 895–905.

Mizrahi, J., Braun, Z., Najenson, T., and Graupe, D. (1985). Quantitative weight bearing and gait evaluation of paraplegics using functional electrical stimulation. *Med. Biol. Eng. Comput.*, **23**, 101–107.

Mortimer, J.T. (1981). Motor prostheses. In: *Handbook of Physiology—The Nervous system II*, pp. 155–187. Baltimore: Williams & Wilkins.

Mortimer, T. (1983). Functional neural stimulation—Neural Prosthesis Program. *Contract #No1-NS-0-2330*, Washington, DC: NIH, Prog. Rep., September 1.

Mortimer, T. (1987). Intramuscular electrodes—Neural Prosthesis Program. *Contract #No1-NS-4-2362*, Washington, DC: NIH, Prog. Rep., August 1.

Mulder, A.J., Boom, H.B.K., Hermens, H.J., and Zilvold, G. (1991). Artificial reflex stimulation for FES induced standing with minimum quadriceps force. *Med. Biol. Eng. Comput.*, in press.

Nannini, N., and Horsh, K. (1990). Muscle recruitment with intrafascicular electrodes. *IEEE Trans. Biomed. Eng.*, **38**, 122–128.

Naples, G.G., Mortimer, J.T., Schreiner, A., and Sweeney, J.D. (1988). A spinal nerve cuff electrode for peripheral nerve stimulation. *IEEE Trans. Biomed. Eng.*, **35**, 905–916.

Perry, J. (1981). Rehabilitation of spasticity. In: R.G. Feldman, R.R. Young, and W.P. Koella, eds. *Spasticity, Disordered Motor Control*, p. 87. Chicago: New Book Medical Publishers.

Petrofsky, J.S., and Phillips, C.A. (1983). Computer controlled walking in the paralyzed individual. *J. Neurol. Orthop. Surg.*, **4**, 153–164.

Petrofsky, J.S., Heaton, H.H., and Phillips, C.A. (1984). Leg exerciser for training of paralysed muscle by closed-loop control. *Med. Biol. Eng. Comput.*, **22**, 298–303.

Petrofsky, J.S., Phillips, C.A., Larson, P., and Douglas, R. (1985). Computer synthesised walking. *J. Neurol. Orthop. Med. Surg.*, **6**, 219–230.

Petrofsky, J.S., and Phillips, C.A. (1986). Closed-loop control of movement of skeletal muscle. *CRC Crit. Rev. Biomed. Eng.*, **13**, 35–96.

Phillips, C.A., Petrofsky, J.S., Hendershot, D.M., and Stafford, D. (1984). Functional electrical exercise—a comprehensive approach for physical conditioning of the spinal cord injured patients. *Orthopedics*, **7**, 1112–1114.

Phillips, C.A. (1989). An interactive system of electronic stimulators and gait orthosis for walking in the spinal cord injured. *Automedica*, **11**, 247–261.

Phillips, G.F. (1990). Finite state description language: A new tool for writing stimulator controllers. In: D. Popovic, ed., *Advances in External Control of Human Extremities X*, pp. 39–54. Belgrade: Nauka.

Popovic, D. (1986). Technical and clinical evaluation of the self fitting modular orthoses. *Final Report, Project No 432*, Washington, DC: NIDRR.

Popovic, D., Tomovic, R., and Schwirtlich, L. (1989). Hybrid assistive system—neuroprosthesis for motion. *IEEE Trans. Biomed. Eng.*, **36**, 729–738.

Popovic, D., Schwirtlich, L., and S. Radosavljevic. (1990). Powered hybrid assistive system. In: D. Popovic, ed., *Advances in External Control of Human Extremities X*, pp. 177–187. Belgrade: Nauka.

Popovic, D., Tomovic, R., Tepavac, D., and Schwirtlich, L. (1991). Control aspects of active above-knee prosthesis. *Int. J. Man Machine Studies*, **35**, 751–767.

Rafil, M., Firosnia, M., Golimbu, C., and Sokolow, J. (1982). Bilateral acetabular stress fractures in a paraplegic patient. *Arch. Phys. Med. Rehabil.*, **63**, 240–246.

Rushton, D.N. (1990). Choice of nerves or roots for multichannel leg-controller implant. In: D. Popovic, ed., *Advances in External Control of Human Extremities X*, pp. 99–108. Belgrade: Nauka.

Schwirtlich, L., and Popovic, D. (1984). Hybrid orthoses for deficient locomotion. In: D. Popovic, ed., *Advances in External Control of Human Extremities VIII*, pp. 23–32. Belgrade: ETAN.

Solomonow, M., Eldred, E., Lyman, J., and Foster, J. (1983). Control of muscle contractile force through indirect high-frequency stimulation. *Am. J. Physiol.*, **62**, 71–82.

Solomonow, M.R., Baratta, R., Shoji, D., D'Ambrosia, N., Rightar, W., Walker, R., and Beandette, R. (1989). FES powered reciprocating gait orthosis for paraplegic locomotion. *Proc. Vienna Int. Workshop on Electrical Stimulation*, 81.

Stefanovska, A., Vodovnik, L., Gros, N., Rebersek, S., and Acimovic-Janezic, R. (1989). FES and Spasticity. *IEEE Trans. Biomed. Eng.*, **36**, 738–745.

Stein, R.B., Nichols, T.R., Jhamandas, J., Davis, L., and Charles, D. (1977). Stable long-term recordings from cat peripheral nerves. *Brain Res.*, **128**, 21–38.

Stein, R.B., and Oguztoreli, M.N. (1984). Modification of muscle responses by spinal circuitry. *Neuroscience*, **11**, 231–240.
Stein, R.B., and Capaday, C. (1988). The modulation of human reflexes during functional motor tasks. *Trends Neurosci.*, **11**, 328–332.
Stein, R.B., Prochazka, A., Popovic, D., Edamura, M., Llewellyn, M.G.M., and Davis, L.A. (1990). Technology transfer and development for walking using functional electrical stimulation. In: D. Popovic, ed., *Advances in External Control of Human Extremities X*, pp. 161–176. Belgrade: Nauka.
Sweeney, J.D., and Mortimer, J.T. (1986). An asymmetric two electrode cuff for generation of unidirectionally propagated action potentials. *IEEE Trans. Biomed. Eng.*, **33**, 541–549.
Thoma, H., Benzer, H. Bruber, H., Holle, J., Kern, H., Reiner, E., Schwanda, G., and Stoehr, H., (1983). First implantation of a 16-channel electric stimulation device in human. *Trans. Am. Soc. Artif. Int. Organs*, Toronto.
Thoma, H., Frey, M., Hole, J., Kern, H., Mayr, W., Schwanda, G., and Stoehr, H. (1987). Functional neurostimulation to substitute locomotion in paraplegia patients. In: J.D. Andrade, ed., *Artificial Organs*, pp. 515–529. New York: VCH Publishers Inc.
Tomovic, R. (1984). Control of assistive systems by external reflex arcs. In: D. Popovic, ed., *Advances in External Control of Human Extremities IX*, pp. 7–21. Dubrovnik.
Tomovic, R., Popovic, D., and Tepavac, D. (1987). Adaptive reflex control of assistive systems. In: *Advances in External Control of Human Extremities IX*, pp. 207–214. Belgrade: ETAN.
Tomovic, R., Popovic, D., and Tepavac, D. (1990). Rule based control of sequential hybrid assistive systems. In: D. Popovic, ed., *Advances in External Control of Human Extremities X*, pp. 11–20. Belgrade: Nauka.
Veltink, P.H., Koopman, A.F.M., and Mulder, A.J. (1990). Control of cyclical lower leg movements generated by FES. In: D. Popovic, ed., *Advances in External Control of Human Extremities X*, pp. 81–90. Belgrade: Nauka.
Vodovnik, L., and McLeod, W.D. (1965). Electronic detours of broken nerve paths. *Med. Electr.*, **20**, 110–116.
Vodovnik, L., Crochetiere, W.J., and Reswick, J.B. (1967). Control of a skeletal joint by electrical stimulation of antagonists. *Med. Biol. Eng.*, **5**, 97–109.
Vossius, G., Mueschen, U., and Hollander, H.J. (1987). Multichannel stimulation of the lower extremities with surface electrodes. In: D. Popovic, ed., *Advances in External Control of Human Extremities IX*, pp. 193–203. Belgrade: ETAN.
Waters, R.L., McNeal, D.R., Fallon, W., and Clifford, B. (1985). Functional electrical stimulation of the peroneal nerve for hemiplegia. *J. Bone Joint Surg.*, **67**, 792–793.
Waters, R.L. (1977). Electrical stimulation of the peroneal and femoral nerve in man, In: F.T. Hambrecht and J.B. Reswick, eds. *Functional Electrical Stimulation: Application in Neural Prostheses*, pp. 55–64. Marcel Dekker, New York.
Wilhere, G.F., Crago, P.E., and Chizeck, H.J. (1985). Design and evaluation of a digital closed-loop controller for the regulation of muscle force by recruitment modulation. *IEEE Trans. Biomed. Eng.*, **32**, 668–676.

12

Control of Multijoint Lower Limb Motor Tasks with Functional Neuromuscular Stimulation

SCOTT TASHMAN AND FELIX E. ZAJAC

Functional neuromuscular stimulation (FNS) of paralyzed muscles can restore standing, walking, and other mobility tasks to spinal cord injured (SCI) individuals. Current FNS systems are, however, not yet clinically implementable, partly because they demand high metabolic energy consumption from the SCI user. For example, these systems are unable to provide fast enough walking for long-enough distances with little muscle fatigue. These existing FNS systems rely on open-loop control only. Storing muscle stimulation patterns in computer memory for later recall by a computer-based open-loop controller is, therefore, inadequate by itself to control intermuscular coordination and multijoint movement. Feedback (closed-loop) control systems are designed to generate (or augment ongoing) muscle stimulation strategies during task execution by monitoring limb position and other variables with sensors. These feedback data are interpreted during task execution within a framework of musculoskeletal biomechanics and controller objectives. Tasks should be executed more efficiently with feedback than with open-loop FNS-control systems, giving SCI individuals greater walking speed and range with less muscle fatigue. Computer models of the complex dynamical musculoskeletal system are required, however, to design feedback FNS-control systems. The computer-simulated performance of a feedback of FNS controller can be assessed by how well a model of the body responds to unexpected perturbations and to modeling errors (e.g., walking over uneven terrain, and underestimation of body weight, respectively). Only the most promising FNS-control systems, therefore, will have to be built and clinically tested. Recent musculoskeletal modeling and simulation studies suggest that hybrid-FNS systems, which supplement FNS with external orthoses, can reduce controller complexity, enhance stability, and protect joints. We believe hybrid-FNS systems have the greatest potential in the near term for restoring functional ambulation.

Researchers study the control of lower limb motor tasks primarily for two reasons. First, there is the quest for knowledge about the intact human control system—a system capable of performing a myriad of complex tasks smoothly and precisely. The ability of the human to perform complex tasks in an uncertain environment is unmatched by the most sophisticated robot. Second, there is a need to develop systems utilizing functional neuromuscular stimulation (FNS) to restore lost function to individuals with paralyzing spinal cord injuries and increase the quality of their life. In 1988, there were about 177,000 spinal-cord-injured (SCI) individuals in the United States alone (PSA, 1990).

The more we understand how the intact human neuromuscular system controls lower limb tasks such as standing and walking, the easier artificial "replacement" control systems can be designed. However, the intact human utilizes information from many sensory modalities to control movement, most of which are not available to FNS system designers. Even if we were capable of developing systems to monitor, for example, joint position, joint velocity, and contact pressure, we would unlikely be able to find satisfactory substitutes for the visual and aural contributions normally used to predict impending environmental obstacles. Muscles have sensors for measuring muscle force (Hasan and Stuart, 1984) for which no substitutes are currently available. Additionally, electrically stimulated muscle recruits motor units in an order reverse to intact CNS-excited muscle (Mortimer, 1981), resulting in FNS muscle that fatigues rapidly. If FNS systems capable of restoring useful function to the SCI individual are to be developed soon, we are restricted to using readily available sensor information, current muscle stimulation methodologies, and modern control-system engineering-design techniques.

This chapter reviews how knowledge of the biomechanics of the musculoskeletal system assists in the design of FNS lower limb control systems. After discussing the performance goals which must be met for the clinical acceptance of FNS standing and walking systems, we review the functional capabilities of current lower limb FNS systems. Next, we argue that improved control systems, designed with the aid of dynamic musculoskeletal models and computer simulation, are needed to meet the performance goals of FNS systems because of the complex nature of multijoint movement. Insight into the lower limb FNS control strategies based on recent computer modeling and simulation-based design efforts will then be presented. Finally, we suggest that hybrid FNS/orthotic systems have the greatest potential for near-term clinical success.

GOALS OF LOWER LIMB FNS SYSTEMS

The primary goal of FNS research has been to restore function to the SCI patient. FNS systems restoring simple reach and grasp in the quadriplegic have been developed and may soon be used outside the research laboratory (Buckett et al., 1988; Handa and Hoshimiya, 1989; Nathan, 1990; Peckham et al., 1980). However, the many tasks that the normal human upper limb can perform challenges the designer of upper limb FNS systems. Lower limb FNS systems, on the other hand, need only to restore a few tasks to be beneficial to the SCI person. For example, if such systems could provide the capabilities of rising from a chair, standing, walking, turning right and left, and stair climbing/descending, the otherwise wheelchair-bound SCI individual would be able to live and work in areas currently inaccessible. In addition to improved mobility, the use of FNS for standing and walking may have other benefits, including improved cardiopulmonary fitness, prevention of muscle contracture, reduction of osteoporosis, improved bowel and bladder function, reduced incidence of decubitus ulcers, improved functional reach, and enhanced self-esteem (Cybulski et al., 1984; Kralj and Bajd, 1989; Lew, 1987; Phillips et al., 1984).

Spinal-cord-injured individuals have a strong desire to stand and walk, as evidenced by the many who have been fitted with passive mechanical long leg braces, also known as knee-ankle-foot orthoses (KAFOs). These devices consist of nearly rigid exoskeletons for the lower limbs which stabilize (and generally immobilize) the ankle and knee joints, allowing crutch-supported standing and limited walking. However, most paraplegic patients fitted and trained with long leg braces do not use them outside the clinic. Crutch axial forces during paraplegic walking using a reciprocal gait and KAFOs can exceed 40% of body weight, placing an undue burden on the upper limbs and contributing to high metabolic energy consumption (Crosbie and Nicol, 1990). Additionally, KAFOs are generally heavy, require excessive donning/doffing time, and are aesthetically unacceptable (Kralj and Grobelnik, 1973). Since wheelchair propulsion is more than twice as fast and five times more energy efficient (per distance traveled) than KAFO walking by low-level (T11 or lower) SCI patients (Cerny et al., 1980), it is not surprising that these patients revert to their wheelchairs after leaving the clinic.

If FNS systems are to be accepted outside of the research laboratory, minimum criteria for standing duration, walking speed, energy consumption, endurance, and upper limb loading must be met. It has been suggested that an FNS gait system should provide continuous standing for 1 hour or more, fast walking at 1.0 to 1.5 m/s for 150 meters, and normal speed walking at 1.0 m/s for 2000 meters, to be acceptable to the typical user (Marsolais and Kobetic, 1988). Additional factors of reliability, comfort, ease of use, safety, and cosmetic acceptability will also play an important role in the ultimate success of FNS systems.

CURRENT STATUS OF LOWER LIMB FNS SYSTEMS

Many FNS systems have been developed to restore lower limb function to SCI individuals. A few representative, state-of-the-art systems for which clinical performance data is available (e.g., standing duration, walking speed, energy consumption) will be discussed. Though these systems are not necessarily the best, we are unaware of others that perform dramatically better. These systems can be divided into two categories: (1) those incorporating FNS alone, or relying only minimally on orthoses (e.g., ankle-foot orthoses to provide ankle stability); and (2) those combining FNS with orthotic devices that limit ankle, knee, and possibly hip motion (usually referred to as *hybrid* FNS systems).

The most basic FNS-only gait systems require a minimum of four channels of surface electrodes. Stepping can be generated by stimulating the stance-leg quadriceps muscles to maintain extension while stimulating the swing-leg peroneal nerve to elicit the flexion-withdrawal reflex, causing simultaneous hip, knee, and ankle flexion. Arm forces (through crutches or a walker) and trunk muscles provide forward propulsion in addition to balance and support. Of 38 SCI patients (injury level T4–T11) fitted with this system, 23 were able to ambulate for limited distances at speeds ranging from 0.2 to 0.45 m/s (Kralj and Bajd, 1989).

Complex FNS-only systems are characterized by large numbers of percutaneous electrodes that stimulate many muscles based on stored (preprogrammed) muscle stimulation patterns. A 32-channel percutaneous FNS system incorporating preprogrammed, switch-activated on/off muscle stimulation patterns was fitted to 11 SCI patients (T4–T11) to restore ambulation (Marsolais and Kobetic, 1987). Trial-and-error was used to determine the preprogrammed stimulation patterns for each patient. Upper limb assistive devices (rolling walkers or occasionally crutches) provided balance and additional propulsive force. With a rolling walker, six of the subjects ambulated for distances of 25 to 330 m at maximum speeds of 0.2 to 0.8 m/s. However, only 2 of the 11 were able to ambulate with crutches, and then only with difficulty. Similar systems rely on footswitches or foot-force detectors to trigger stored stimulation patterns for each of the seven to ten phases of gait (Chizeck et al., 1988; Kobetic and Marsolais, 1988). Though these systems claim to improve synchronization between the body kinematics and the stimulation pattern, clinical performance trials have not been reported.

Hybrid FNS systems generally have fewer channels of muscle stimulation than FNS-only systems. The complexity of the orthoses varies considerably. The least complex one (given our definition of a hybrid FNS system) consists of a floor-reaction orthosis and two channels of stimulation per leg (quadriceps and the peroneal nerve) (Andrews et al., 1988). The floor-reaction orthosis is a rigid ankle-foot orthosis with an anterior strap over the patellar tendon. The brace stabilizes the knee in full extension as long as the body center of mass is anterior to the knee. Foot force, patellar-strap force, knee angle, and trunk inclination are sensed and processed to detect the horizontal position of the body center of mass. The quadriceps are stimulated if the center of mass is computed to be posterior to the knee. During standing, the brace/FNS combination maintains both knees in extension, crutches or parallel bars stabilize the upper body, and anterior pelvic tilt locks the hips in extension. With this system (along with a plastic spinal brace to prevent lordosis and to stabilize the trunk), a subject with a complete T6-7 lesion was able to stand for more than 1 hour with arm support. Limited ambulation was achieved by stimulating the swing-leg peroneal nerve to activate the flexion withdrawal reflex and initiate swing and the stance-leg quadriceps to maintain knee extension.

A more complex, though common, orthosis incorporated into hybrid systems is the reciprocating gait orthosis (RGO) (Douglas et al., 1983). The RGO consists of bilateral long leg braces designed to prevent ankle and knee motion. The braces are coupled to a pelvic band with pin joints, allowing hip motion in only the sagittal plane. A cable system couples the two hip joints, such that extension of one hip generates flexion of the other, facilitating leg reciprocation. A C7 quadriplegic patient fitted with an RGO and six handswitch-controlled FNS channels was able to walk at speeds up to 0.56 m/s for distances up to 800 m (Phillips, 1989). Six SCI patients (injury level C6–T11) were fitted with a similar RGO system that had four switch-controlled FNS channels (Solomonow et al., 1989; see also Chapter 10, this volume). Only the hamstrings and quadriceps muscles were stimulated. These individuals were able to rise unassisted from a chair and walk at speeds up to 0.37 m/s, for a maximum distance averaging 800 m. A two-position locking hip joint enabled patients to walk up gentle inclines. Other systems, incorporating stored patterns of FNS and long leg braces with pelvic support, have also been described (Stallard et al., 1986), but performance of these systems has not been reported.

IMPROVING CONTROL OF LOWER LIMB FNS SYSTEMS

Existing hybrid or FNS-only systems are incapable of meeting the speed and endurance criteria outlined above. One factor limiting the performance of these systems is the use of preprogrammed stimulation patterns. Preprogrammed control is probably adequate for tasks such as rising from a chair. However, it is inadequate for restoring other tasks such as walking, or even for providing long-duration standing, because errors in performance arising from unexpected forces acting on the body cannot be corrected. Feedback control compensates for errors because sensors (e.g., joint-angle sensors) are employed to detect body movement, and the control system applies FNS stimulation to correct for the computed deviations from the desired movement. Control theory is reviewed next, followed by a discussion of FNS control systems.

Control Systems Overview

The mechanical system being controlled is referred to as the *plant* (e.g., the human musculoskeletal system). The configuration of the system at any instant in time comprises the plant *states* (e.g., body segment positions and velocities). The devices that power the system are called *actuators* (e.g., muscles). The signals driving the actuators are the *controls* (e.g., neural pulse trains in intact humans and electrical stimuli in FNS systems). The *controller* is the process by which the controls are generated (e.g., the CNS in the intact human, and the stimulus pulse-train controller in the FNS system). The time histories of the plant states in response to the control signals is referred to as the system *trajectory* (e.g., the joint-angle time histories).

Controllers can be designed to function without sensors and therefore without knowledge of the actual plant trajectory (*open-loop* control), since trajectory information is not fed back to the controller (see Figure 12–1A). *Reference-based* open-loop controllers precompute and store (a priori to task execution) muscle stimulation patterns that will, hopefully, execute the desired motor task. The FNS walking systems described above utilize reference-based open-loop control. Muscle stimulation patterns were developed by combining clinical experience with trial-and-error, and then stored in the controller. Finding muscle stimulation patterns by trial-and-error which generate a smooth, energy-efficient gait is difficult because of the dynamic interactions among the body segments (see below) (Zajac and Gordon, 1989).

Muscle stimulation patterns can also be found by mathematically modeling the plant (i.e., the musculoskeletal system) and the tasks to be executed. Computer

CONTROL OF MULTIJOINT LOWER LIMB MOTOR TASKS

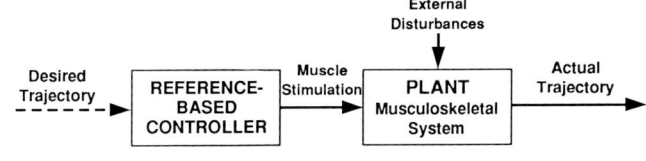

A. Open-Loop Control (Reference-Based)

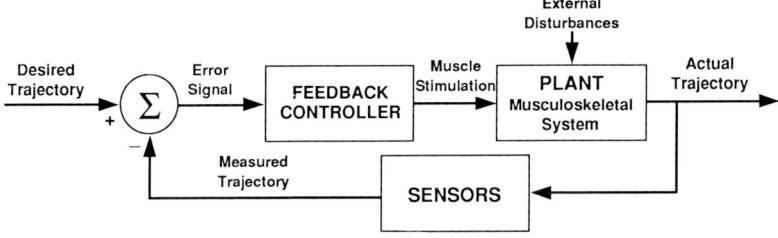

B. Closed-Loop Control (Error-Driven)

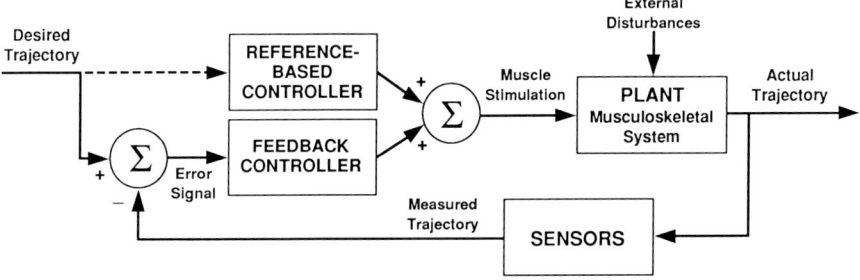

C. Combined Error-Driven and Reference-Based Control

Figure 12–1 Open- and closed-loop control systems. The desired trajectory may be required for the design of the reference-based controller, but does not act as an input during controller operation; this relationship is indicated by the dashed lines in (A) and (C) (see text for further explanation).

algorithms are then used to find stimulation patterns which will generate trajectories believed to fulfill the motor task requirements. One such algorithm uses *inverse dynamics* to calculate muscle stimulation patterns from an inverse of the musculoskeletal system model and a set of trajectories known to accomplish the desired motor task (see below). Muscle stimulation patterns may be determined by inverse dynamics prior to task execution and stored in a reference-based controller.

Regardless of design method and implementation, the performance of any open-loop control system will probably be inadequate, since *disturbances* will cause performance to deviate significantly from that required for proper task execution. A disturbance is any unexpected condition or event encountered by the plant. Functional neuromuscular stimulation systems are likely to encounter such disturbances; for example, from walking on uneven, inclined, or rough surfaces; from forces due to voluntary arm movements or wind; and from unexpected actuator performance,

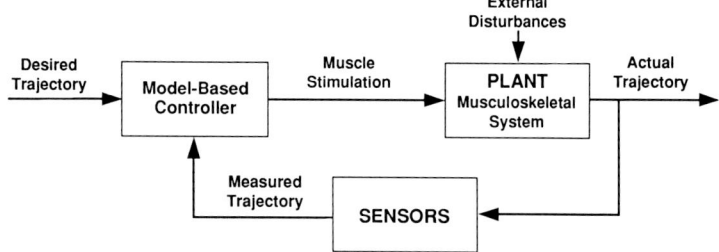

Figure 12–2 The model-based or computed-torque control system (see text for explanation).

such as may arise from muscle fatigue. Even in the absence of disturbances, open-loop control will probably be inadequate, since musculoskeletal properties will never be fully understood or perfectly modeled.

To correct for disturbances and musculoskeletal modeling errors, a *feedback controller* with ongoing knowledge of the effects of the disturbance must be designed. *Sensors* (e.g., joint-angle sensors) provide measurements from which the current state of the system (e.g., the actual joint angles and velocities) can be estimated. These estimates are fed back to the controller, resulting in a feedback, or *closed-loop* control system (Figure 12–1B). Closed-loop controllers are sometimes referred to as *error driven*, since they respond to the trajectory error, determined by subtracting the measured trajectory from the desired trajectory. Error-driven systems are particularly well suited to tasks where the desired trajectories are constant or slowly changing, such as the maintenance of vertical posture in standing.

To control tasks where trajectories must change rapidly but predictably (such as walking), reference control is sometimes employed in addition to error-driven feedback (Figure 12–1C). These controllers utilize open-loop control to generate an approximate trajectory (Figure 12–1A). A feedback controller similar to that shown in Figure 12–1B is employed in-parallel to correct for trajectory errors resulting from disturbances and modeling errors. If the body deviates too far from the desired trajectory, however, the stored controls may actually interfere with the recovery being provided by the feedback controller. This situation can arise because the reference-based controller functions independently from the feedback controller and cannot adjust its stored stimulation patterns during the task.

A more robust system for walking could be developed with *model-based* control (Figure 12–2). Model-based controllers utilize sensors and a dynamic model of the system to continuously recalculate the best trajectory to complete the desired task. During walking, if the body is following the desired path, the model-based controller generates the same muscle stimulation pattern as a reference-based controller designed with inverse dynamics. If the body deviates from the desired path, the model-based controller calculates a new path and generates a new muscle stimulation pattern which, according to the dynamic model, should maintain or restore stable walking. Though this sounds attractive, the complexity and computational requirements of model-based control continue to limit its application to simple problems.

Closed-loop control has many advantages for FNS systems. A closed-loop control system can automatically compensate for small disturbances and consequent trajectory errors. Closed-loop control can also regulate system behavior more precisely than open-loop control, for example, by smoothing the motion during walking and reducing the amount of stimulation (Marsolais and Edwards, 1988). Such regulation may then result in efficient FNS-controlled walking systems, since overstimulation and excessive torque production may be responsible for the high energy cost observed during FNS tasks (Marsolais and Kobetic, 1987). Closed-loop control also lets the designer specify system response characteristics. For example, a closed-loop system with both position and force feedback could be designed to provide *stiffness* control. Stiffness control specifies not only the desired position for a joint, but also the amount of force required to move the joint from that position. Though stiffness control may be energetically inefficient because of cocontraction of muscles, stiffness control may reject disturbances and regulate limb interaction with the environment well (Crago et al., 1990; Durfee, 1989; Hogan, 1985). Feedback can also be used to detect potential falls, and either act to compensate and correct the condition, or shift to a "safety" mode to reduce the chance of injury. In summary, closed-loop control lets the designer develop systems with a level of performance and flexibility well beyond that possible with open-loop control.

Why Dynamic Models are Needed

The benefits of closed-loop (feedback) control are clear. However, these benefits are not without cost. Closed-loop FNS control systems require sensors and are more complex to design and implement. Improper design can lead to instability, resulting in excessive stimulation and unpredictable (and potentially dangerous) performance. Although controllers for "simple" (single-input, single-output) systems can be designed without knowledge of the plant, more complex systems (e.g., the human musculoskeletal system) generally require *dynamic models* for control-system design (Franklin et al., 1986). A dynamic model is a set of equations that emulate the behavior of the physical system. Unlike static models, dynamic models specify how the current states of the system (e.g., body trajectories) depend on the past (e.g., the prior body trajectories and muscle forces). The inputs to a dynamic model of a human motor task are the muscle stimulation patterns, and the outputs are the computed body trajectories.

A dynamic model of a human lower limb task consists of three parts (Figure 12–3A). *Muscle dynamics* are specified by a set of differential and constraint equations that describe how neural (or FNS) stimulation patterns produce force in *musculotendon actuators* [muscle and tendon act together inextricably to produce force; thus we use the term musculotendon actuator; see Zajac (1989)]. Muscle force to joint-torque conversion is specified by a set of algebraic equations based on *musculoskeletal geometry* (i.e., the physical arrangement of bones and joints and the attachment points of muscles and tendons to the skeleton). Finally, joint torques produce motion of the limb segments and the external objects connected to the body as dictated by *segmental dynamics*, which are specified by another set of differential and constraint equations (sometimes these equations are referred to as the *equations of motion* of the system).

Dynamic models are required because the motion of multibodied systems, such as the human body, is so complex that even the qualitative effects of muscle forces cannot be predicted without the use of such models. For example, each muscle in

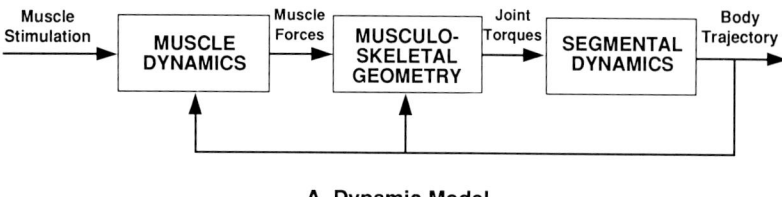

A. Dynamic Model

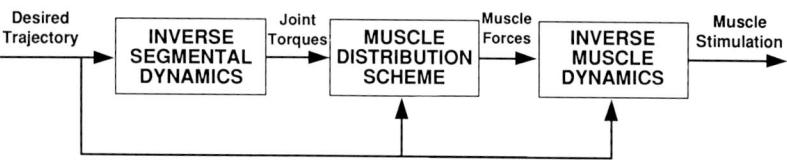

B. Inverse Dynamic Model

Figure 12–3 The dynamic model and its inverse (see text for explanation).

general acts to cause an angular acceleration of every joint in the body because of the *dynamic coupling* of forces acting on one segment to accelerate another due to the articulations among the segments. Consider the equations of motion (or segmental dynamics) describing the motion of the body segments during standing and walking (Khang and Zajac 1989a; Yamaguchi and Zajac, 1990). There are n equations, where n equals the number of *degrees of freedom* (DOF) of the system. The number of DOF is equal to the number of coordinates required to fully specify the position and orientation of all the segments of the body and all the objects touching the body, as determined by the number of segments and objects and the nature of the connections (joints) among the segments and objects (Kane and Levinson, 1985). The n equations can be represented in vector form:

$$\ddot{\theta} = M^{-1}(\theta)[T_m + T_v(\theta,\dot{\theta}) + T_g(\theta)]$$

where,

θ = vector of joint angles

$\dot{\theta}$ = vector of joint angular velocities

$\ddot{\theta}$ = vector of joint angular accelerations

M^{-1} = inverse system mass matrix

T_m = vector of direct muscle torques

T_v = vector of torques due to centrifugal and Coriolis forces

T_g = vector of torques due to gravity

The acceleration of each joint $\ddot{\theta}_i$ depends on the sum of three terms: the contributions from the muscle torque vector T_m, the velocity-dependent torque vector T_v, and the gravity torque vector T_g. We will concentrate on the muscle torque contributions, ignoring those from T_v and T_g. T_m is a vector of the torques produced by muscles

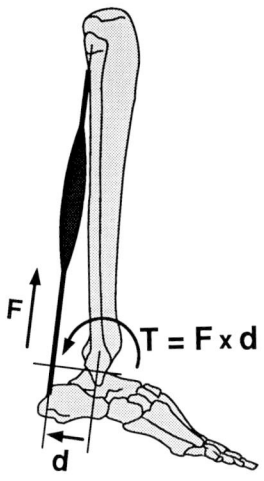

Figure 12–4 Muscle joint-torque generation. The joint torque, T, produced by a muscle at a rotary joint is determined by taking the cross-product of the muscle force vector, F, and the vector, d, from the center of rotation of the joint to the line of action of the force.

spanning the joints (Figure 12–4). These torques are multiplied by M^{-1}, which is the inverse of M, the $n \times n$ system mass matrix. M depends only on the mass properties of the system and the joint angle vector θ; it is independent of velocity.

If M (and therefore M^{-1}) had only diagonal elements, then a muscle would cause angular acceleration of only the joint (or joints) it spans. However, M and M^{-1} are generally full matrices, with significant off-diagonal terms, and therefore, a muscle induces an angular acceleration of every joint of the body. The direction and absolute magnitude of the angular acceleration induced by a muscle at each joint at a specific instant can be found from the equations of motion for the system and the torque produced by the muscle at that instant. However, the direction and the relative magnitudes of joint angular accelerations induced by a muscle can be found from just the equations of motion (Zajac and Gordon, 1989).

Because of dynamic coupling, biarticular muscles (muscles crossing two joints) may accelerate a joint it spans in a direction opposite to its torque at that joint. For example, gastrocnemius muscle, which develops an ankle plantarflexor (extensor) torque and a knee flexor torque, accelerates the ankle toward dorsiflexion at times during standing, and the knee toward extension at other times (Khang, 1988; Zajac and Gordon, 1989). The reason is that its ankle extensor torque accelerates all the leg joints toward extension and its knee flexor torque accelerates all the joints toward flexion. The net direction of the angular acceleration of each joint is the direction of the sum of the two accelerations of that joint caused by the two torques, and thus can be either flexion or extension. The net direction depends on body posture, body morphometry, and the relative magnitude of the two joint torques.

Dynamic coupling can also alter the apparent action of a muscle crossing a single joint, if the joint has more than one DOF. For example, muscles crossing ball-and-socket joints (three DOF) can generate an angular acceleration in a direction different from the direction of the muscle torque (Mansour and Pereira, 1987; Zajac and Gordon, 1989). Thus, the precise action of a muscle in a multijoint, multi-DOF system is not always obvious, and can change during a task as the angles of the joints change. Models of multijoint movement allow us to understand these dynamic interactions and can be used to design FNS controllers.

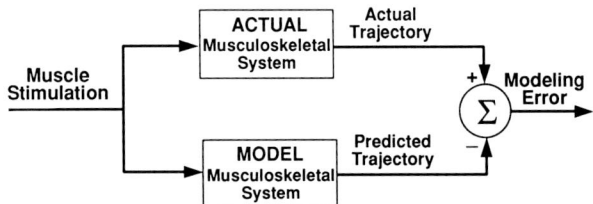

Figure 12-5 Errors in the dynamic model can cause differences between the trajectories predicted by the model and exhibited by the actual system.

Using Dynamic Models to Design FNS Controllers

Control-system design methods for complex systems depend on dynamic models. For example, reference-based or feed-forward controllers (Figures 12-1A and 12-1C) can be developed by inverting the dynamic model to determine the muscle stimulation pattern that will produce a desired trajectory (Figure 12-3B). This process is called *inverse dynamics*, since the inputs and outputs are reversed (Figure 12-3A to 12-3B). The resulting stimulation pattern could theoretically drive the system along the desired trajectory in the absence of disturbances. However, some degree of modeling error is unavoidable, since dynamic models can never perfectly represent physical systems, and the trajectory of the actual musculoskeletal system will be different than predicted by the model (Figure 12-5). Modeling errors can be overcome by using error-driven feedback controllers in combination with reference-based or feed-forward controllers (Figure 12-1C).

Developing a reference-based controller with inverse dynamics is not straightforward, because the controller equations cannot be determined merely by "flipping around" the dynamic model, since musculoskeletal geometry is generally noninvertible. That is, muscle forces are not uniquely determined from joint torques (Figures 12-3B, *muscle distribution scheme*), though joint-torques are uniquely specified by muscle forces (Figure 12-3A, *musculoskeletal geometry*). If the human lower limb had only one muscle pulling in each direction at each joint, then the muscle forces required to produce a specified set of joint torques would be unique. However, the required joint torques can be met by different muscle force combinations. The task of distributing a net joint torque among all the muscles crossing the joint is referred to as the *muscle redundancy*, or *muscle force distribution* problem. For review, see Zajac and Gordon (1989).

One solution to the muscle redundancy problem is to choose only one muscle to generate each required torque and ignore the rest. Because muscle strength and endurance is limited (particularly for FNS muscle), this approach is unfeasible. Another, more common approach is to use *static optimization* methods, which require that a *cost function* be specified. The cost function is a mathematical quantity (usually based on some combination of muscle size, force, and activation level) which is calculated for each of the muscles and summed. It is generally chosen to represent the stress and/or rate of fatigue of muscle. The principle of static optimization is to find at each instant of the motor task, independent of the other instants, the muscle forces that produce the desired torques while minimizing the cost function, thereby avoiding excessive stress or rapid fatigue in any one muscle at that instant. Since static optimization problems can be solved relatively easily, this approach may soon be feasible for designing control systems, especially as microprocessor speeds increase. Static optimization has been limited to date to simulation studies, where the objective is to determine individual muscle forces, for example, from gait laboratory measurements of joint and force-plate trajectories (Crowninshield and Brand, 1981; Pederson et al., 1987), and to the theoretical design of an FNS feedback controller for standing (Khang and Zajac, 1989a).

Static optimization is limited by its failure to account for the dynamic characteristics of musculotendon actuators. Muscle forces cannot be generated instantaneously, and force output depends on the dynamic state and the recent history of stimulation of the muscle. Since static methods cannot account for these factors, the consequences of the current optimization results on future performance is not considered. What is desired, of course, is for the cost to be minimized over all time.

To obtain a solution that guarantees optimality over the entire task, *dynamic* optimization must be used, where a *performance criterion* applicable to the entire task is minimized. The performance criterion can be chosen to provide the desired tradeoff between muscular effort and trajectory errors. Using a dynamic model of the whole system, including a model of the musculotendon actuator dynamics (Figure 12–3A), a dynamic optimization algorithm finds the muscle stimulation pattern that provides the best performance. Though methods to solve dynamic optimization problems are few, and computations needed to find a solution many, dynamic optimization is conceptually very powerful and has been used to study lower limb tasks, including gait (Davy and Audu, 1987; Hatze, 1976; Pandy et al., 1990; Yamaguchi and Zajac, 1990).

Dynamic optimization can assist in the design of reference-based controllers. Muscle stimulation patterns providing the best performance, as determined by the dynamic optimization algorithm, would be stored in the controller before implementation of the FNS system. These stimulation patterns should provide smooth, efficient movement, since they would have been designed to account for the dynamic interactions of the musculoskeletal components. Error-driven closed-loop control would still have to be implemented to compensate for modeling errors and disturbances (Figure 12–1C).

Dynamic optimization can provide the basis to design a model-based *optimal controller* (Figure 12–2). An optimal controller is like a continually updated reference-based controller. If sensors indicate significant deviations from the desired trajectory, the controller solves a dynamic optimization problem to determine a new path which will bring the body from its current position back to the desired trajectory, while maintaining balance and stability. The future muscle stimulation pattern is computed based on the newly determined path. This scheme requires many dynamic optimizations and other computations at speeds beyond current software and hardware capabilities.

Dynamic models can also assist in the design of simpler feedback controllers. Many algorithms are available to the design engineer which will generate feedback control laws given a dynamic model and the desired performance characteristics (see below) (Franklin et al., 1986). A dynamic model can also be used to design an *estimator*, which estimates all the states from a few sensors. These estimates are then used in feedback control. State estimation may be very beneficial to FNS systems because some states are impossible to measure in humans (e.g., muscle fiber length), and because reduction in FNS hardware (e.g., the number of sensors) is desired.

Simulating FNS Controller Performance

Dynamic models allow body-segment trajectories to be determined from muscle stimulation patterns. This process is known as *simulation* or *forward dynamics*. Simulation provides the designer with a tool for evaluating the performance of different controller designs and predicting the response of the controlled system to disturbances. Dynamic modeling and simulation permit the designer to ask, "What if. . .?" and explore many options without the time and expense of actually implementing the systems in hardware. Once a system has been selected, simulation can help predict its stability and behavior under various conditions (e.g., disturbances), and sensitivity of performance to parameter and modeling errors.

Linear control theory and reduced-order nonlinear models are frequently employed to simplify the control system design process. Since the dynamic model then used to design a controller is simplified, the performance of the controller should always be tested with simulations based on the full, nonlinear model of the human motor task. In this way, fine tuning of the feedback parameters can be made to give even better performance, or if performance is unsatisfactory, the control design can be discarded before hardware implementation.

Dynamic modeling and simulation can provide benefits beyond the design and testing of FNS control systems. All elements of the model can be explored in great detail, revealing information about internal forces and movements which cannot be directly measured from the human body. For example, improper use of FNS can result in the generation of excessive joint forces and bone stresses, possibly leading to injury (Kralj and Bajd, 1989). Though these forces cannot be measured directly, they can be predicted via simulation, and potentially hazardous situations can be identified.

Simulation provides a faster, cheaper alternative to hardware implementation and initial testing of FNS systems. Though the final evaluation must be done in hardware and with human subjects, we believe that humanitarianism and safety of SCI patients will best be served by evaluating controllers thoroughly with simulation before patient testing. The predictive capability of the simulated control system, however, depends on the accuracy of the musculoskeletal model.

MODELING THE MUSCULOSKELETAL SYSTEM

The human lower limb is generally modeled as a set of rigid limb segments, whose motion relative to each other is defined by the joint articulations (i.e., skeletal geometry and ligamentous constraints). The interaction of external forces (e.g., gravity) and environmental constraints (e.g., ground) with the body segments also has to be modeled. The modeled segments and how they interact with the environment together define the body segmental dynamics. Human-generated power is provided to the segments via an assumed set of musculotendon actuators, which generate forces that act on the segments (musculotendon dynamics). How much

CONTROL OF MULTIJOINT LOWER LIMB MOTOR TASKS

force is generated by an actuator depends on the relative position and motion of the segments, which is defined by musculoskeletal geometry. The direction of each musculotendon force relative to the segments (again defined by musculoskeletal geometry) affects the direction the segments will accelerate due to that force. The musculoskeletal system (i.e., the plant, Figure 12-3A) thus consists of three major elements: body segmental dynamics, musculoskeletal geometry, and musculotendon actuator dynamics.

Body Segmental Dynamics

The complexity of a body-segment dynamical model depends on the number and types of body segments, the joints connecting the segments, and the interaction among the segments and the environment. How complex a model is required for dynamic analysis of FNS standing and walking? A rather complex one is required to predict human response to all lower limb motor tasks. However, an overly complex model may so complicate the control system design process that good solutions are difficult or impossible to find. Also, the predictive quality of a model depends not only on model complexity, but also on the accuracy with which model parameters (e.g., lengths, masses, moments of inertia) and structure (e.g., of the joints) can be determined. The biomechanist must decide, for each task to be studied, the model that is believed to represent the best tradeoff between accuracy and complexity.

Some decisions on how complex the model should be are simple; others are not. For instance, lower limb body segments can be assumed rigid during standing and walking, since bone deformations within a segment are small compared to intersegmental movement. More controversial is the decision on how many segments should be assumed (especially for the trunk and the foot), or how many DOF should be assumed for each joint. For example, models have ranged from a 1-segment, 1-DOF (Jaeger, 1986) to a 17-segment, 44-DOF model (Hatze, 1980). These decisions on model complexity have important implications to the design of FNS control systems.

Two-dimensional models have been used to study standing and walking. For example, a one-segment (Jaeger, 1986) and a three-segment (head/arms/trunk, one thigh, one shank) (Gordon, 1990; Khang, 1988) model has been to study sagittal plane standing and to design FNS systems when both feet are assumed to be flat and stationary on the floor. However, additional segments may be required to adequately model FNS-controlled standing and walking. For example, arm movements are significant during FNS-controlled standing (Khang, 1988). During gait, the pelvis may need to be modeled separately from the trunk (Hatze, 1977; Townsend and Seireg, 1973; Yamaguchi, 1990), and the foot may need to be modeled as multiple segments (Yamaguchi, 1990).

Most FNS systems will require control of motion in all three planes, not just in the sagittal plane. For example, coronal as well as sagittal plane control at the hip is probably required for postural stability (Chizeck et al., 1988). Of the ten types of joint movement suggested to be most important to normal gait (Yamaguchi, 1990), only half are in the sagittal plane: hip flexion/extension, knee flexion/extension, ankle plantar/dorsiflexion, foot rotation about the metatarsals, and sacral-pelvic flexion/extension. Three are in the frontal plane: hip abduction/adduction, ankle inversion/eversion, and sacral-pelvic lateral bending. Least significant are transverse plane rotations (e.g., hip external/internal rotation and axial trunk rotation). Frontal plane motion at the ankle, hip, and sacral-pelvic joints to keep the body center of mass over the stance foot is needed to reduce muscular effort and energy consumption (Yamaguchi, 1990). Models with only one-DOF sagittal-plane hip joints cause the fore-aft ground reaction force to be poorly predicted during the single-support phase of gait, because multiple-DOF hips reduce the mechanical coupling between the swing and stance legs (Pandy and Berme, 1988). Also, paraplegic FNS-generated gait will probably not induce normal gait motion. Low-level thoracic SCI individuals will probably take advantage of trunk muscles under voluntary control to generate a rotational pelvic thrust in order to assist in the initiation of swing, as observed when they use non-FNS orthotic walking aids (e.g., the RGO). These movements can only be analyzed with a three-dimensional (3-D) model.

The number of DOF being controlled during gait changes, and this poses another complication to modeling gait. During the swing phase (in the absence of upper body support), the body is an *open kinematic chain*, since only one foot is contacting the ground. The number of net joint-torques then equals the number of degrees of freedom, and the system is determinate. This means that the trajectory of the body segments uniquely determines the net torques acting at the joints (see earlier section). However, contact of the other foot or a crutch makes the body a *closed kinematic chain* and the number of degrees of freedom is less than the number of net joint torques. Thus, segmental trajectories no longer uniquely determine the net joint torques, and the system is indeterminate. Many different combinations of joint torques can therefore be selected, and finding a reference-based controller is more difficult. Different models (and associated equations of motion) must be developed for each phase (Onyshko and Winter, 1980). Additionally, foot impact must be modeled to determine how the segment velocities change at the transition from one model to the other. Optimal control algorithms cannot be applied to the entire movement, since they require a single set of equations. Although each phase could be optimized independently, the resulting movement may not be optimal, since the state of the system at the transition points would have to be specified arbitrarily. An alternative is to develop a set of artificial constraint forces that "hold" the foot on the ground during double support, allowing one set of equations to represent motion at all times (Hatze and Venter, 1981). Though this may be theoretically convenient, the artificial constraints must be carefully developed to predict natural movement and avoid mathematical instability.

In summary, models to be employed in FNS control system design of unsupported standing and walking should be structured as follows. For standing, models should have at least two leg segments (shank and thigh), a two-segment trunk (pelvis and upper trunk/head), and a 3-D hip and pelvis. Arm movement (and the resulting forces) must also be accounted for. If posture switching (weight-shifting from one leg to the other) is employed to reduce fatigue, each leg will have to be modeled separately. Models for walking will probably require three segments per leg (foot, shank, and thigh), a two-segment trunk, and a 3-D hip and pelvis, assuming the system is used in conjunction with ankle-foot orthoses to limit ankle motion to the sagittal plane. Additionally, models of walking must account for voluntary upper limb assistance from crutches or walkers. Control system design techniques will be difficult to use with models of this complexity. Though controllers designed from simpler models are possible, more complex models are still required to simulate the expected, real-life performance of these controllers. Finally, the complexity of these models, and the implementation of the control laws resulting from complex models, can be reduced when orthotic devices are employed (see discussion below).

Musculoskeletal Geometry

Muscles do not produce pure torques at the joints. Instead, they exert forces on the body segments to which they attach. For frictionless, rotary joints, these muscle forces have a net effect on body segmental motion that can be found by the joint torques these muscles exert (Zajac and Gordon, 1989). The conversion of a muscle force to a joint torque, in such cases, is dictated by musculoskeletal geometry and is conceptually straightforward. The joint torque, T, produced by a muscle is determined by taking the cross-product of the muscle force vector, F, and the vector, d, from the center of rotation of the joint to the line of action of the force (Figure 11–4). In actuality, muscles are not straight lines and joints are not hinges. Muscles and their tendons may attach over a wide area and wrap around or slide over bone, making determination of "the line of force" difficult. Joints may exhibit rolling and sliding motion (e.g., the knee), proscribing the use of fixed joint centers, or precluding the use of joint torques altogether (Yamaguchi and Zajac, 1989). Failure to properly account for these and other factors in the dynamic model may result in considerable errors in joint-torque calculations (Delp et al., 1990; Hoy et al., 1990; Zajac and Gordon, 1989), and thus inadequate controller designs. Nevertheless, much anthropometric data have been collected that can be used to specify muscle lines of action and musculoskeletal geometry (Yamaguchi et al., 1990).

Musculotendon Actuator Dynamics

Musculotendon actuators, consisting of contractile muscle fibers and connecting tissue and tendon, have important dynamic characteristics inherent to their ability to develop force, including time delays, nonlinear elasticity, and nonlinear dependencies on the current muscle state (e.g., length and velocity of the muscle fibers) and past muscle states (e.g., history of the shortening/lengthening and activation of the muscle fibers). Two fundamental classes of mathematical models of actuators, based on normally innervated muscle, but with widely varying complexity, have been developed; macroscopic models, and microscopic models. Several good reviews of these models are available (Winters and Stark, 1987; Zahalak, 1990; Zajac, 1989; see also Chapter 2, this volume).

Macroscopic models are not necessarily derived from the actual microscopic biophysical and biochemical mechanisms responsible for muscular contraction, though the A.V. Hill macroscopic model (Hill, 1938) had long been considered consistent with such mechanisms (Zahalak, 1990). Instead, these phenomenological models attempt to describe the observed mechanical input-output behavior of muscle with comparatively simple *ordinary* differential equations (see reviews by Winters, 1990; Zajac, 1989), and thus require less computational effort and fewer parameters than the microscopic models.

Microscopic models are derived from the biophysical and biochemical molecular

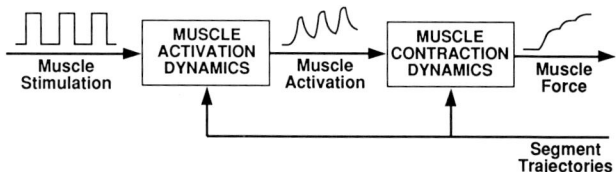

Figure 12–6 Block diagram of general musculotendon actuator model, showing low-pass filtering action of muscle dynamics (see text for explanation).

mechanisms of sarcomere force production [e.g., the cross-bridge and sliding-filament models of contraction (Hill et al., 1975; Huxley, 1957)]. These microscopic models of sarcomere contraction have many parameters, which, for human tissue, are now unmeasurable and difficult to estimate, and require that *partial* differential equations be solved. Since partial differential equations require much more computation to solve than ordinary differential equations, microscopic models will probably not be used to design FNS control systems. However, the "distribution-moment" model, which is a mathematical approximation to the cross-bridge model (see review by Zahalak and Ma, 1990), offers hope in relating macroscopic to microscopic properties, and its computational efficiency may be sufficient to be employed in models of multimuscle motor control.

Models of muscle under neural pulse stimulation (e.g., models of a normally innervated motor unit, or of a FNS-excited muscle), whether developed from microscopic or macroscopic properties, have similar fundamental input-output properties; that is, they all recognize that muscle is basically a second-order low-pass filter (Figure 12–6). Muscle stimulation (neural excitation or FNS) is considered to be pulse-like, with varying frequency. These pulses initiate a chemical reaction which stimulates the contractile elements within the muscle, producing muscle force. Both macroscopic and microscopic models divide this process into two phases: activation dynamics (the chemical process associated with stimulation-contraction coupling) and contraction dynamics (the generation of force by activated contractile elements). Each of the two phases acts as a *low-pass filter*, with the output responding slower and more smoothly than the input. Though all models treat muscle as a low-pass filter, the complexity of the equations used to describe the filter varies greatly.

Only macroscopic models have been used to model FNS-excited muscle. Though Hill-based models have been used to study design issues related to FNS-controlled standing and walking (Khang and Zajac, 1989a; Yamaguchi and Zajac, 1990), simpler models may suffice and are particularly attractive for control-system design. Two such models (Figure 12–7) use a nonlinear static recruitment curve (isometric force versus pulse-width curve), which models how much muscle tissue is being excited

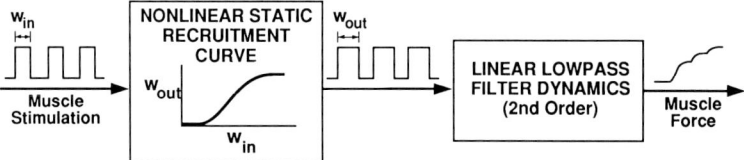

Figure 12–7 A musculotendon actuator model for predicting isometric force in electrically stimulated muscle (see text for explanation).

by the electrode pulses, followed by second-order linear dynamics, which models the basic filtering property of muscle (Bernotas et al., 1986; Durfee and MacLean, 1989). The simulated isometric (or near-isometric) force trajectories to a train of pulses computed from these models compared well with the actual trajectories developed by the electrically stimulated cat muscles. The performance of these models during movement may not be as good, however, since the models do not account for the dependence of force on muscle fiber length and velocity.

A significant weakness in the application of all muscle models to FNS systems is their failure to account for muscle fatigue. Muscle force output of electrically stimulated muscle has been shown to decrease due to fatigue. This effect becomes more significant as the duration and intensity of the stimulation increases (Kuntzman et al., 1990). Since FNS systems for standing and walking may involve stimulation for long periods of time, models of muscle fatigue must be developed.

INSIGHTS FROM RECENT MODELING WORK

Designing FNS control systems to produce standing and walking in paraplegics is no easy task because many body segments are involved and because the dynamical interactions among them are complex (see above). Attempts to develop multijoint dynamic models and multimuscle FNS controllers applicable to standing and walking are now discussed.

Standing

Moderate duration standing by paraplegics is possible with a simple open-loop FNS system (Kralj and Bajd, 1989). Continuous bilateral FNS of the quadriceps locks the knees in extension. With the aid of crutches or a walker, complementary voluntary arm and trunk muscle contractions produce a C-shaped body posture (i.e., by moving the pelvis forward and extending the trunk, the body center of mass is kept posterior to the hip joint, maintaining hip extension). More complex systems may be able to provide unsupported standing, allowing functional use of the arms and a more natural posture. The control of unsupported standing is analogous to the task of stabilizing a multisegment inverted pendulum with a large mass sitting on top. Although the system is inherently unstable, relatively small forces are required to maintain this posture as long as the body segments stay at or near vertical and no external forces other than gravity are acting on the body. If the body is perturbed, however, large forces must be generated quickly, in the proper directions, and in the right sequence, to restore upright posture and prevent a fall. Obviously, feedback control, which excites muscles based on measured body segmental deviations from the vertical, is needed.

One design of such a feedback control system applicable to standing in the sagittal plane was based on *linearizing* the equations of motion of a five-segment (foot, shank, thigh, trunk/head, and arms) model about the upright position and applying the well-developed theory of *linear* optimal control (Khang, 1988; Khang and Zajac, 1989a; Khang and Zajac, 1989b). First-order activation dynamics and a linear, first-order approximation to the two-element Hill-type muscle/tendon model represented the 13 musculotendon actuators of the lower limb. A two-step process was used to design a feedback controller. First, the torque-generating capabilities of all muscles crossing a joint were combined into an "equivalent joint-torque actuator," so that the total number of joint-torque actuators was equal to the number of joints, temporarily avoiding muscle redundancy. With the problem thus simplified, linear dynamic optimization was used to design a constant-gain, multi-input/multioutput feedback controller. That is, the amount of joint-torque activation needed at each joint was based on a weighted sum of all the deviations in segmental position and velocity from the resting upright posture and the amount of joint-torque effort expended. Second, the redundancy problem was solved at each instant by distributing each joint-torque activation among the individual musculotendon actuators via static optimization so as to minimize metabolic energy consumption by the muscles at that instant. Simulations were conducted to assess how well this two-step controller can be expected to perform. The simulations assumed a complex model of the musculoskeletal system, and showed that the controller can restore upright posture even when the body is initially extremely flexed, and can maintain this posture during fast arm movements (Khang and Zajac, 1989b). This type of controller can probably be designed and implemented to effect 3-D control of FNS-induced standing, without reliance on arms for balance and support, by additionally accounting for frontal plane leg movement and pelvic-trunk movement.

Though such controllers may function well in keeping the body vertical most of the time, they will undoubtedly be unable to prevent the body from falling when large disturbances are encountered. Modeling can again assist in designing strategies to detect when falls are imminent, and then to alert the paraplegic to take corrective (hopefully) upper body action. Simultaneous with the alert, the controller could be designed to effect an alternate strategy to drive the body as best as it can toward the upright position. In fact, such corrective action requires (generally) full activation of some muscles, though the muscles that need to be activated depend on the disturbed posture (Gordon, 1990). A number of nonintuitive strategies may be required, including one where the initial acceleration of the hip has to be in the "wrong" direction (e.g., flexor acceleration of the hip when the hip is already flexed) (Gordon, 1990). It may be possible to design a controller with acceptable performance that utilizes these strategies all the time, in which case controller switching would be unnecessary and the controller would be robust to all disturbances. Extreme situations could be identified where restoration of upright position would be impossible; a different strategy could be then employed to provide a safe, controlled fall.

Walking

The control of walking is more difficult than the stabilization of a multisegment inverted pendulum. No stationary position to move toward exists; instead, the target is a trajectory of the body segments. The body is at great risk of falling at specific times during the gait cycle, because the heavy trunk mass is subject to large accelerations and the base of ground support is small. Modeling is more challenging because the gait cycle consists of distinct phases (e.g., swing and stance), which are inextricably linked. Further, the joints move through ranges of motion and positions that may prohibit linearization.

A feasibility study to see how a limited number of muscles could be controlled (e.g., by FNS) to restore a near-normal gait pattern illustrates the challenge of modeling gait and designing FNS controllers (Yamaguchi, 1989; Yamaguchi, 1990; Yamaguchi and Zajac, 1990). An eight-DOF, 3-D model, consisting of seven rigid bodies (two feet, two shanks, two thighs, and a trunk) was developed to simulate both the single- and double-support phases of walking. Ankle-foot orthoses were assumed to limit ankle motion to the sagittal plane and prevent excessive dorsiflexion. A Hill-type model (Zajac, 1989), including force-length and force-velocity properties of muscle and an elastic tendon, was used to model 14 lower limb muscle groups. Dynamic optimization (a dynamic programming algorithm) found the controls (the muscle stimulation patterns, in increments of 10%) to minimize a performance criterion based on trajectory errors and cubed muscle stresses. The stimulation patterns were then manually fine-tuned until simulations produced the desired gait pattern.

Dynamic coupling among segments was found to be important. For example, rectus femoris (RF), which develops a knee extensor torque, actually acted to accelerate the knee into flexion during swing. A net knee flexor acceleration arose because the hip flexor torque generated by RF produced a knee flexion acceleration large enough to overpower the knee extension acceleration induced by the RF knee extensor torque. Critical points in the gait cycle were identified where precise synergistic muscle control is necessary. For example, (1) the soleus and vasti muscles must prevent collapse of the stance-side knee and ankle during early to mid single-leg support, (2) abductor muscles must maintain lateral stability of the stance-side hip during single-leg support, and (3) many muscles must work together to ensure ground clearance of the swing foot, since both the height of the swing-leg ankle and the orientation of the foot at its lowest point are critical. Unfortunately, the model predicted that some of the muscles (e.g., the plantarflexors) need to produce forces in excess of 50% of normal strength, which exceeds the current force generation capacity of FNS-reconditioned paralyzed muscles (Kralj and Bajd, 1989).

The control schemes described above for standing and walking are based on the concept of *global* control, where the state of the entire system determines the control of each muscle. The control process would certainly be much easier if the stimulation of each muscle could be determined by examining only the state of one joint spanned by the muscle (*local* control). As discussed previously, dynamic coupling among the body segments precludes this simplistic approach. Biarticular muscles, by spanning two joints, act to further couple lower limb joints (Chizeck et al., 1988). Local joint control, combined with limited global control (called *hierarchical* control) has been attempted in the effort to overcome these obstacles (Andrews and Kirkwood, 1989; Furusho and Masabuchi, 1987). A hierarchical system combining open-loop FNS with local stiffness control at the knee has been proposed where knee position and ground-reaction-force feedback are used to improve gait and reduce knee hyperextension (Willemin and Chizeck, 1989). Another suggested hierarchical system would generate standing and walking by combining local position feedback at the lower limb joints with global foot-force feedback for trunk control (Vukobratovic and Stokic, 1980).

Though hierarchical control has potential, no good evidence exists to suggest that it will be more successful at controlling FNS-generated gait than global control. Simulation showing how a hierarchical control system performs is therefore the next logical step. Regardless, dedicating some portion of the control system to the maintenance of trunk position has considerable merit. Because the trunk represents a large mass sitting on top of an unstable support, recovery of stability is very difficult if the trunk deviates substantially from vertical. In fact, trunk stability has been identified as a major obstacle to gait restoration in SCI persons (Marsolais and Kobetic, 1987), and the maintenance of posture and balance of the trunk in both the sagittal and frontal planes is believed to be one of the primary tasks confronting the human during gait (Winter, 1988). Though some trunk support can be provided by upper limb assistance, trunk position maintenance must be addressed regardless of the specific control methodology used.

THE CASE FOR HYBRID SYSTEMS

Clinical systems, capable of restoring stable walking to paraplegics while meeting the required speed and efficiency goals, are not yet available. Modeling, simulation, and control-system design applied to the development of FNS systems have begun, but a satisfactory solution is not even evident from these data. The primary reason for the slow progress is due to the biomechanical complexity of the human musculoskeletal system, which demands that many new frontiers be explored to evolve toward a solution.

Hybrid FNS systems were developed to simplify FNS control. The orthosis complements the FNS, improving performance by reducing the number of DOF to be controlled and the forces required from stimulated muscle. A hybrid FNS system consisting of an RGO, a simple control scheme, and only a few FNS channels can provide performance as good or better than the most complex FNS-only system (see above). By reducing energy consumption and upper limb (crutch) support forces, hybrid FNS systems also perform significantly better than mechanical orthotic systems alone (Nene, 1989; Solomonow et al., 1989; Stallard et al., 1986).

The amount by which FNS control is simplified depends on the orthotic device employed in the hybrid FNS system. Ankle-foot orthoses are common because foot and ankle rotation is either limited to rotation about the ankle only, or eliminated all together. Conventional KAFOs eliminate almost all knee and ankle rotation, although devices have been developed that allow limited knee rotation, controlled by an electrically activated friction brake (Schoenberg and Long, 1987). Hip guidance orthoses further reduce the DOF by restricting hip rotation to the sagittal plane (Stallard et al., 1986), and RGOs remove one more DOF by coupling the rotation of the two hips (Douglas, 1986; Phillips and Hendershot, 1988; Solomonow et al., 1989). The posterior pelvic band of some RGOs extends vertically beyond the pelvis to assist with trunk stabilization (Douglas et al., 1983). System simplification does come with a cost, however, since each DOF removed from the human reduces the capability of the hybrid FNS system. The movement exhibited by patients ambulating with RGOs resembles walking only because leg reciprocation and forward progression is imparted to the human. Because no knee, ankle, or nonsagittal plane hip rotation is provided, considerable rotary and lateral pelvic motion is required for foot clearance during swing, and step length is reduced significantly.

Active orthotic devices can supplement FNS by providing (or dissipating) power without necessarily reducing the DOF of the body. Active braking of knee rotation is one example (Schoenberg and Long, 1987). Controlled mechanical braking at the joints may be able to replace eccentric muscle contractions, providing limb deceleration and cocontraction for stiffness control with reduced muscular effort, and possibly fine control even when muscle stimulation is loosely regulated (Durfee and Hausdorff, 1990). A "self-fitting modular orthosis" (SFMO) has been developed that combines FNS and motor-powered actuators with a lightweight, modular brace. The SFMO is designed to limit joint rotation to the sagittal plane while it dynamically aligns itself (i.e., "self-fits itself") to the joint during walking (Popovic, 1990; see also Chapter 11, this volume). An expert system using foot-force and joint-angle information as inputs to a set of 23 rules determines the desired motor task (level walking, ramp walking, standing up, sitting down, backward walking, and turning) (Popovic et al., 1989). For each task and for each patient, the open-loop control signals to both the FNS system and the motor-powered actuators are determined by trial-and-error. A 3-D, eight-segment body model has been developed to study walking with the SFMO and assist in the development of advanced control strategies (Popovic, 1990). Although externally powered joint actuators have appeal to the control engineer, since they are much better understood and easier to control than muscles, their implementation should be approached cautiously. These devices may prove to be unacceptable to the clinical SCI population unless they can be made highly reliable, efficient, lightweight, and unobtrusive.

Hybrid FNS systems may have other benefits in addition to control simplification. Spinal-cord-injured patients using FNS systems can be subject to joint injury due to excessive forces or inappropriate movements. Such injuries can go undetected, since these patients may have little or no sensation from their lower limbs. Lower limb bracing can protect the joints by restricting motion (Marsolais, 1989; Muccio and Marsolais, 1987). Also, orthotics allow convenient attachment of force and joint-angle sensors required for feedback control. Finally, complete orthotic systems, such as the RGO, can provide support, protection, and even some degree of mobility should FNS fail.

CONCLUSIONS

Multijoint lower limb biomechanics is complex. The human musculoskeletal system is nonlinear, coupled, and contains many degrees of freedom. Functional neuromuscular stimulation systems with simple, open-loop control will probably be unable to afford a high enough level of performance and functionality to gain general acceptance among the SCI population. The development of sophisticated control systems depends on the use of computer models capable of representing the essential behavior of the system. We believe that these models will have to be complex. Control engineers equipped with the most powerful design tools available are expected to be so challenged that ingenious solutions may be necessary.

Ideally, the FNS system should be implantable, including the electrodes, the feedback sensors, and possibly even the control system itself. The ideal control system should mimic the intact neurocontrol system as closely as possible, in which case it could then provide for walking and standing in the presence of virtually every conceivable disturbance. Further, the FNS system must be easy to use and completely reliable. Clearly, such a system demands the development of new technologies. Although progress is being made in many areas, it is uncertain when all of these technologies will become available. As work progresses towards this idealistic goal, however, existing technologies may soon be capable of providing a clinically functional system. In this regard, we believe hybrid systems currently exhibit the most promise.

Hybrid FNS systems may be able to meet the near-term goal of providing functional standing and mobility. Modeling and simulation are tools that can be used to determine how performance is expected to vary among potential FNS hybrid systems. However, design criteria other than functionality are equally (and perhaps more) important, such as cosmesis, portability, and time to don and doff the system. Control engineers and biomechanists must work closely with clinicians and SCI patients to further develop and refine the minimum requirements of FNS systems necessary for patient acceptance and use outside the research laboratory.

ACKNOWLEDGMENTS

This work was supported by the Rehabilitation Research and Development Service, Department of Veterans Affairs. We thank Dr. William K. Durfee for his comments on the manuscript.

REFERENCES

Andrews, B.J., Baxendale, R.H., Barnett, R., Phillips, G.F., Yamazaki, T., Paul, J.P., and Freeman, P.A. (1988). Hybrid FES orthosis incorporating closed loop control and sensory feedback. *J. Biomed. Eng.*, **10**, 190–195.

Andrews, B.J., and Kirkwood, C.A. (1989). Control of hybrid FES orthoses. *Proc. IEEE EMBS 11th Annual Conference, Seattle, WA.* 1473–1474.

Bernotas, L.A., Crago, P.E., and Chizeck, H.J. (1986). A discrete-time model of electrically stimulated muscle. *IEEE Trans. Biomed. Eng.*, **33**, 829–837.

Buckett, J.R., Peckham, P.H., Thrope, G.B., Braswell, S.D., and Keith, M.W. (1988). A flexible, portable system for neuromuscular stimulation in the paralyzed upper extremity. *IEEE Trans. Biomed. Eng.*, **35**, 897–904.

Cerny, K., Waters, R., Hislop, H., and Perry, J. (1980). Walking and wheelchair energetics in persons with paraplegia. *Phys. Ther.*, **60**, 1133–1139.

Chizeck, H.J., Kobetic, R., Marsolais, E.B., Abbas, J.J., Donner, I.H., and Simon, E. (1988). Control of functional neuromuscular stimulation systems for standing and locomotion in paraplegics. *Proc. IEEE*, **76**, 1155–1165.

Crago, P.E., Lemay, M.A., and Liu, L. (1990). External control of limb movements involving environmental interactions. In: J.M. Winters and S.L.-Y. Woo, eds., *Multiple Muscle Systems—Biomechanics and Movement Organization*, pp. 343–359. New York: Springer-Verlag.

Crosbie, W.J., and Nicol, A.C. (1990). Reciprocal aided gait in paraplegia. *Paraplegia*, **28**, 353–363.

Crowninshield, R.D., and Brand, R.A. (1981). A physiologically based criterion of muscle force prediction in locomotion. *J. Biomech.*, **14**, 793–801.

Cybulski, G.R., Penn, R.D., and Jaeger, R.J. (1984). Lower extremity functional neuromuscular stimulation in cases of spinal cord injury. *Neurosurgery*, **15**, 132–146.

Davy, D.T., and Audu, M.L. (1987). A dynamic optimization technique for predicting muscle forces in the swing phase of gait. *J. Biomech.*, **20**, 187–201.

Delp, S.L., Loan, J.P., Hoy, M.G., Zajac, F.E., Topp, E.L., and Rosen, J.M. (1990). An interactive graphics-based model of the lower extremity to study orthopaedic surgical procedures. *IEEE Trans. Biomed. Eng.*, **37**, 757–767.

Douglas, R. (1986). *LSU Reciprocating Gait Orthosis: Description and Application Manual.* Louisiana State University/Durr-Fillauer Medical, Inc.

Douglas, R., Larson, P.F., D'Ambrosia, R., and McCall, R.E. (1983). The LSU reciprocation-gait orthosis. *Orthopedics*, **6**, 834–838.

Durfee, W.K. (1989). Task-based methods for evaluating electrically stimulated antagonist muscle controllers. *IEEE Trans. Biomed. Eng.*, **36**, 309–321.

Durfee, W.K., and Hausdorff, J.M. (1990). Regulating knee joint position by combining electrical stimulation with a controllable friction brake. *Ann. Biomed. Eng.*, **18**, 575–596.

Durfee, W.K., and MacLean, K.E. (1989). Methods for estimating isometric recruitment curves of electrically stimulated muscle. *IEEE Trans. Biomed. Eng.*, **36**, 654–667.

Franklin, G.F., Powell, J.D., and Emami-Naeini, A. (1986). *Feedback Control of Dynamic Systems.* Reading, MA: Addison-Wesley.

Furusho, J., and Masabuchi, M. (1987). A theoretically motivated reduced order model for the control of dynamic biped locomotion. *J. Dyn. Syst. Meas. Control Trans. ASME*, **109**, 155–163.

Gordon, M.E. (1990). *An Analysis of the Biomechanics and Muscular Synergies of Human Standing.* Ph.D. Thesis. Stanford University.

Handa, Y., and Hoshimiya, N. (1989). Multichannel FES for motor control of the disabled. *Proc. IEEE EMBS 11th Annual Conference, Seattle, WA.* 1002–1003.

Hasan, Z., and Stuart, D.G. (1984). Mammalian muscle receptors. In: R.A. Davidoff, ed., *Handbook of the Spinal Cord, Volumes 2 and 3: Anatomy and Physiology*, pp. 559–607. New York: Marcel Dekker.

Hatze, H. (1976). The complete optimization of a human motion. *Math. Biosci.*, **28**, 99–135.

Hatze, H. (1977). A complete set of control equations for the human musculo-skeletal system. *J. Biomech.*, **10**, 799–805.

Hatze, H. (1980). Neuromusculoskeletal control systems modeling—a critical review of recent developments. *IEEE Trans. Autom. Control*, **25**, 375–385.

Hatze, H., and Venter, A. (1981). Practical activation and retention of locomotion constraints in neuromusculoskeletal control system models. *J. Biomech.*, **14**, 873–877.

Hill, A.V. (1938). The heat of shortening and the dynamic constants of muscle. *Proc. Roy. Soc. Lond.* [*Biol.*], **126**, 136–195.

Hill, T.L., Eisenberg, E., Chen, Y., and Podolsky, R.J. (1975). Some self-consistent two-state sliding filament models of muscle contraction. *Biophys. J.*, **15**, 335–372.

Hogan, N. (1985). The mechanics of multi-joint posture and movement control. *Biol. Cybern.*, **52**, 315–331.

Hoy, M.G., Zajac, F.E., and Gordon, M.E. (1990). A musculoskeletal model of the human lower extremity: The effect of muscle, tendon, and moment arm on the moment-angle relationship of musculotendon actuators at the hip, knee, and ankle. *J. Biomech.*, **23**, 157–170.

Huxley, A.F. (1957). Muscle structure and theories of contraction. *Prog. Biophys. Biophys. Chem.*, **7**, 257–318.

Jaeger, R.J. (1986). Design and simulation of closed-loop electrical stimulation orthoses for restoration of quiet standing in paraplegia. *J. Biomech.*, **19**, 825–835.

Kane, T.R., and Levinson, D.A. (1985). *Dynamics: Theory and Applications*. New York: McGraw-Hill.
Khang, G. (1988). *Paraplegic Standing Controlled by Functional Neuromuscular Stimulation: Computer Model, Control-System Design, and Simulation Studies*. Ph.D. Thesis. Stanford University.
Khang, G., and Zajac, F.E. (1989a). Paraplegic standing by functional electrical stimulation: Part I—computer model and control-system design. *IEEE Trans. Biomed. Eng.*, **36**, 873–884.
Khang, G., and Zajac, F.E. (1989b). Paraplegic standing by functional electrical stimulation: Part II—computer simulation studies. *IEEE Trans. Biomed. Eng.*, **36**, 885–894.
Kobetic, R., and Marsolais, E.B. (1988). Control of paraplegic gait by detection of discrete events. *Proc. ICAART '88, Montreal, Canada*. 346–347.
Kralj, A., and Grobelnik, S. (1973). Functional electrical stimulation: A new hope for paraplegic patients? *Bull. Pros. Res.*, **20**, 75–102.
Kralj, A.R., and Bajd, T. (1989). *Functional Electrical Stimulation: Standing and Walking after Spinal Cord Injury*. Boca Raton, FL: CRC Press.
Kuntzman, A.J., Glaser, R.M., Shively, R.A., Rodgers, M.M., and Ezenwa, B.N. (1990). Muscle fatigue characteristics with FNS-induced contractions. *Proc. RESNA 13th Annual Conference, Washington, D.C.* 161–162.
Lew, R.D. (1987). The effects of FNS on disuse osteoporosis. *Proc. 10th Annual Conference on Rehabilitation Technology, San Jose, CA.* 616–617.
Mansour, J.M., and Pereira, J.M. (1987). Quantitative functional anatomy of the lower limb with application to human gait. *J. Biomech.*, **20**, 51–58.
Marsolais, E.B. (1989). FNS application for restoring function in stroke patients. *Proc. IEEE EMBS 11th Annual Conference, Seattle, WA.* 829–830.
Marsolais, E.B., and Edwards, B.G. (1988). Energy costs of walking and standing with functional neuromuscular stimulation and long leg braces. *Arch. Phys. Med. Rehabil.*, **69**, 243–249.
Marsolais, E.B., and Kobetic, R. (1987). Functional electrical stimulation for walking in paraplegia. *J. Bone Joint Surg.*, **69-A**, 728–733.
Marsolais, E.B., and Kobetic, R. (1988). Design considerations for a practical functional electrical stimulation systems for restoring gait in the paralyzed person. *Proc. ICAART '88, Montreal, Canada.* 338–339.
Mortimer, J.T. (1981). Motor Prostheses. In: V.B. Brooks, ed., *Handbook of Physiology: The Nervous System. Vol. II, Motor Control*, pp. 155–187. Bethesda, MD: American Physiological Society.
Muccio, P.E., and Marsolais, E.B. (1987). Experience with ankle-foot orthoses and paraplegic subjects using functional neuromuscular stimulation. *Proc. RESNA 10th Annual Conference, San Jose, CA.* 613–615.
Nathan, R.H. (1990). Upper limb functions regained in quadriplegia: A hybrid computerized neuromuscular stimulation system. *Arch. Phys. Med. Rehabil.*, **71**, 415–421.
Nene, A.V. (1989). An assessment of the orlau parawalker-electrical stimulation powered orthosis. *Proc. IEEE EMBS 11th Annual Conference, Seattle, WA.* 1016–1017.
Onyshko, S., and Winter, D.A. (1980). A mathematical model for the dynamics of human locomotion. *J. Biomech.*, **13**, 361–368.
Pandy, M.G., and Berme, N. (1988). Synthesis of human walking: A planar model for single support. *J. Biomech.*, **21**, 1053–1060.
Pandy, M.G., Zajac, F.E., Sim, E., and Levine, W.S. (1990). An optimal control model for maximum-height human jumping. *J. Biomech.*, **23**, 1185–1198.
Peckham, P.H., Marsolais, E.B., and Mortimer, J.T. (1980). Restoration of key grip and

release in the C6 tetraplegic through functional electrical stimulation. *J. Hand Surg.*, **5**, 462–469.

Pederson, D.R., Brand, R.A., Cheng, C., and Arora, J.S. (1987). Direct comparison of muscle force predictions using linear and nonlinear programming. *J. Biomech. Eng.*, **109**, 192–199.

Phillips, C.A. (1989). Functional electrical stimulation and lower extremity bracing for ambulation exercise of the spinal cord injured individual: A medically prescribed system. *Phys. Ther.*, **69**, 842–849.

Phillips, C.A., and Hendershot, D.M. (1988). The EMS-RGO: A physician prescribable FES ambulation exercise system. *Proc. IEEE EMBS 10th Annual Conference, New Orleans, LA*. 1573–1574.

Phillips, C.A., Petrofsky, J.S., Hendershot, D.M., and Stafford, D. (1984). Functional electrical exercise—a comprehensive approach for physical conditioning of the spinal cord injured patient. *Orthopedics*, **7**, 1112.

Popovic, D. (1990). Dynamics of the self-fitting modular orthosis. *IEEE J. Robotics Automation*, **6**, 200–207.

Popovic, D., Tomovic, R., and Schwirtlich, L. (1989). Hybrid assistive system—the motor neuroprosthesis. *IEEE Trans. Biomed. Eng.*, **36**, 729–736.

PSA. (1990). Estimates of SCI prevalence. *Paralysis Soc. Am. Research Briefs*, **4**, 1–7.

Schoenberg, A., and Long, J. (1987). Design of a quickly-assembled, light-weight leg orthosis for FES assisted paraplegic mobility. *Proc. RESNA 10th Annual Conference, San Jose, CA*. 633–635.

Solomonow, M., Baratta, R., Hirokawa, S., Rightor, N., Walker, W., Beaudette, P., Shoji, H., and D'Ambrosia, R. (1989). The RGO generation II: Muscle stimulation powered orthosis as a practical walking system for thoracic paraplegics. *Orthopedics*, **12**, 1309–1315.

Stallard, J., Major, R.E., Poiner, R., Farmer, I.R., and Jones, N. (1986). Engineering design considerations of the ORLAU parawalker and FES hybrid system. *Eng. Med.*, **15**, 123–129.

Townsend, M.A., and Seireg, A.A. (1973). Effect of model complexity and gait criteria on the synthesis of bipedal locomotion. *IEEE Trans. Biomed. Eng.*, **20**, 433–444.

Vukobratovic, M., and Stokic, D. (1980). Significance of force-feedback in controlling artificial locomotion-manipulation systems. *IEEE Trans. Biomed. Eng.*, **27**, 705–713.

Willemin, D.E., and Chizeck, H.J. (1989). Feedback control of the knee during the stance phase of paraplegic gait, using a stiffness regulator. *Proc. RESNA 12th Annual Conference, New Orleans, LA*. 399–400.

Winter, D.A. (1988). Motor control of human gait—a multitask movement. *Proc. IEEE EMBS 10th Annual Conference, New Orleans, LA*. 612–613.

Winters, J.M. (1990). Hill-based muscle models: A systems engineering perspective. In: J.M. Winters and S.L.-Y. Woo, ed., *Multiple Muscle Systems—Biomechanics and Movement Organization*, pp. 69–93. New York: Springer-Verlag.

Winters, J.M., and Stark, L. (1987). Muscle models: What is gained and what is lost by varying model complexity. *Biol. Cybern.*, **55**, 403–420.

Yamaguchi, G.T. (1989). *Feasibility and Conceptual Design of Functional Neuromuscular Stimulation Systems for the Restoration of Natural Gaits to Paraplegics Based on Dynamic Musculoskeletal Models*. Ph.D. Thesis. Stanford University.

Yamaguchi, G.T. (1990). Performing whole-body simulations of gait with 3-D, dynamic musculoskeletal models. In: J.M. Winters and S.L.-Y. Woo, eds., *Multiple Muscle Systems—Biomechanics and Movement Organization*, pp. 663–679. New York: Springer-Verlag.

Yamaguchi, G.T., Sawa, A.G.U., Moran, D.W., Fessler, M.J., and Winters, J.M. (1990). A survey of human musculotendon actuator parameters. In: J.M. Winters and S.L.-Y.

Woo, eds., *Multiple Muscle Systems—Biomechanics and Movement Organization*, pp. 717–773. New York: Springer-Verlag.

Yamaguchi, G.T., and Zajac, F.E. (1989). A planar model of the knee joint to characterize the knee extension mechanism. *J. Biomech.*, **22**, 1–10.

Yamaguchi, G.T., and Zajac, F.E. (1990). Restoring unassisted gait to paraplegics via functional neuromuscular stimulation: A computer simulation study. *IEEE Trans. Biomed. Eng.*, **37**, 886–902.

Zahalak, G.I. (1990). Modeling muscle mechanics (and energetics). In: J.M. Winters and S.L.-Y. Woo, eds., *Multiple Muscle Systems—Biomechanics and Movement Organization*, pp. 1–23. New York: Springer-Verlag.

Zahalak, G.I., and Ma, S.-P. (1990). Muscle activation and contraction: Constitutive relations based directly on cross-bridge kinetics. *J. Biomech. Eng.*, **112**, 52–62.

Zajac, F.E. (1989). Muscle and tendon: Properties, models, scaling, and application to biomechanics and motor control. In: J.R. Bourne, ed., *CRC Crit. Rev. Biomed. Eng.*, **17**(4), 359–411. Boca Raton, FL: CRC Press.

Zajac, F.E., and Gordon, M.E. (1989). Determining muscle's force and action in multi-articular movement. In: K. Pandolf, ed., *Exercise Sport Sci. Rev.*, **17**, 187–230. Baltimore: Williams & Wilkins.

IV
Adaptive Control and Technology Transfer

13
Feedback Control of Normal and Electrically Induced Movements

RICHARD B. STEIN

This chapter traces the development of ideas about the role of sensory receptors in the control of movement. Over the years proposals have been made that a particular physical variable is controlled by the nervous system during movement (e.g., the "follow-up length servo" of Merton or the "stiffness regulation" of Houk and his colleagues). The richness of sensory receptors in mammalian limbs would allow control of a number of physical variables. Instead of precisely controlling a particular variable, a flexible control strategy seems to have evolved which uses sensory information differently in different tasks and even from time to time within a given task. Functional electrical stimulation (FES), intended to replace movements that have been lost as a result of accident or disease processes, has often been implemented without explicit control mechanisms involving sensory feedback. In addition, spasticity and other common symptoms of these conditions may represent a loss of the flexibility of the natural feedback. Understanding the adaptive control that nature has evolved and the deficits that are typically caused by injury may help to guide future improvements in FES systems. Hopefully, improved systems will adapt more easily to different tasks and different environmental conditions in a way that will improve patient acceptance.

Sensory receptors have long been known to provide feedback via reflexes and voluntary reactions for the control of posture and locomotion. However, nearly 40 years ago, Merton (1953) first suggested an explicit control strategy for producing normal human movements. Thirty years ago, Liberson et al. (1961) developed the first practical method for replacing movements by electrical stimulation in the limbs of patients suffering partial paralysis. This chapter will trace the subsequent devel-

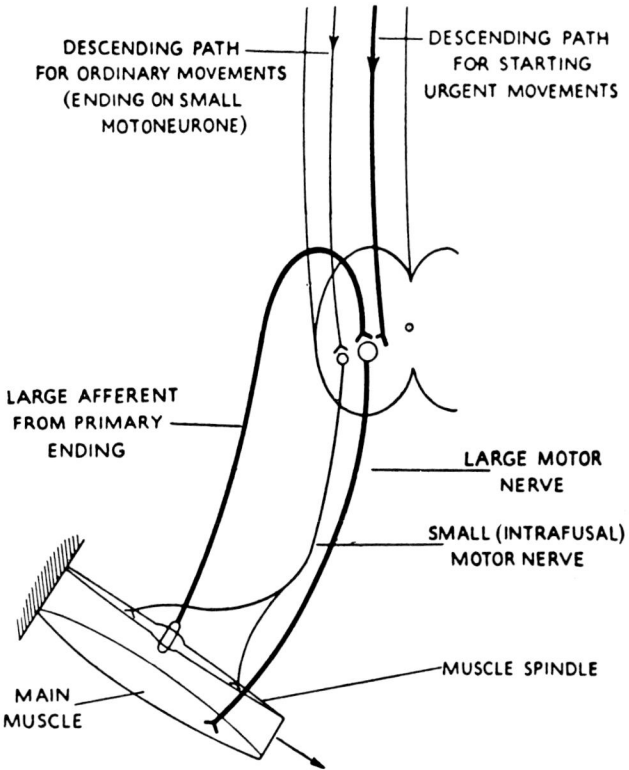

Figure 13–1 Diagram from Merton (1953) suggesting that primary spindle afferents function as a "follow-up length servo" in the control of movement, by analogy with the simple feedback system shown in Figure 13–2A. Further explanation in the text.

opment of ideas on the control of normal movements and the attempts to replace these in paralyzed patients. The two have developed in-parallel in some respects, but have diverged in others. In my view, attempts to replace motor function have to be at least consonant with the normal methods that are used by the body, if they are to succeed.

CONTROL OF LENGTH

Merton (Figure 13–1) emphasized the role of a particular type of receptor, the primary ending of the muscle spindle (Matthews, 1981). The sensory or afferent nerve fibers from the muscle spindle are unique among sensory receptors in being influenced by a private motor supply (the small or γ-motor neurons) which innervate the specialized muscle fibers that lie within the muscle spindle (intrafusal muscle fibers). The larger α-motor neurons innervate the bulk of the muscle which lies outside this sensory structure.

Merton suggested that descending inputs from the brain would activate the γ-motor neurons in a manner similar to the control input to a length feedback system or length-servo (Figure 13–2A). The large afferent nerve fibers (group Ia) from the

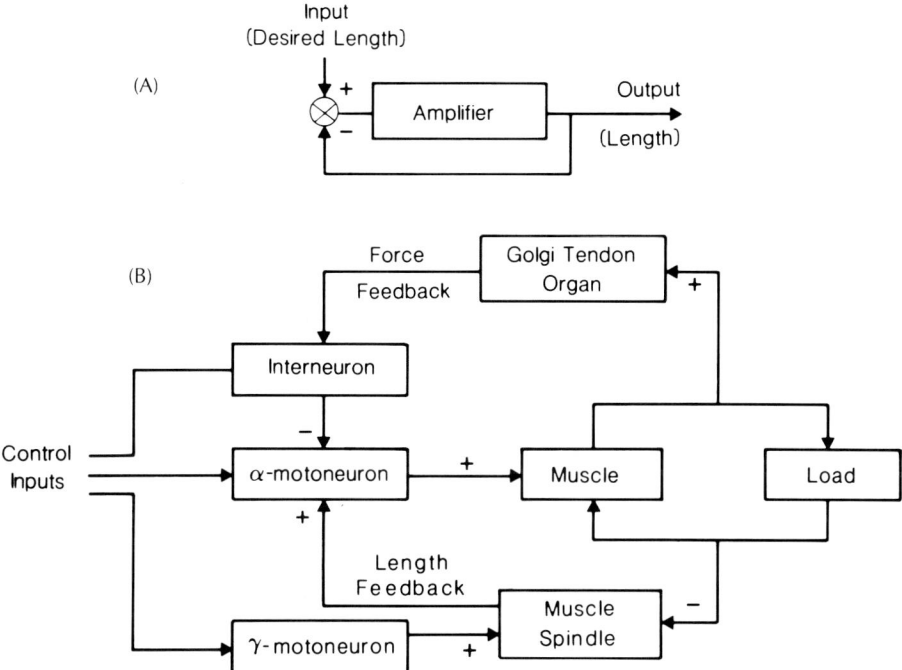

Figure 13–2 (A) A simple feedback system. (B) A more realistic model would require that control from the central nervous system be exerted at several points. Both length and force feedback are available to modify the motor output. (Modified from Kandel and Schwartz, 1985, with permission.)

primary endings of the muscle spindles were known to be sensitive to muscle length and to have monosynaptic connections onto the α-motor neurons. This reflex would then serve as an amplifier to produce the motor output. The resultant muscular contraction would shorten the intrafusal as well as the extrafusal muscle fibers, since they lie essentially in-parallel. This shortening would remove the tension on the sensory endings of the afferent nerve fibers which lie on the intrafusal muscle fibers and their activity would decrease and provide the negative feedback signal for comparing with the control input (desired length) in the diagram of Figure 13–2A.

Merton's suggestion generated numerous experiments and, based on experimental findings, has been modified several times in the intervening years. For example, there are significant time delays in conduction of nerve signals, and in contraction of muscle fibers. Merton realized (Figure 13–1) that urgent movements might have to be initiated by pathways directly onto the α-motor neurons. However, using the technique of microneurography (Vallbo et al., 1979), nerve impulses can be recorded from primary afferents in normal human subjects during ordinary movements. The postulate from Figure 13–1 that activity in the afferent fibers should precede activity in α-motor neurons has not been verified (Vallbo, 1971). The two tend to fire more or less at the same time, which suggests that there is coactivation of pathways onto α- and γ-motor neurons, rather than preferential activation of either pathway. The relative degree of activation in the two pathways may be altered for different movements, but the feedback loop can still be used to assist in the movement.

This suggestion has been referred to as "servo-assistance" to distinguish it from

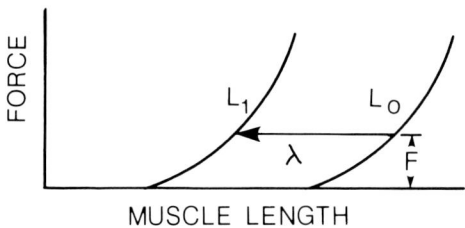

Figure 13–3 Feldman's equilibrium point hypothesis. Contraction producing a force, F, will move a load from length L_0 to length L_1 if central inputs shift the threshold of an invariant relationship between length and force by an amount λ. This relationship is determined by a combination of active muscle and reflex properties. (Modified from Berkenbilt et al., 1986, with permission.)

the simple feedback or "servo-control" scheme of Figure 13–1. The idea was proposed in slightly different forms by several investigators in the early 1970s (Matthews, 1972; Houk, 1972; Stein, 1974) and is shown in Figure 13–2B. Central control inputs to the α-motor neurons cause the muscle to shorten against its load and remove some length feedback from the muscle spindle. If the load is heavy, less contraction will occur and hence less feedback will be removed. The α-motor neurons and the muscle will continue to be excited until the desired length is approached. Similarly, control signals to the γ-motor neuron will further excite the muscle spindle and produce extra length feedback and further contraction. Thus, inputs to γ-motor neurons can modify the desired length in a manner analogous to that proposed by Merton.

STIFFNESS REGULATION

Figure 13–2B also suggests a role for another sensory receptor, the Golgi tendon organ. These receptors sense the force generated in the tendon of the muscle and feed back information (via group-Ib nerve fibers) to interneurons which then inhibit α-motor neurons. The Golgi tendon organs are not themselves under central control, but the interneurons in the feedback pathway (known as group-Ib interneurons) do receive a number of other inputs (Harrison and Jankowska, 1985). From this scheme Houk suggested that neither force nor length would be independently controlled, but rather their ratio, stiffness (Houk and Rymer, 1981).

These ideas were developed further by Feldman (1986) as the "equilibrium point hypothesis," which is illustrated in Figure 13–3. According to this hypothesis, muscle properties together with the feedback loops shown in Figure 13–3 determine the relation between force and length of a muscle, which Feldman termed the "invariant characteristic." Note that the slope of the relationship may increase at higher force levels, because the stiffness of a muscle increases proportionally with the number of force-generating cross-bridges that are formed (reviewed by Kearney and Hunter, 1990). At the same time, the reflexes may eliminate some of the highly nonlinear properties of muscle so that the combination is more easily controlled (Nichols and Houk, 1976). The role of the central nervous system is then simply to shift the threshold of the invariant relation between force and length (a translation along the length axis) so that the muscle will contract against a given load to bring it to a new position.

Feldman extended his hypothesis to antagonistic pairs of muscles in which the equilibrium point is formed between two invariant characteristics (Feldman et al.,

1990). Since each can be activated to some extent independently by the central nervous system (Kearney and Hunter, 1990), cocontraction can be used to increase stiffness without producing movement. This would be useful, for example, to stabilize a load against unexpected perturbations. Flanagan et al. (1990) also extended the hypothesis to make predictions about time-varying contractions, including rhythmic contractions. Further discussion of the control of stiffness during movements under various external conditions is found in Chapter 6.

Crago et al. (1991) had good success in using both length and force feedback in the control of grasping by spinal-cord-injured subjects. Force sensors are attached to the thumb and goniometers measure the angle between the thumb and the other fingers. In grasping an object, length feedback but no force feedback is present until the hand actually contacts the object. If the object is rigid, length feedback does not change, but force feedback increases as the object is grasped more tightly. Using the combination of length and force feedback permits a smooth transition at the discontinuity between the phase of no resistance (before contact) and the phase of very high resistance (after contact). Grasping objects of differing stiffness is also facilitated, since a combination of length and force feedback will be available as the object is grasped more tightly. Although these ideas seem promising, implementing them in a practical device for quadriplegics still remains a task for the future. Reliability is difficult because of the need to put external sensors on the hand and the fact that the placement will vary from day to day. An alternative is to record nerve activity from the body's own sensors using cuff electrodes or other techniques (the pros and cons of this alternative approach are outlined in Chapter 5.)

GAIN OR EFFICACY OF THE REFLEXES

Although this scheme may be effective for external control during grasping, its efficacy during normal control of movements remains uncertain. Houk et al. (1970) attempted to measure the gain of the feedback loop from Golgi tendon organs in a decerebrate cat (one in which the higher brain structures had been removed). These animals show a rather rigid, extended posture. Stimulating a small nerve filament to generate extra tension led to some inhibition, but the gain of the feedback loop was typically between 0.2 and 0.8 in different preparations. More recent attempts to measure the gain have given even lower values (Rymer and Hasan, 1980). These authors suggested that the interneuron in the pathway (Figure 13–2B) may be strongly inhibited and therefore force feedback is largely blocked, but it would be nice to demonstrate a higher gain in other preparations.

Matthews (1959) also questioned the gain of the length feedback pathway. He stretched soleus muscle (an ankle extensor) through its entire physiological range, again in a decerebrate cat. Even with this degree of stretch the muscle only generated a fraction of its maximum force output. In these experiments the muscle was held rigidly and not allowed to shorten so the feedback loop was effectively opened. With length as an input and force as an output, one can not calculate a dimensionless gain for the feedback loop. However, if the gain were high, even a small length change would be expected to generate a large force.

Yang et al. (1991) recently reexamined this question in normal human subjects walking on a treadmill. A pneumatic device was attached to the foot, and at a random time during the period when the foot was on the ground (stance phase), it lifted the forefoot and flexed the ankle by about 5°. Primary muscle spindle afferents are sensitive to velocity as well as length, with a break point in their frequency response curve at 1 to 2 Hz (Matthews and Stein, 1969). The electrical activity of the α-motor neurons [the electromyogram (EMG)] produced by these perturbations was also well fitted by a combination of length and velocity inputs. The best fit was typically obtained with a breakpoint near the expected frequency and an average time delay of 38 msec, which corresponds to the known latency of the monosynaptic pathway from primary muscle spindle afferents in this muscle.

The magnitude of the response was small early in the stance phase, but increased progressively during stance. In human locomotion, the ankle extensors such as soleus are stretched throughout much of the stance phase. Knowing the magnitude and velocity of that stretch and the response of a given subject to comparable perturbations at each phase of the step cycle, one can predict how much of the EMG is being generated by the reflex. From these calculations 30 to 60% of the EMG activity appears to be produced by the stretch reflex over the period the muscle is being stretched, with the balance being generated centrally by other inputs onto the motor neurons.

This contrasts with attempts to reproduce locomotion by functional electrical stimulation (FES) in spinal-cord-injured patients, which have often operated without feedback (e.g., Marsolais and Kobetic, 1987). Since the amount of force to keep the knees from buckling during stance is not measured, the knee extensors are generally stimulated maximally to ensure safety. This will obviously increase energy consumption during walking and limit endurance (see Chapter 10), since the muscles will fatigue more rapidly than with lesser amounts of stimulation.

Mayagoitia and Andrews (1990) attempted to overcome this problem by using an "artificial reflex" (see also Prochazka and Wiles, 1983). Force sensors were placed in a floor-reaction orthosis (FRO). This differs from a conventional ankle-foot orthosis (AFO) in that it has a piece in front of the tibia which prevents forward rotation over the ankle (Figure 13–4). As long as the center of gravity of the body is in front of the knee, pressure on this front piece pushes the tibia back and tends to passively lock the knee joint. Stimulation is only needed when the center of gravity moves behind the knee. The pressure sensor in the FRO was used to detect these shifts and only apply stimuli to the knee extensors (quadriceps muscles) as required. With this system subjects can stand for long periods of time (>30 minutes) without fatiguing the muscles. These same principles are being extended to the control of locomotion (Andrews, 1990).

ADAPTIVE GAIN CONTROL

I pointed out above that the magnitude of the response to a given perturbation is greater at different times during the stance phase of locomotion. This suggests that the reflex gain is changed adaptively. This can be studied more precisely by stimulating a muscle nerve at a strength that mainly excites group-IA afferents. Some α-motor neurons will also be stimulated, which will produce an EMG wave in the

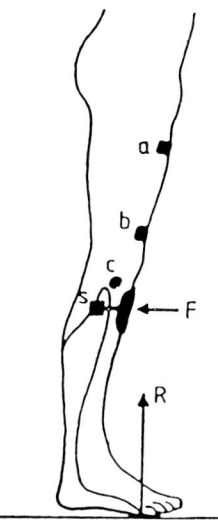

Figure 13–4 "Artificial reflex" system using a floor-reaction orthosis (FRO). If the ground reaction force, R, is in front of the knee, the orthosis will provide a force, F, to keep the knee locked. A strain guage (S) measures the force, and if it drops below a threshold value (e.g., the patient sways backward), stimuli are applied to the quadriceps to keep the knee locked. (From Mayagoitia and Andrews, 1990, with permission.)

muscle, referred to as a motor or M-wave (Figure 13–5A). The magnitude of this wave can be monitored to check that a constant fraction of α-motor neuron fibers and presumably a constant fraction of group-IA afferents are being stimulated throughout the step cycle (Figure 13–5B). Changes in reflex gain will therefore be evident from the later reflex EMG wave, which is known as the Hoffmann or H-wave, after the German neurologist who first described it (Figure 13–5C). With these stimuli, a certain fraction of group-Ib afferents may also be stimulated, but this volley will arrive a bit later at the motor neurons, because of the interneuron in this pathway. Also, because this pathway is inhibitory, it can not account for the excitatory response seen (the H-wave).

The beginning of the traces in Figure 13–5 is at the time in the step cycle when the heel strikes the ground and the duration of the traces corresponds to one step cycle. The stance phase occupies approximately 60% of the duration and the swing phase the final 40%. The H-wave is small during the beginning of stance and increases progressively during this phase. The response becomes very small during the swing phase of locomotion. This variation is well adapted to the requirements of normal stepping. During early stance, the center of gravity of the body is behind the foot, but its momentum is carrying it forward over the foot. A reflex response in the ankle extensors at this time would generate torque that would impede this forward movement. Once the body is in front of the foot the reflex will push the body upward and forward, which will maintain the forward momentum and assist in the subsequent swing phase. During the swing phase the ankle is actively flexed so that the toes will clear the ground. This will again stretch the ankle extensors and a reflex response would be inappropriate. It would in fact tend to lower the foot (footdrop), and the foot may then drag along the ground.

What is the mechanism of this variation in H-waves during the step cycle? One simple explanation would be that as the central control signal increases, as evidenced by the increasing soleus EMG in Figure 13–5, more motor neurons are active and hence can be excited by the sensory input. One might therefore expect a parallel increase in the H-wave with EMG activity as is in fact seen in Figures 13–5 and

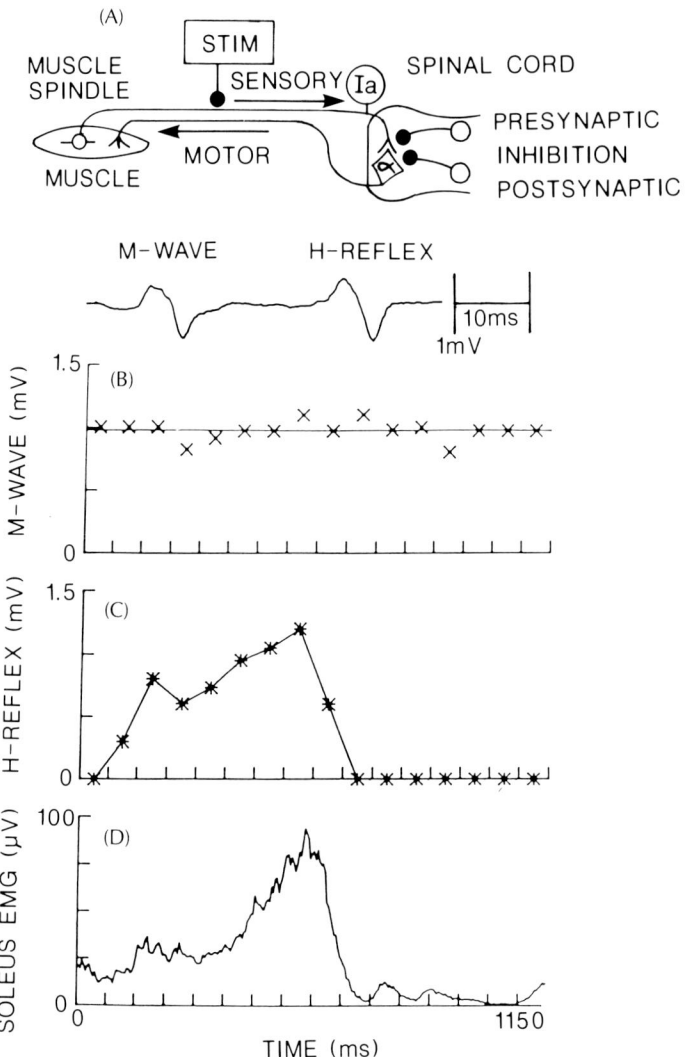

Figure 13–5 (A) A stimulus to the human tibial nerve produces two EMG responses in the soleus muscle: an M-wave from direct excitation of motor axons and an H-reflex from stimulation of group-Ia fibers from muscle spindles. The effect of this stimulation can be modified by inputs postsynaptically onto the α-motor neuron or presynaptically onto the terminals of the group-Ia fibers. During walking, even if the stimulus produces a constant M-wave over the step cycle (B), the H-reflex varies dramatically (C), approximately in parallel with the activity (D) in the muscle. (From Stein and Capaday, 1988, with permission.)

13–6. However, also shown in Figure 13–6A are the H-waves recorded from one subject on the same day while he was quietly standing or generating various constant levels of EMG. Note that for a given level of EMG activity the reflexes during walking and standing can be quite different. Since the muscle stiffness is the same and the reflex stiffness varies, this task-dependent reflex change is not consistent

FEEDBACK CONTROL OF NORMAL AND ELECTRICALLY INDUCED MOVEMENTS

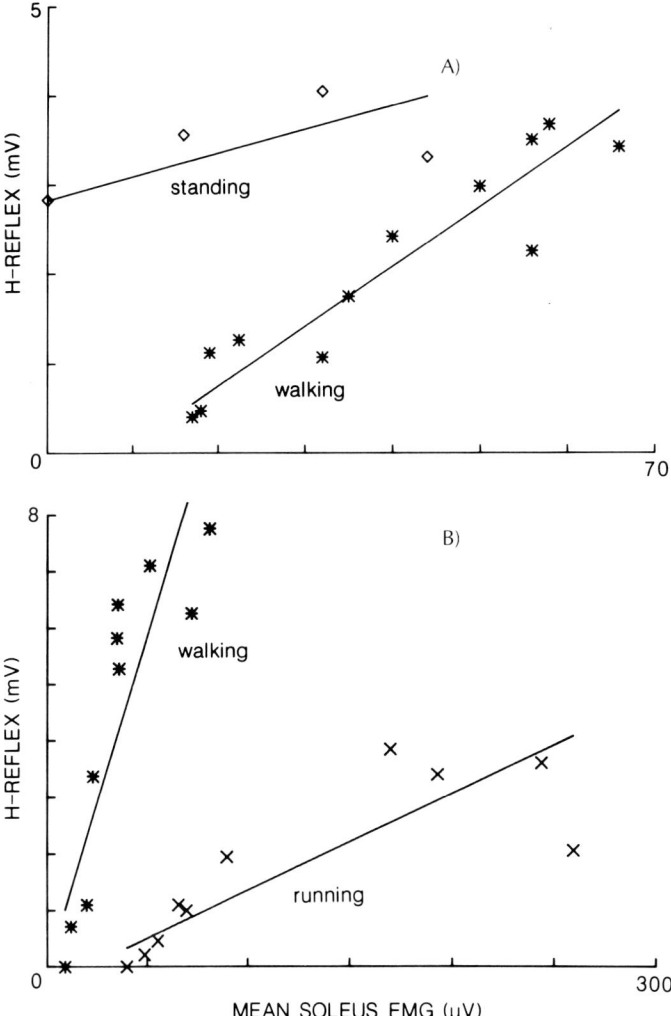

Figure 13–6 Comparison in two subjects of the changes in H-reflex (at a constant M-wave) for (A) standing and walking with (B) walking and running. (From Stein and Capaday, 1988, with permission.)

with Feldman's idea of an invariant characteristic. However, the magnitude of the deviation has not been measured accurately.

The speed with which a subject can change from one reflex gain to another is quite remarkable. If a subject is quietly standing and is given a tone as a signal to begin walking, the reflex response will decrease within a reaction time from that expected for standing to that expected for walking with little or no change in EMG activity in the soleus muscle (Edamura et al., 1991). Clear task-dependent differences at a given level of activity are also seen between walking and running (Figure 13–6B), although the effect is mainly a change in slope, whereas the change between standing and walking (Figure 13–6A) is mainly a change in the y-intercept.

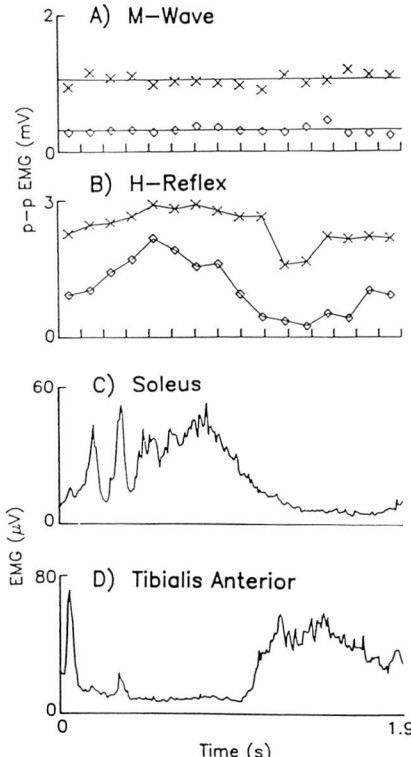

Figure 13–7 Two levels of stimulation were used with a spastic patient. With a level of stimulation comparable to the normal subject in Figure 13–5 (×'s) little modulation was observed in the H-reflex. With a much lower stimulus (◊) a clear modulation was evident. (From Stein et al., 1991, with permission.)

A mechanism which is consistent with a number of animal and modeling studies (Capaday and Stein, 1987, 1989) is also shown in Figure 13–5A. In addition to the excitatory and inhibitory inputs from various sources in the central nervous system which impinge on the motor neuron, control can be exercised presynaptically. Synapses end on presynaptic terminals of the group-IA afferent fibers, which can reduce the amount of transmitter this muscle spindle afferent will release and hence reduce the reflex gain of this pathway selectively. Presynaptic inhibition can therefore account for the task-specific reflex changes observed at a given level of EMG activity, whereas postsynaptic effects cannot (Capaday and Stein, 1989).

DISORDERED CONTROL

The H-reflex method can also be used to measure the reflex responses in patients with brain or incomplete spinal cord injuries. These patients, although often able to walk to some extent, may have trouble with footdrop and spasticity. Figure 13–7 shows data from such a patient who walked relatively slowly (compare the time scales in Figure 13–5 and 13–7). With a stimulus at a strength that produced an M-wave of about 1 mV, little modulation is evident in the H-wave. However, with a lower stimulus strength that produced a very small M-wave, a relatively normal modulation of the H-wave was produced. The simplest explanation of this data is that the reflex gain is abnormally high, so that with the usual level of stimulation the reflex response was saturated. This explanation is consistent with the usual observation in spasticity where a movement of the limb produces an abnormally large reflex response.

Another indication of high reflex gain is evident from the alternating bursts of activity in soleus muscle and tibialis anterior (an ankle flexor) muscle in Figure 13–7. If the ankle of a spastic patient at rest is flexed, it often goes into an oscillation known as clonus. Depending on its severity, the clonus may be damped or may be maintained for long periods of time. Clonus is generally viewed as an instability due to the high gain of a feedback loop with time delays (Stein and Lee, 1981). From the known reflex delays, the low-pass properties of muscle (see Chapter 3), and the high-pass properties of muscle spindles (from its velocity sensitivity), the frequency of oscillation can be calculated (Stein and Lee, 1981). The alternating bursts of activity at the onset of stance are consistent with the stretch of the ankle muscles early in stance phase, coupled with the abnormally high gain at that time.

However, recent studies from Rymer's lab (reviewed by Katz and Rymer, 1989) did not find enhanced reflex gain under laboratory conditions in patients with evidence of spasticity clinically. Instead, there was a clear change in threshold (i.e., the length-tension relation was shifted to the left, as indicated in Figure 13–3). Rymer's measurements were on the upper limb in a postural task using constant velocity stretches, whereas the measurements shown in Figure 13–7 were in the lower limb of a walking subject and used electrical stimuli. Further work is clearly required to determine which differences are important in explaining the discrepancies between the two sets of results.

Whatever the mechanism turns out to be, the abnormal reflexes underlying spasticity and clonus are a problem for attempts to produce locomotion or other movements by FES in spinal-cord-injured patients. The most common way of treating this problem is pharmacologically. The presynaptic inhibitory pathway described above (Figure 13–5A) releases a chemical transmitter, gamma-aminobutyric acid (GABA), and an agonist of this transmitter (baclofen) can be taken by mouth. In many patients, this drug produces enough inhibition to reduce reflexes to acceptable levels. In patients with extreme spasticity, however, the drug may not be effective taken by mouth, but an infusion pump can be implanted so that the drug is applied directly to the spinal cord. Implantation can produce dramatic improvements in patients with otherwise intractable spasticity (Latash et al., 1989). Either by oral or implanted administration, a steady level of presynaptic inhibition will be produced by the drug. Task-dependent changes in reflex gain may still not be possible, but at least the spasms and clonus can be controlled to the point that they do not interfere with the use of FES to replace movements.

OTHER CONTROL STRATEGIES

The natural control system has other elements which further increase its degree of sophistication. In addition to the Golgi tendon organs and primary muscle spindle afferent, there is a smaller, secondary muscle spindle afferent. Whereas the primary afferent is sensitive to velocity and length, the secondary afferent is more of a pure length sensor under most conditions. There are also two types of γ-motor neuron (static and dynamic) and different types of intrafusal fibers (nuclear bag and nuclear chain). I will not give details of this complexity here, but the pattern of connections

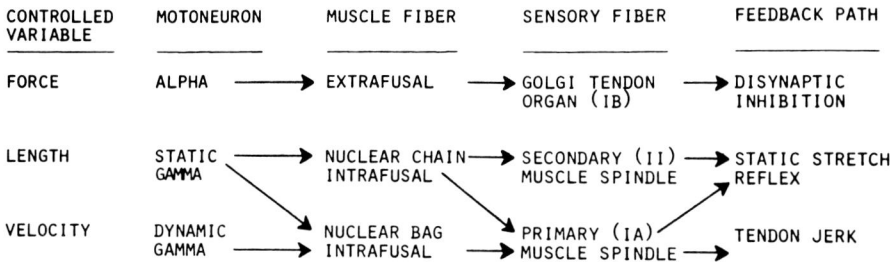

Figure 13–8 Possible schemes by which some muscle variables could be controlled. Arrows indicate known anatomical connections. Further discussion of these and other possibilities is found in the text and in Stein (1982).

suggests that three distinct pathways could exist for control of different variables such as force, length, and velocity (Figure 13–8). Combinations of these variables could be used to control stiffness (force/length) or viscosity (force/velocity).

Whether one or more of these possible strategies is actually used by the body is still unsettled (see, for example, the open commentary in Stein, 1982), but some data have accumulated more recently on how the two types of γ-motor neurons are used during behavior. This is illustrated in Figure 13–9, taken from a paper by Murphy et al. (1984) in which γ-motor neurons were recorded from a high decerebrate cat. The cat was suspended over a moving treadmill belt. After a second or two of foot contact the animal began to show rhythmic walking movements, as indicated by the bursts of EMG activity in soleus muscle and the corresponding force traces generated by the muscle. The bottom traces in parts (A) and (B) show the

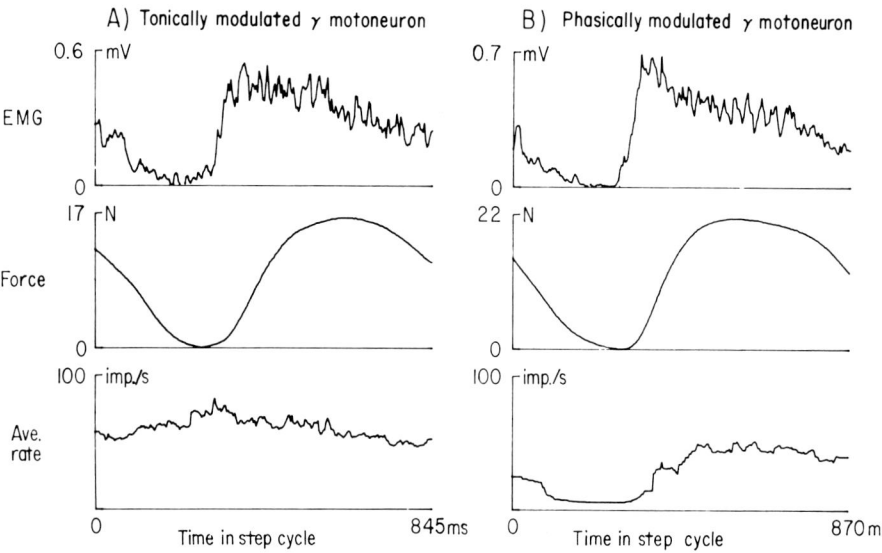

Figure 13–9 Average rate of nerve impulses from a tonically modulated (A) and a phasically modulated (B) γ-motor neuron during the step cycle. EMG and force were recorded from soleus muscle in a mesencephalic, decerebrate cat. These animals show rhythmic walking movements when suspended over a moving treadmill. (From Murphy et al., 1984, with permission.)

responses of two different types of γ-motor neurons. The one in (A) gradually increased its firing rate in the interval between the onset of treadmill motion and the onset of walking, but its rate was only weakly modulated with each step. In contrast, the γ-motor neuron in (B) showed no change in its firing rate until the animal began to walk, but the rate was then deeply modulated with each step. Further experiments indicated that the tonically modulated units such as in (A) were static γ-motor neurons, while the phasically modulated units such as in (B) were dynamic γ-motor neurons (Taylor et al., 1985).

Figure 13-8 indicates that only the static γ-motor neuron affects the discharge of the secondary muscle spindle afferent. This motor neuron increases its discharge rate, but has little effect on its sensitivity to stretch (Matthews, 1981). Since the static γ-motor neuron fires relatively steadily during walking, it will produce a high rate of firing in the secondary muscle spindle afferent which will be modulated only by the length changes taking place in the muscle. The secondary afferent could then act as a good length transducer. Interestingly, these afferents have relatively weak reflex effects, compared to the primary afferents (Stauffer et al., 1976), but have strong connections to the cortex. They would therefore be ideally suited to inform the brain of the length changes taking place in the muscles during each step.

In contrast, the dynamic γ-motor neuron only affects the primary afferent. These motor neurons increase the firing rate of muscle spindles, their sensitivity to small amplitudes of stretch, and their response to the velocity of larger stretches (Matthews, 1981). Because of the phasic nature of the discharge in dynamic γ-motor neurons during walking, the rate of firing and the sensitivity of the primary muscle spindle afferent is turned up during stance when the muscle is active and turned down during the swing phase when it is inactive. These peripheral changes at the level of the receptor will reinforce the central reflex changes in the adaptive control of reflex gain (see the earlier section on this topic). Thus, the two types of muscle spindle receptor appear to be used differently during walking, at least in the decerebrate cat. The primary afferent is used in the modulation of reflex gain within each step cycle, while the secondary afferent is signaling length changes to the cortex, so that corrections can be made from one cycle to the next.

It has not been possible to record γ-motor neurons in intact cats (or people) during behavior, but muscle spindle afferents have been recorded (summarized in Prochazka et al., 1989). Using data from a wide range of motor behaviors, Hulliger et al. (1987) imposed the same pattern of length changes to muscles in an anesthetized cat, using a muscle puller, as occurred in the behaving animal. They then determined iteratively what pattern of stimulation to γ-motor neurons would be required to account for the discharge of the afferent. Some of the results are consistent with those described for the decerebrate cat, but a variety of patterns of dynamic and γ-motor neuron activation were required to match the observed pattern of afferent activity during the different behaviors of the intact animal (Hulliger et al., 1989).

From this work emerged the idea of "fusimotor set" (Prochazka, 1989), namely that in preparing for a movement, not only is the posture of an animal and the program for its movement "set" by the activity of α-motor neurons, but the γ-motor neurons (also called fusimotor motor neurons) are set as well to provide sensory feedback from the muscle spindles that is appropriate for the specific movement to be carried out.

CUTANEOUS REFLEXES

Up to this point we have only considered muscle afferents, but the body has a wide variety of receptors in its skin and joints (see also Chapter 5). The effects of stimulating these receptors is often lumped under the terms "flexor reflex" or "withdrawal reflex" and the receptors giving rise to this reflex are often referred to as "flexor reflex afferents." The role of this reflex is evident, for example, if you step on a tack while walking. The limb is flexed reflexly to withdraw it from the painful stimulus, often before the sensation of pain reaches the brain. It was this reflex that was used by Liberson et al. (1961) to produce a flexion of the limb for stepping in stroke patients who could not adequately flex the limb voluntarily. Many others have used it since (see review by Kralj and Bajd, 1989).

At the beginning of the century, Sherrington (1906) already pointed out several distinctive features of the flexion reflex. The reflex habituates (the response is less with repetition) and does not vary smoothly with increases in stimulus strength. Even at a given strength of stimulus, reproducibility is poor from trial to trial and the reflex takes a period of time to recover after each trial (refractoriness). Recently, Andrews et al. (1990) have tried to find ways around these problems (see also Chapter 10), but they may be inherent in the reflex. The only real advantage of using the reflex is that with one surface electrode, flexion can be obtained at several joints. Otherwise, several electrodes would be needed, some of which may have to be implanted (Stein et al., 1990).

Cutaneous afferents are of course involved in other reflexes such as the "placing reaction" with gentle, non-noxious skin contact (Bard, 1933). Recent experiments with electrical stimuli to cutaneous nerves have demonstrated that cutaneous reflexes are even more dramatically modulated during walking (Yang and Stein, 1990; Duysens et al., 1990). The same stimulus to the same nerve can produce an excitation in a given muscle during one part of the step cycle and an inhibition to the same muscle in another part of the step cycle. This "reflex reversal" is typically seen in muscles such as tibialis anterior or rectus femoris which have two bursts of activity with different functional roles in the step cycle.

Attempts to utilize cutaneous signals in FES (see Chapter 5) may need to consider the complex way in which these reflexes are normally used in control. Cutaneous as well as muscle receptors form part of an intriguing natural feedback system. Rather than particular physical variables being controlled, as suggested in Figure 13–8, a sophisticated and highly adaptive system has apparently developed with evolution for control of movements. Hopefully, we can develop effective artificial systems to replace these movements on a much shorter time scale than was required for the natural system to evolve.

REFERENCES

Andrews, B.J. (1990). A prototype modular hybrid FES orthotic system for paraplegics. In: D. Popović, ed., *Advances in External Control of Human Extremities X*, pp. 187–196. Belgrade: Nauka.

Andrews, B.J., Baxendale, R.H., Granat, M.H., and Nicol, D.J. (1990). Flexion withdrawal reflexes in spinal cord-injured man. *J. Physiol.*, **429**, 50P.

Bard, P. (1938). Studies on the cortical representation of somatic sensibility. *Harvey Lect.*, **33**, 143–169.

Berkinblit, M.B., Feldman, A.G., and Fukson, O.I. (1986). Adaptability of innate motor patterns and motor control mechanisms. *Behav. Brain Sci.*, **9**, 585–638.

Capaday, C., and Stein, R.B. (1987). A method for simulating the reflex output of a motoneuron pool. *J. Neurosci. Methods.*, **21**, 91–104.

Capaday, C., and Stein, R.B. (1989). The effects of postsynaptic inhibition on the monosynaptic reflex of the cat at different levels of motoneuron pool activity. *Exp. Brain Res.*, **77**, 577–584.

Crago, P.E., Nakai, R.J., and Chizeck, H.J. (1991). Feedback regulation of hand grasp opening and contact force during stimulation of paralysed muscle. *IEEE Trans. Biomed. Eng.*, **38**, 17–28.

Duysens, J., Trippel, M., Horstmann, G.A., and Dietz, V. (1990). Gating and reversal of reflexes in ankle muscles during human walking. *Exp. Brain Res.*, **82**, 351–358.

Edamura, M., Yang, J.F., and Stein, R.B. (1991). Factors that determine the magnitude and time course of human H-reflexes in locomotion. *J. Neurosci.*, in press.

Feldman, A.G., Adamovich, S.V., Ostry, D.J., and Flanagan, J.R. (1990). The origin of electromyograms—explanations based on the equilibrium point hypothesis. In: J.M. Winters, and S.L.-Y. Woo, eds., *Multiple Muscle Systems: Biomechanics and Movement Organization*, Berlin: Springer-Verlag.

Feldman, A.G. (1986). Once more on the equilibrium-point hypothesis (λ-model) for motor control. *J. Motor Behav.*, **18**, 17–54.

Flanagan, J.R., Ostry, D.J., and Feldman, A.G. (1990). Control of human jaw and multi-joint arm movements. In: G. Hammond, ed., *Cerebral Control of Speech and Limb Movements*, pp. 29–58. London: Springer-Verlag.

Harrison, P.J., and Jankowska, E. (1985). Sources of input to interneurons mediating group I non-reciprocal inhibition of motoneurones in the cat. *J. Physiol. (Lond.)*, **361**, 379–401.

Houk, J.C. (1972). The phylogeny of muscular control configurations. In: H. Drischel, and P. Dettmar, eds., *Byocybernetics IV*, pp. 125–144. Jena: Gustav Fischer Verlag.

Houk, J.C., and Rymer, W.Z. (1981). Neural control of muscle length and tension. In: V.B. Brooks, ed., *Handbook of Physiology, Sect. I., Vol. II: Motor Control*, pp. 257–323. Baltimore: Williams & Wilkins.

Houk, J., Singer, J.J., and Goldman, M.C. (1970). An evaluation of length and force feedback in decerebrate cats. *J. Neurophysiol.*, **33**, 784–811.

Hulliger, M., Horber, F., Mevded, A., and Prochazka, A. (1987). An experimental simulation method for iterative and interactive reconstruction of unknown (fusimotor) inputs contributing to known (spindle afferent) responses. *J. Neurosci. Methods*, **21**, 225–238.

Hulliger, M., Dürmüller, N., Prochazka, A., and Trend, P. (1989). Flexible fusimotor control of muscle spindle feedback during a variety of natural movements. *Prog. Brain Res.*, **80**, 87–101.

Kandel, E.R., and Schwartz, J.H. (1985). *Principles of Neuroscience, 2nd edition*. New York: Elsevier.

Katz, R.T., and Rymer, W.Z. (1989). Spastic hypertonia: Mechanisms and measurement. *Arch. Phys. Med. Rehabil.*, **70**, 144–155.

Kearney, R.E., and Hunter, I.W. (1990). System identification of human joint dynamics. *Crit. Rev. Biomed. Eng.*, **18**, 55–87.

Kralj, A., and Bajd, T. (1989). *Functional Electrical Stimulation, Standing and Walking after Spinal Cord Injury*. Boca Raton, FL: CRC Press.

Latash, M.L., Penn, R.D., Corcos, D.M., and Gottlieb, G.L. (1989). Short-term effects of intrathecal baclofen in spasticity. *Exp. Neurol.*, **103**, 165–172.

Liberson, W., Holmquest, H.J., Scot, D., and Dow, A. (1961). Functional electrotherapy stimulation of the peroneal nerve synchronized with the swing phase of the gait of hemiplegic patients. *Arch. Phys. Med. Rehab.*, **42**, 101–105.

Marsolais, E.B., and Kobetic, R. (1987). Functional electrical stimulation for walking in paraplegia. *J. Bone Joint Surg.*, **69A**, 728–733.

Matthews, P.B.C. (1959). The dependence of tension upon extension in the stretch reflex of the decerebrate cat. *J. Physiol. (Lond.)*, **184**, 450–472.

Matthews, P.B.C. (1972). *Mammalian Muscle Receptors and their Central Actions*. London: Arnold.

Matthews, P.B.C. (1981). Review lecture: Evolving views on the internal operation and functional role of the muscle spindle. *J. Physiol. (Lond.)*, **320**, 1–30.

Matthews, P.B.C., and Stein, R.B. (1969). The sensitivity of muscle spindle afferents to small sinusoidal changes in length. *J. Physiol. (Lon.)*, **202**, 59–82.

Mayagoitia, R.E., and Andrews, B.J. (1990). Stability during standing for 30 minutes in a hybrid FRO. In: D. Popović, ed., *Advances in External Control of Human Extremities X*, pp. 119–130. Belgrade: Nauka.

Merton, P.A. (1953). Speculations on the servo-control of movement. In: G.E.W. Wolstenholme, ed., *The Spinal Cord*, pp. 247–255. Churchill Livingstone London.

Murphy, P.R., Stein, R.B., and Taylor J. (1984). Synaptic transmission from muscle afferents during fictive locomotion in the mesencephalic cat. *J. Neurophysiol.*, **53**, 341–360.

Nichols, T.R., and Houk, J.C. (1976). Improvement in linearity and regulation of stiffness that results from actions of stretch reflex. *J. Neurophysiol.*, **39**, 119–142.

Prochazka, A. (1989). Sensorimotor gain control: A basic strategy of motor systems. *Prog. Neurobiol.*, **33** 281–307.

Prochazka, A., Trend, P., Hulliger, M., and Vincent, S. (1989). Ensemble proprioceptive activity in the cat step cycle: Towards a representative look-up chart. *Prog. Brain Res.*, **80**, 61–74.

Prochazka, A., and Wiles, C.M. (1983). Electrical stimulation of paretic leg muscles in man, allowing feedback-controlled movements to be generated from the wrist. *J. Physiol.*, **343**, 20–21P.

Rymer, W.Z., and Hasan, Z. (1980). Absence of force-feedback regulation in soleus muscle of the decerebrate cat. *Brain Res.* **184**, 203–209.

Sherrington, C.S. (1906). *The Integrative Action of the Nervous System*. New Haven, CT: Yale University Press.

Stauffer, E.K., Watt, D.G.D., Taylor, A., Reinking, R.M., and Stuart, D.G. (1976). Analysis of muscle receptor connections by spike-triggered averaging. 2. Spindle group II afferents. *J. Neurophysiol.*, **39**, 1393–1402.

Stein, R.B. (1974). The peripheral control of movement. *Physiol. Rev.*, **54**, 215–243.

Stein, R.B. (1982). What muscle variable(s) does the nervous system control in limb movements? *Behav. Brain Sci.*, **5**, 535–577.

Stein, R.B., and Capaday, C. (1988). The modulation of human reflexes during functional motor tasks. *Trends Neurosci.*, **11**, 328–332.

Stein, R.B., and Lee, R.G. (1981). Tremor and clonus. In: V.B. Brooks, ed., *Handbook of Physiology, Sect. I. Vol. 2: Motor Control*, pp. 325–343. Baltimore: Williams & Wilkins.

Stein, R.B., Prochazka, A., Popović, D., Edamura, M., Llewellyn, M.G.A., and Davis, L.A. (1990). Technology transfer and development for walking using functional electrical stimulation. In: D. Popović, ed., *Advances in External Control of Human Extremities*, pp. 161–175. Belgrade: Nauka.

Stein, R.B., Yang, J., Edamura, M., and Capaday, C. (1991). Reflex modulation during normal and pathological human locomotion. In: M. Shimamura, et al., eds., *Neurobiological Basis of Human Locomotion*, pp. 335–346. Tokyo: Japan Scientific Society Press.

Taylor, J., Stein, R.B., and Murphy, P.R. (1985). Impulse rates and sensitivity to stretch of muscle spindle afferent fibers during locomotion in the premammillary cat. *J. Neurophysiol.*, **53**, 341–360.

Vallbo, Å.B. (1971). Muscle spindle response at the onset of isometric voluntary contractions in man. Time difference between fusimotor and skeletomotor effects. *J. Physiol. (Lond.)*, **218**, 405–431.

Vallbo, Å.B., Hagbarth, K.-E., Torebjörk, H.E., and Wallin, B.G. 1979). Somatosensory, proprioceptive and sympathetic activity in human peripheral nerves. *Physiol. Rev.*, **59**, 919–957.

Yang, J.F., and Stein, R.B. (1990). Phase-dependent reflex reversal in human leg muscles during walking. *J. Neurophysiol.*, **64**, 607–616.

Yang, J., Stein, R.B., and James, K.B. (1991). Contribution of peripheral afferents to the activation of the soleus muscle during walking in humans. *Exp. Brain Res.*, in press.

14

Adaptive and Nonlinear Control Methods for Neural Prostheses

HOWARD J. CHIZECK

An important tool for the improvement of the performance of functional neuromuscular stimulation (FNS) technology is the use of sensor-derived feedback signals to modulate the electrical stimulation of muscle. The use of feedback control provides enhanced repeatability and predictability of muscle responses, and endows a neural prosthesis with the ability to adjust to both external disturbances (such as changing loads on limbs) and internal time variations (such as fatigue). Feedback controllers of stimulation are currently being developed and tested in experimental neural prostheses for upper extremity and lower extremity functions. The nonlinear and time-varying nature of electrically stimulated muscle (and the associated biomechanical system), as well as the discrete-event nature of many upper and lower extremity functional tasks, provide significant challenges to controller design. A particular complicating factor is that accurate predictive models of stimulated muscle and biomechanical interactions are often unavailable. Although new research is underway to obtain more precise dynamic models, the development of improved FNS assistive devices requires designs that are either robust to modeling and parameter errors, or that adapt to them. Control systems that use methods of adaptive control, nonlinear control theory, rule-based "intelligent" control, control using artificial neural nets, and the control of discrete-event driven systems are currently under investigation. Recent results in FNS control are described here, including new theoretical approaches, and animal model tests of controllers and applications in the human upper and lower extremity.

This chapter addresses the design of automatic control subsystems for motor neural prostheses, within an overall framework of systems engineering. In particular, the use of nonlinear and adaptive control methods is examined. Controllers that have been developed (or are under consideration) for neural prostheses to partially restore functions of the lower extremity (such as standing and locomotion) and of the upper extremity (such as grasping tasks) will be considered.

Before beginning this task, however, it is important to accurately assess the dilemma facing the designers of motor neural prostheses. It is similar to (but perhaps more difficult than) the following situation. Suppose that, in 1940, a top team of multidisciplinary scientists and engineers were miraculously presented with two contemporary aircraft (perhaps Stealth fighters), one damaged and one not, and that this team was highly motivated to restore the functions of the broken one. The purposes of most of the major subsystems of the aircraft would be understood, but the details of the component parts would be quite mysterious. It would require extensive experimentation and study to characterize their properties, structures, and functions. Any repair would have to be made using technology that was significantly inferior to the original. Perhaps the most mysterious part would be the "fly-by-wire" automatic control system that allows an essentially unstable aircraft to fly.

The design of motor neural prostheses is like this "reverse engineering" repair problem. It is complicated by our lack of detailed quantitative understanding of the original equipment, and by our inability to use the same technologies. In most respects, the communication, stimulation, sensor, sensor signal processing, and controller hardware available to contemporary engineers is quite primitive when compared to biological components. In addition, details of the methods of biological control are only partially understood. The biomechanical subsystems to be controlled are inherently nonlinear and possess time-varying input-output properties. Thus standard control engineering methods involving the assumption that components are linear (and, for transform-based methods, that they are time invariant) are unlikely to yield high performance. For this reason, the use of nonlinear control methods and adaptive control techniques is of interest.

Of necessity, the discussion here cannot be limited solely to topics of controller design. Motor neural prostheses controllers must be considered as part of the larger system. The automatic controllers for neural prostheses are not hardware components; rather, they are the "smarts" of a system, residing in a microprocessor. They serve to integrate, coordinate, and manage the functions of the other components of a "patient-neural prostheses system." Therefore the exposition presented here will follow a "top-down" systems approach to controller specification and design.

A conceptual diagram representing the structure and information flow in a "patient-plus-neural prostheses system" is contained in Figure 14–1. Boxes indicate component subsystems, and arrows indicate information flows between them. The patient is represented by the three boxes labeled supraspinal CNS, biomechanical system, and physiological sensors. The biomechanical system, which comprises the skeleton, muscles, tendons, ligaments, and all other tissues, has quantities of motion (such as joint positions and velocities, accelerations, and contact forces) as its outputs. The individual controls the biomechanical system via motor commands from the central nervous system, based on information provided by physiological sensors. Motor commands and sensory feedback signals are carried through spinal cord pathways, as indicated on the right of Figure 14–1A. If these pathways are damaged, then the individual does not have control of certain biomechanical systems outputs,

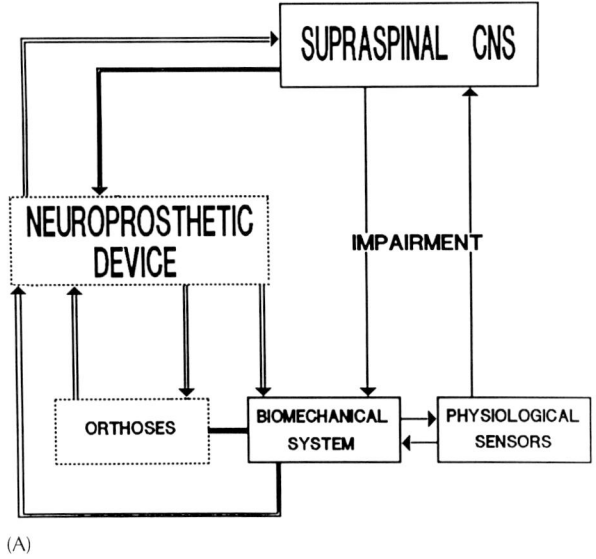

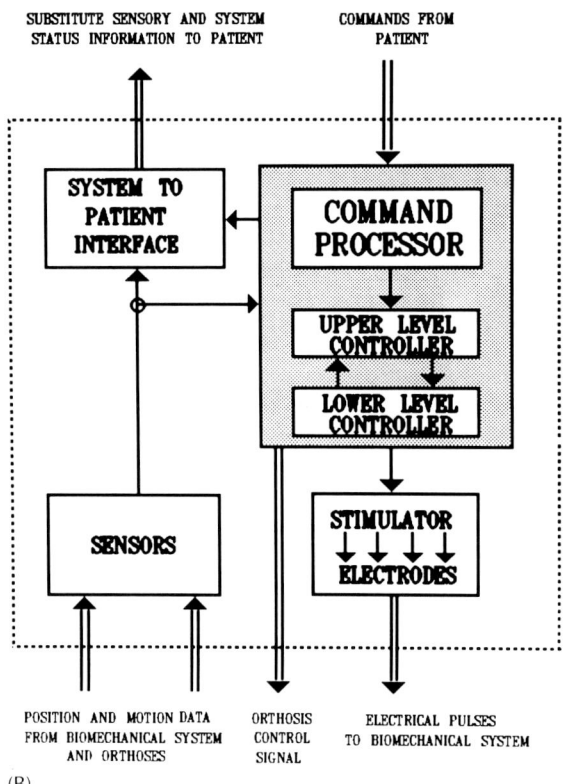

Figure 14–1 (A) Conceptual diagram of the impaired neuromusculoskeletal system and assistive devices. (B) Conceptual diagram of neural prosthetic system. (From Chizeck et al., 1988b, with permission.)

or sensation of them. In this situation a motor neural prosthesis may be used to substitute for loss of function resulting from the damaged pathways.

Major subsystems of a hypothetical motor neural prosthesis are contained within the dotted-line rectangles in Figure 14–1B. These may include electrodes, a stimulator, sensors, a system-to-patient interface, a command and control subsystem (the grey box in Figure 14–1B), and orthoses. There are three information feedback paths in the combined patient-neural prosthesis system. One is the remaining intact sensory information of the individual (e.g., visual, proprioceptive, vestibular). The other two paths involve information measured by sensors and delivered either to the command and control subsystem, or to the patient via the system-to-patient interface.

Artificial sensors used to obtain this information might include transducers of contact forces, slippage, joint position, acceleration, and proximity. A review of sensor needs for neural prostheses appears in Crago et al. (1986), and a description of many available sensors appears in Chapter 4. Ideally, intact natural sensors might be used by the motor neural prosthesis, just as intact muscles are. Important steps in the development of the technology to do this are described in Chapter 5.

Information obtained from the processing of these sensor signals may be used in a system-to-patient interface. This is a device providing communication between the motor neural prosthesis and the patient. So-called "substitute sensory" information and information about the device status (e.g., low battery) can be delivered by audible tones, lights, displays, or tactile stimulation [e.g., Szeto and Riso (1987); see also Chapter 8, this volume].

The command control subsystem box in Figure 14–1B represents all of the computation and signal processing that is used to convert patient commands and sensor information into electrical stimulation (and, possibly, signals to active brace components, as in Tomovic et al. (1972) and Durfee and Hausdorff (1990)). Its structure will be described in the remainder of this chapter, following this introduction.

Command inputs from the patient allow for selection of desired motor tasks and scaling of effort (e.g., of walking speed, height of step, grasping force). They may require voluntary action (e.g., finger-mounted switches and joysticks (Marsolais et al., 1985) for lower extremity motor neural prostheses, shoulder-motion activated switch (Mortimer et al., 1974) for upper extremity systems, or voice activation (Handa et al., 1985)). Alternatively, they may be generated from electromyograph (EMG) signals derived from neurologically intact muscles (Graupe et al., 1983, 1984). Command input devices and protocols should be designed to require as little conscious effort as possible, and to permit rapid and reliable command transmission. The translation of command inputs into specific desired tasks is the function of the command processor.

The electrodes deliver one or more channels of electrical-stimulation waveforms produced by the stimulator. Several types of electrodes have been developed for use in motor neural prostheses. Each type of electrode introduces nonlinearities and time variations in the response of the stimulated muscle. These complicate control. Although surface electrodes are the simplest to apply and are the most commonly used, significantly greater selectivity can be obtained using implanted electrodes. These include intramuscular electrodes (Caldwell and Reswick, 1975; Marsolais and Kobetic, 1986), either surgically installed or percutaneously entering, via implantation using a hypodermic needle; epineural (Holle et al., 1984; Thoma et al., 1983) and nerve cuff electrodes (Brindley et al., 1979; Naples, 1987; Wilemon et al. 1970) implanted on or around nerves; and epimysial electrodes (Grandjean and Mortimer, 1986; McNeal et al., 1977) surgically attached to the surface of the muscle. For the control of complex and precise movements, the ability to individually address different muscles is essential, and is best accomplished using implanted electrodes. The use of surface electrodes might be compared to playing the piano with one's fist, instead of using the fingers.

The stimulator converts specified stimulation parameters for each output channel (such as pulse width, pulse frequency, and amplitude) into electrical signals. In most implementations, only one channel is actively stimulating at any instant of time; during one "cycle" (typically 25–50 msec), each channel in turn is active. This asynchronicity does not present problems for the controller, since each muscle is stimulated at or above its fusion frequency (where a 10% ripple in output force between stimulus pulses is obtained), and the biomechanical system acts as a low-pass filter to remove these oscillations. Several research groups are developing completely implantable stimulators, where all power and control information is broadcast to an implanted unit (e.g., Smith et al., 1987). For many (if not most) motor neural prostheses, the use of implantable stimulators will greatly enhance ease of use, cosmesis, and practicality. However, control systems for motor neural prostheses should now be designed with the "quanta" of available channels provided by these implantable stimulators in mind (8, 16, and perhaps 24 and 32).

Orthoses directly modify the biomechanical system. They exert forces on it, restrict its motion, and change its mass and dynamic properties. For individuals with only minor impairments, orthoses alone may provide adequate function (although they may be cosmetically unacceptable). Brace systems may be combined with FNS in hybrid orthosis systems for lower extremity use (Andrews and Bajd, 1984; Andrews et al., 1987; Schwirtlich and Popovic, 1984; see also Chapter 10, this volume). They can also be used with FNS for upper extremity neural prostheses, perhaps combined with surgically-accomplished bracing (as described in Chapter 8).

There is a synergy between electrical stimulation, orthoses, and feedback control. One can think of both orthoses and feedback as reducing the amount of electrical stimulation that is required to perform certain tasks. Feedback modulation of stimulation can accomplish this reduction by using less stimulation when there is less need (i.e., when the system outputs are close to target values). Insensitivity to disturbances can be attained through adjustment of stimulation levels, rather than by excessive open-loop stimulation. Orthoses can reduce the stimulation required by physically constraining certain motions, in order to provide biomechanical stability and support. Alternately, electrical stimulation can be thought of as providing motors for hybrid orthoses, with feedback-controlled stimulation yielding more precise torque generation. In addition, bracing can provide stable mounting sites for sensors of various quantities, allowing for improved measurements and thus enhanced feedback control effectiveness.

MOTOR NEURAL PROSTHESIS CONTROLLER STRUCTURE AND DESIGN

In this section we first address the controller design process for motor neural prostheses. Then the overall structure of these control systems will be considered. Because of the complexity of motor neural prostheses, the design of their control systems is perhaps best carried out as an iterative multistage process, using analytical methods, computer simulation, experimental evaluation, and repeated redesign. The four stages of design can be summarized as follows.

1. *Analytical design.* From first principles and mathematical models of the system, a controller design is arrived at. This process depends on the quality of models that are available. For some subsystems, such as electrically stimulated muscle (see Chapter 2), walking biomechanics (see Chapter 9) and reflex actions during walking (see Chapter 13), models are available. However obtaining parameter values of these models for specific individuals may require a significant effort (as in Chapter 3, for muscle-model identification). For some subsystem models, subject-specific parameters may be unavailable.

    If good models are available, and they are of a mathematical form for which contempoary control theory is up to the task, then analytical controller design methods can be applied directly. More often, simplified linearizations of models are used to obtain initial controller designs, via "classical" methods (e.g., root locus) or state space techniques [e.g., linear quadratic controllers as in Peterson and Chizeck (1987)]. If adequate models are not available, then very simple controller designs [e.g., digital proportional-integral-derivative (PID) controllers] can be applied.

2. *Computer simulation.* The next step, whenever possible, is to test the controller performance using computer stimulation. The systems to be controlled are complex, involving multiple degrees of freedom, nonlinearities, time variations and, for gait, static instability (see Chapters 11 and 12). Models of these factors can be used in the computer simulations to evaluate the performance of controllers that were designed without formally taking them into account. An excellent example of this is the work of Khang and Zajac (1989a,b).

    Computer simulation evaluation of controllers should first verify that the controller performs well when the assumed models are, in fact, true. The "tuning" of controller parameters can be done in large part in computer simulation (e.g., see Lemay, 1991; Liu, 1989). The controller design should next be made robust to modeling errors or, if necessary, endowed with an adaptive capability to adjust model parameters. Computer simulations that include parameter uncertainties or changes in parameter values, as well as noise, can be carried out to confirm robustness.

3. *Experimental evaluation in animal models.* When appropriate, controller performance should be evaluated in animal models. The motivation here is human safety. Following computer simulation trials and prior to testing in human subjects, evaluations with animal models can be used to modify controller tuning and to verify that computer simulation errors (resulting from poor mathematical models) have not inadvertently supported bad controller designs.

4. *Experimental evaluation in human subjects.* The next stage is experimental evaluation of the controller performance. Often, analysis of experimental results may lead to a return to the first two steps above.

We next consider the overall structure of control systems for motor neural prostheses and the types of control action that might be used. The controller can be thought of as having a two-level hierarchical structure, as shown in Figure 14–1B. The lower level is responsible for the control of one or more joints, enabling them to follow desired trajectories (e.g., of positions, forces, velocities) that are specified by the upper level. The upper level of the controller directs and coordinates the lower level controllers, during each particular task segment. By task segment, we mean a particular "piece" of a task; for example, a phase of gait or a portion of a maneuver. The upper level controller supervises the accomplishment of a task by leading the overall system through a sequence of task segments, on the basis of discrete events, which include detected events (e.g., heel strike or toe-off in locomotion) or patient commands (e.g., from the hand switch). During each task segment, the lower level controllers are instructed to perform their jobs, with target positions and trajectories as well as controller tuning parameters being specified by the upper level of control.

At both levels of the control system, sensor information can be used to modify stimulation. There are four types of potential benefits of using this feedback control or closed-loop control in a motor neural prosthesis. The first type results from *attainment of more precise positions and motion.* Stabilization of otherwise unstable systems, such as in upright posture (Cybulski et al., 1986; Chizeck et al., 1988b) is an example of this benefit of feedback. The use of feedback control to reduce knee hyperextension during the stance phase of gait is another example of this benefit of closed-loop control (Willemin and Chizeck, 1989).

A second benefit of feedback control is *compensation for internal disturbances.* Phenomena such as the time-varying properties of muscle, length-dependent muscle dynamics and recruitment, biomechanical coupling across joints, and muscle fatigue all limit the accuracy of open-loop stimulation. Feedback control can reduce the deviations from desired positions and movements that may result from these factors.

A third benefit of feedback control is the potential *reduction of stimulation* that results from the adjustment of stimulation to reflect what is needed to carry out the task. This may translate into increased endurance.

Finally, closed-loop control may provide *improved ease of use* of motor neural prostheses. One property of feedback is that it tends to increase the linearity of the system that is controlled. Linear relationships between patient command inputs and the resulting output may make the operation of the device easier and may simplify patient training.

Terminology regarding the "open-loop" or "closed-loop" nature of motor neural prosthesis controller designs has unfortunately become somewhat confused in the literature. One reason is that all motor neural prostheses involve at least the residual sensory feedback path described earlier, resulting in modification of patient-generated commands by the supraspinal central nervous system (CNS). Considering the hierarchical structure of Figure 14–1, controller designs for motor neural prostheses can be classified into four broad categories.

1. *"Open-loop" stimulation control.* In this situation, there is essentially no lower level of control in Figure 14–1B. All of the stimulation parameters are based upon prestored values that are selected by patient input commands. There is no automatic triggering or modification of these stimulator patterns, although

for repetitive tasks such as gait, a timer may be used to switch between different values (instead of using patient command inputs only). The upper extremity system described in Chapter 8, the "withdrawal reflex" surface electrode walking systems reported by Kralj et al. (1980, 1983) and others, and the percutaneous electrode walking system described in Marsolais and Kobetic (1983), are of this type.

2. *Sensor-triggered open-loop stimulation control.* In this approach, sensor signals are also used to switch between prestored stimulation patterns. For example, foot switches can be used to trigger stimulation for different phases of gait, as described in Kobetic and Marsolais (1985). This method has been used in surface FNS gait systems (Petrofsky and Phillips, 1983), and in hybrid FNS/orthosis systems by many groups. For further details, see Chapters 10 and 11.

3. *Sensor-modulated control of stimulation.* This type of control takes place at the lower level of the controller in Figure 14–1B. Sensor-derived signals are used to continually modify stimulation to one or more sets of (possibly antagonistic) muscles. Controller designs to do this are described in the next section of this chapter. They include digital fixed-parameter controllers (such as PID controllers and lead-lag compensators), controllers based upon linear models of the subsystem being regulated (e.g., as pole-placement controllers), and controllers based on nonlinear models (e.g., feedback linearization controllers). Instead of using fixed-parameter feedback control laws, adaptive controllers that include an on-line estimation of model parameters can also be implemented.

4. *Sensor-modified patterns.* This type of control takes place at the upper level of the controller structure shown in Figure 14–1B. It refers to the use of sensor-derived measurements of system quantities of motion to modify the stored stimulation parameters (that are used in 1 and above), and also to modify tuning parameters or instructions to lower level controllers. For grasp function systems, this might be an "automatic recalibration" process that alters stored stimulation patterns for the next task, based upon the last one. In this way, some automatic compensation for daily patient variations, external disturbances (such as offset forces due to position of objects), or internal disturbances to the system (such as sensor drift or muscle fatigue) might be obtained. In gait systems, performance of the system in previous cycles can be used to modify stimulation in future cycles. This can allow for adjustment to changes in slope and walking surfaces. In motor neural prostheses for gait, the inherent delays in muscle response to stimulation may permit only this type of closed-loop compensation for many variables of interest.

In the following two sections, methods for lower level controllers and for upper level controllers will be considered separately. Application of controllers to upper and lower extremity neural prostheses will be discussed throughout. Given the author's experiences, the description of the applications will focus on work done using intramuscular and epimysial electrodes by the Cleveland group (at Case Western Reserve University, the Cleveland VA Medical Center, and MetroHealth Medical Center).

LOWER LEVEL CONTROLLERS

The lower level control of Figure 14–1B involves the regulation of muscle stimulation for specific subsystems of the overall motor neural prosthesis-patient system (such as the muscles acting on a particular joint). During stimulation, the relationship between the stimulus parameters (inputs to the muscles) and the force and/or position output is highly nonlinear. Overall input/output nonlinearities arise, in part, from the nonlinear relationship between stimulus parameters and the active muscle force or joint angles (Crago et al., 1980; Gorman and Mortimer, 1983). In open-loop systems, some compensation for these nonlinearities can be obained by multiplicative cancellation. However, the cancellation cannot be exact due to the dependence on factors such as muscle length (and hence joint position and unknown load properties). There are also significant time dependencies of muscle activation and force production: electrode movement, potentiation and fatigue, and effects which cannot be canceled on a predictive basis.

Feedback control is complicated by these nonlinear and time-varying system properties. In addition, there are several other factors that complicate lower-level controller design. Stimulation "spillover" to unintended muscles, and its dependence on joint position, is one such phenomenon. Precise models of the dynamic effects resulting from joint geometries, biomechanical couplings, and multiple muscle stimulation are often not available.

In the following discussion, several different approaches to the design of lower level controllers will be described. At one extreme are "classical" digital controllers that depend very little on models of the system. They do not require or exploit detailed models of system input-output properties. However, they therefore are not sensitive to incorrect models of these properties. At the other extreme are feedback linearization controller designs that take full advantage of good models of the system. In addition, adaptive methods that adjust model parameters based upon observed system inputs and outputs will also be described.

Stiffness Controller Configuration

Prior to a discussion of different lower level controller types, we briefly consider a "configuration" of force and position (or torque and angle) signals that allow one controller (of any of the types we will discuss below), to simultaneously control both output quantities. This stiffness controller configuration is described briefly here, and in more detail in Crago et al. (1991).

The stiffness control configuration, shown in Figure 14–2, has two important features. First, the properties of the load determine the relative importance of the feedback from force and position transducers. Thus, the controller need not switch between position of force control modes. Such switching otherwise could be a source of oscillations. Second, only a single command signal is needed to control force and position. In the unloaded condition, the command directly controls position (here the force feedback signal is zero). Under rigid loading, the command directly controls force (here the position feedback signal is a constant offset). Both quantities will vary with the command when the load is compliant, viscous, or inertial.

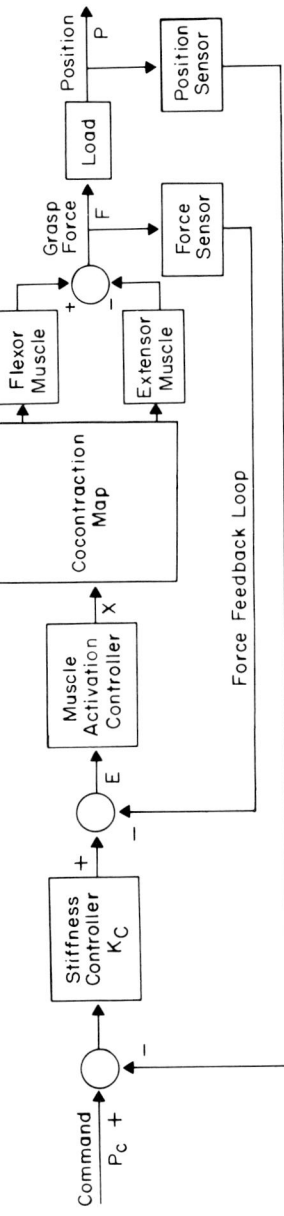

Figure 14–2 Block diagram of grasp stiffness regulation system. The input command specifies the virtual position of the grasp. The difference between the virtual position and the actual position is multiplied by the regulated value of stiffness to determine the input to the force regulator. A muscle activation controller specifies the pulse width and stimulus period for the muscles according to the mapping scheme shown in Figure 14–3. The flexor and extensor muscles exert torques in opposite directions at the joint. It is the difference between these torques that determines the force exerted on the external load. The interaction between the external load and the regulated stiffness determines the actual grasp position and force. (From Crago et al., 1991, with permission.)

307

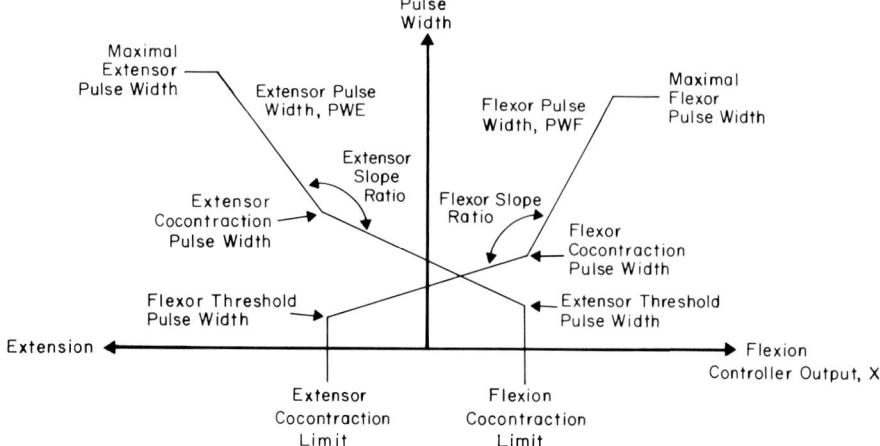

Figure 14–3 Co-stimulation (or cocontraction) mapping for the control of two antagonist muscles. The maps determine the stimulus pulse widths for each muscle as a function of the activation controller output. The overlap between the outputs for the two muscles determines the degree of coactivation. At either side are regions of single-muscle activation. (From Crago et al., 1991, with permission.)

The stiffness controller configuration regulates the ratio of force change to position change, rather than force or position alone. Under constant input conditions, the steady-state relationship is given by.

$$[F = K(C\text{-}P)] \qquad (1)$$

where F and P are force and position, respectively, K is the regulated stiffness, and C is the command input. Only the net force produced by contact with the external load is assumed to be available for feedback. The joint position and contact force depend on the balance between the mechanical properties of the stimulated muscle system and the mechanical properties of the load.

The muscle activation controller in Figure 14–2 uses the error signal from the force and position feedback loops. It is followed by a co-stimulation map which converts this digital controller output into stimulation signals for each electrode. In Figure 14–2, two antagonist muscles are used to control movement at a single joint: one to provide flexion and the other to provide extension. Each muscle is excited by a separate train of stimulus pulses. The two muscles are activated simultaneously, although they oppose each other, to provide continuity of control at low levels of activation. Figure 14–3 illustrates such a co-stimulation map. It translates the controller output into stimulus parameters for a set of muscles. Note that flexors and extensors have an overlapping region. This allows for avoidance of the deadband inherent in single-muscle recruitment characteristics. It permits two-way muscle action, and increases linearity over the controller operating range. Methods for the tuning of these cocontraction maps are addressed in Crago et al. (1990) and Lemay (1991).

Fixed-Parameter Digital Feedback Controllers

We first consider simple digital muscle stimulation controllers that handle nonlinearities and time variations in the system by ignoring them. Very little modeling

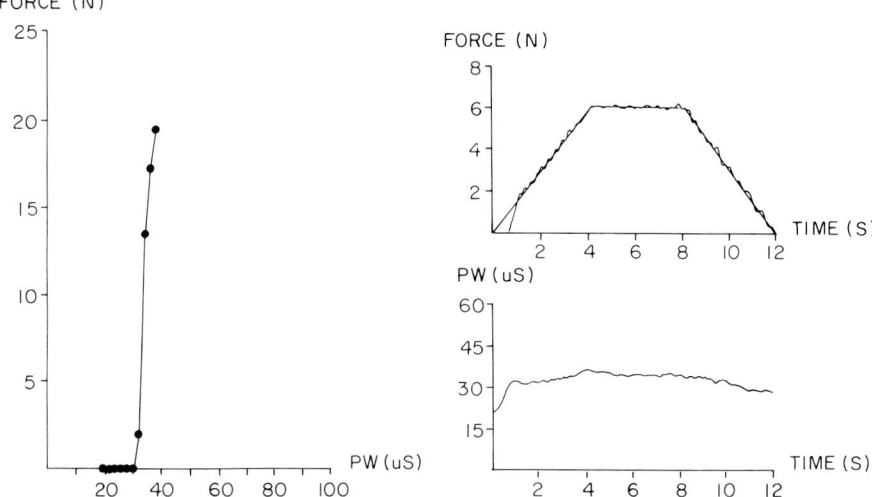

Figure 14-4 Controller performance in cat plantaris muscle. Stimulation is at a stimulus period of 30 msec. (A) Recruitment characteristic (steady-state force versus pulse width). (B) Ramp response (top) and input (bottom) with controller gain = 0.1 and m = 0.6. Solid line is the target force trajectory (From Chizeck et al., 1988a, with permission.)

information about the system is needed to implement such controllers (only the sign of the gain, and the input-output delay). If additional information is not available, the use of this type of controller is often a good choice.

As described in Chizeck et al (1988a), regulation of a single output (net muscle force, or joint position, or stiffness) can be obtained by modulating the pulse width of a constant-amplitude electrical stimulation pulse train according to the very simple compensator design:

$$D(z) = (\text{gain}) \, (z\text{-}m)/(z\text{-}1) \qquad (2)$$

This z-domain transfer function $D(z)$ has one "pole" (at $z = 1$) that provides the discrete time equivalent of integral action, and one controller "zero" (at $z = m$, where $0 < m < 1$). It can be implemented by the difference equation:

$$x(k) = x(k-1) + \text{gain} * [e(k-1)] \qquad (3)$$

where time index k is incremented at each stimulus period. The quantity $x(k)$ is the controller output (before normalization) and $e(k)$ is the error at the start of the kth stimulus period. The controller gain is normalized and unitless. The integral action ensures that there will be no steady-state error in response to a step intput. The controller zero, m, modifies the transient response of the controlled system.

An example of the performance of this controller in tracking a ramping reference force trajectory (in an isometric trial) is shown in Figure 14-4. Experimental tests of this controller in isometric animal models (Chizeck et al., 1988a) have shown that good performance can be obtained despite tenfold changes in loop gain (loop gain is the product of all component gains around the complete feedback loop, from either the system or its controller).

Equations (2) and (3) above represent a special tuning of a digital proportional-integral-derivative controller, that can be written as

$$x(k) = K_I * [x(k - 1) + e(k)] + K_D * [e(k) - e(k - 1)] + K_P * e(k) \quad (4)$$

The controller output at each time is a linear combination of the current tracking error (weighted by tuneable parameter K_P, the difference between the current and most recent error (weighted by K_D), and the sum of past tracking errors (weighted by K_I). Versions of this controller in animal models have shown that with the proper selection of the controller parameters, overall stability and good transient behavior can be obtained (Chang, 1984), over a wide variation of recruitment gains.

One reason that the simple digital controllers described above work well is that electrically stimulated muscle under constant pulse-frequency (i.e., stimulus period) stimulation can be modeled as a low-order linear autoregressive moving average (ARMA) model in discrete time (Bernotas et al., 1986). Although the force output of muscle is continuous in time, it is natural to represent a constant stimulus period stimulation input signal (with varying pulse widths or amplitudes) as a discrete time signal.

From collected input and output data (i.e., pulse widths and forces), the parameters of these ARMA models, and consequently the poles, zeros, and gain of the associated transfer function models or ARMA model parameters, can be obtained (Bernotas et al., 1986; see also Chapter 3, this volume). These parameters can be used to choose the controller tuning parameters, analytically or through computer simulation. When this identification and controller adjustment is done on line, the result is an adaptive controller (see below). The system parameters can also be used to design controllers using standard classical techniques such as pole-placement and lead-lag compensation, that require the assumption of a linear system model.

Adaptive Controllers of Linear Systems

If the linear model parameters are time varying or are not well known in advance, or if the linear model is an approximation of the nonlinear system that changes in accuracy as the system operates, then adaptive linear controllers may be more effective than fixed-parameter digital feedback controllers (Astrom and Wittenmark, 1989). Conceptually, these controllers work as follows: parameters of the linear input-output model are fit "on line," during system operation, on the basis of applied inputs and measured outputs. These parameters are then used in the linear controller. Adaptive controllers may involve pole placement, or the minimization of various objective functions (such as a weighted combination of output tracking error and input effort). What is important is the ability of the model to predict future outputs, which allows for the determination of inputs by the controllers.

A second-order deterministic autoregressive moving-average model of isometric muscle response (Bernotas et al., 1986) has been used to develop a simple adaptive muscle activation controller (Bernotas et al., 1987). This controller demonstrated the ability to adapt to changing conditions, such as fatigue and excursions into different regions of the muscle recruitment nonlinearity. An example of this controller, used in the stiffness configuration of Figure 14–2, is shown in Figure 14–5.

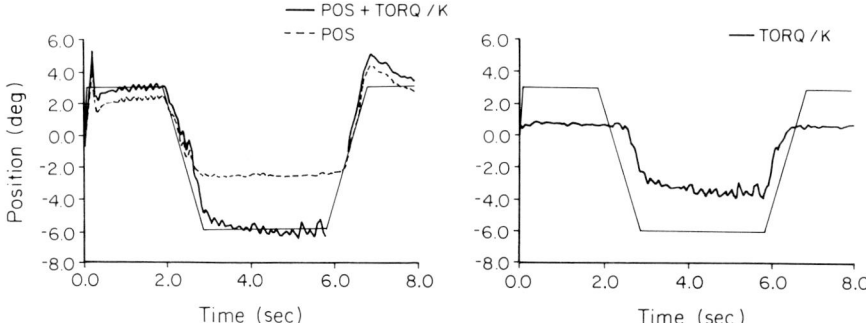

Figure 14–5 Performance of the adaptive controller, in chronically implanted cat TA and MG muscles, during control of load transitions with a ramp rate of 9°/s. The broken line in the plot represents the joint position. The solid line is the controlled variable (position = torque/K). Torque/K is also shown separately. The joint position was the variable under control during the unloaded portion of the movement. It remains constant after the load transition (in this case, the cat's paw contacts a barrier), as shown by the broken line. After this load transition, the joint torque becomes the controlled variable. (Adapted from Lan et al., 1991b, with permission.)

A similar adaptive controller was used, with surface stimulation, in the human upper extremity (Allin and Inbar, 1986).

Real-time identification of the muscle input-output parameters for nonlinear systems can be used to develop adaptive nonlinear controllers. For example, the combined nonlinear recruitment identification and linear dynamics identification (Chia et al., 1991) obtained using recursive least-squares methods on a Hammerstein-type nonlinear model (with a shifted polynomial representing the recruitment curve) has been evaluated in electrically stimulated human quadriceps muscle and found to greatly enhance the predictive performance of the identified model. All that is necessary to use linear adaptive control methods is to invert the identified recruitment nonlinearity (this is possible because it is monotonic).

Adaptive controllers can potentially endow a motor neural prosthesis with the ability to adjust to certain internal and external disturbances. However, the use of adaptive controllers can lead to poor performance if structural assumptions about the system are violated. For example, there may be variations in the "offset" of the output (i.e., a variable baseline value resulting from no input). This could arise, for example, from a drift in a joint-angle sensor. Such variations may lead to real-time misidentification of the system, and result in instability. A method for preventing this is described in Timmons et al. (1991).

In principle, adaptive linear controllers are available for multple-input, multiple-output (MIMO) systems. For most methods, it is necessary that the input-output delay for each input-output pair be known precisely, and that the system be minimum phase (have all its zeros in the unit circle of the z plane). The handling of different input-output delays in the same system, and the minimum phase requirement, have limited the application of adaptive linear controllers to MIMO biomedical applications.

In recent years, adaptive controllers that are less sensitive to unknown or time-varying input-output delays and that can control nonminimum phase systems have been developed (see e.g., Clarke, 1984; Voss et al., 1987). Recently it has been demonstrated that most if not all of these controllers are special cases of a "unified" structure (Dong and Chizeck, 1991a,b), and that proper representation using this structure allows for significant computational savings (Dong and Chizeck 1990a,b).

Simultaneous Pulse Width and Stimulus Period Modulation Control

A different approach to the digital muscle activation controller is the pulse width/stimulus period (PW/SP) controller (Chizeck et al., 1989). The PW/SP controller is an ad hoc combination of the PW controller with SP modulation. Its operation is biologically motivated, in the sense that it is designed to allow for a burst of high-frequency stimulation at the start of a motion, or when large forces must be generated, but to also allow for a relatively low frequency of muscle stimulation when more is not needed.

The controller output is calculated based on the PW control law given in the following difference equations:

$$U(t+kh) = U(t) + G(kh) * E(t+kh) - m * G(kh) * E(t) \quad (5)$$

$$G(kh) = H * [1 + (kh) * (C/2)] \quad (6)$$

$$E(t+kh) = K[C_p(t+kh) - P(t+kh)] - F(t+kh) \quad (7)$$

where t is time of last stimulation, h is observation period, k is an integer, $U(\cdot)$ is controller output, $E(\cdot)$ is controller driving error, $G(kh)$ is controller gain which is dependent on controller's stimulus period ($=kh$), m is controller zero, H and C are two constants corresponding to the continuous time PI controller gain and zero:

$$D(s) = H(s + C)/s \quad (8)$$

Equation (2) can be obtained by bilinear transformation for equation (8). The control law reduces to the PW controller if the SP is constant. Equation (6) allows for adjustment of the gain of $D(z)$ to account for sampling effects; that is, to obtain the same equivalent continuous time controller gain. The controller modulates the SPs of the two antagonistic muscles in push-pull manner; that is, when one muscle's SP is decreased, the SP of its opponent is increased (or remains unchanged). This guarantees that during cocontraction, the net force produced by the antagonist increases in the desired direction. The controller weighs the error accumulated in the past against the number of stimuli applied to the two muscles, and makes decision to stimulate one or both muscles. An example of the effect of adding SP modulation is shown in Figure 14–6.

A comparative evaluation (in animal trials) of the digital PI, the PW/SP, and the adaptive controller appears in Lan et al., (1991b). In general, the PW/SP controller attains the best performance, but at a cost of significant computational complexity relative to the digital PID controller.

Multiple Joint, Multiple Degree of Freedom Control

Motor neural prostheses for standing, locomotion, arm movement, and hand grasp all involve control of multijoint limbs, having multiple degrees of freedom (DOF).

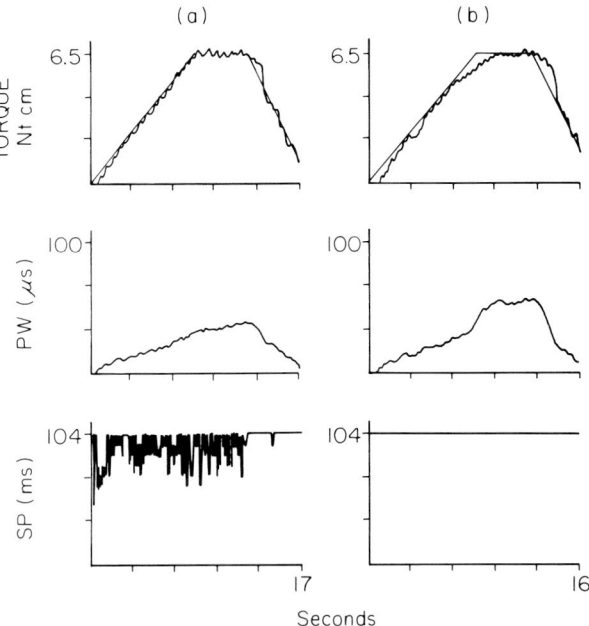

Figure 14-6 Ramp response with simultaneous PW/SP modulation (left) and with PW modulation alone (right). Single muscle trials (cat tibialis anterior) using the same PW controller (gain of .06 and m = .6) at 30% of maximum angle. (A) PW/SP modulation with SP modulation between 48 msec and 104 msec. (B) PW modulation only, at SP = 104 msec. Note that for the increasing ramp, the SP modulation obtains much better tracking. During the decreasing ramp, the SP modulation saturates at the maximum allowable interval 104 msec. (Adapted from Chizeck et al., 1989, with permission.)

Feedback control of them will, in general, require multiple MIMO controllers. Compared to single-joint, single-DOF limbs, significant additional challenges to lower level controllers result. For example, let us compare single-joint and multijoint control. In a single-joint limb, the endpoint force is proportional to the joint torque, scaled by the segment length and endpoint movement of the limb is proportional to the joint's angular motion. However, in a multijoint limb, the forces at the limb's endpoint are determined by the limb geometry, as well as by joint-torque magnitudes. As the limb geometry changes, so does the relationship between endpoint forces and joint torques. Endpoint position and individual joint positions are similarly coupled. These inherently nonlinear, time-varying *geometric coupling* relationships complicate controller design.

Multijoint limb control is also complicated by muscles that cross two or more joints, causing coupled torque production at each. Such *biarticular coupling* can be exploited to provide coordination or to reduce energy consumption; however, it also greatly complicates controller design.

The controllers described in the previous sections can be incorporated, along with feed-forward use of inverse model dynamics, into a perturbation controller structure for the control of multiple-link, multiple-DOF systems. One configuration for doing this is shown in Figure 14-7. A two-input, two-output PI controller was applied in Lan et al., (1990, 1991a) for the control of endpoint force, position, and

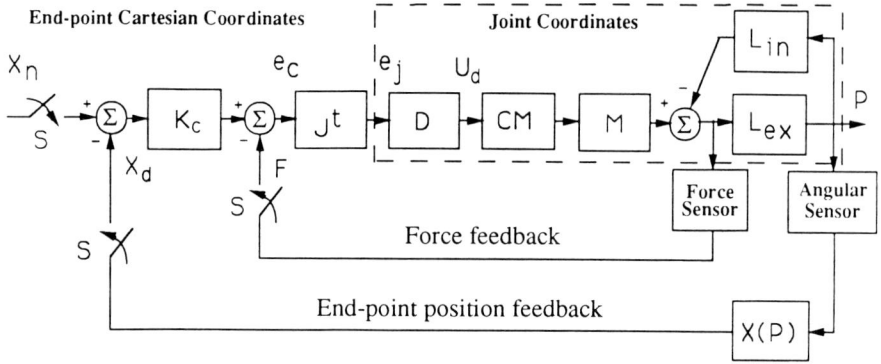

Figure 14–7 Block diagram of the control system for endpoint stiffness regulation. The subsystem within the dashed line operates in the joint space, and the rest operates in endpoint Cartesian space. The input command X_n is compared to the measured endpoint position, to obtain an error. J^t indicates the Jacobian matrix multiplication that transforms this error into joint coordinates, where it acts on controller, D. This output is mapped by the co-stimulation map (CM), to the muscles (M). Note that there is an internal load (L_{in}) that includes the limb inertia, joint viscosity, and passive compliance. The external load (L_{ex}) represents interactions with the environment. The limb movement position P, and the interaction force, F, are measured and fed back to the controller, in order to achieve endpoint stiffness regulation. (Adapted from Lan et al., 1991a, with permission.)

stiffness in a two-link, two-joint animal model. In particular, the use of centralized and decoupling controllers was examined, based on the multivariable PI tuning methods of (Peltomaa and Koivo (1983).

Application of Lower Level Controllers in Motor Neural Prostheses

The controller of equation (2) has been applied and evaluated in a stiffness regulation configuration (force and position control) for grasping tasks in patients having quadriplegia due to spinal cord injury at the C5–C6 level (Crago et al., 1991). Injury at these levels generally leaves patients with the ability to position their hands in space, but without voluntary control of grasp and release. A principal function of the hand is to grasp and manipulate objects. This requires that the position of the digits be controlled prior to contact, that force be controlled when grasping a rigid object, and that both position and force be controlled when grasping compliant objects. In open-loop FNS systems, the user must compensate for errors in grasp by adjusting the command signal, while monitoring performance visually. The use of feedback control to regulate the input-output properties of hand grasp can, in principle, provide linearity and repeatability. This can make control by the patient easier, since prediction of the system behavior on the basis of previous experience becomes more reliable.

The PID version of the controller described above (with minor modifications to prevent integrator "windup") has been investigated for use during FNS standing of paraplegics and hemiplegics. Control of ankle position (Stanic and Trnkoczy, 1974; Jaeger, 1986), knee and ankle position (Rosenthal, 1984), coronal plane hip motion (Donner, 1986; Abbas and Chizeck, 1991), and combined hip and trunk motion (Abbas and Chizeck, 1987, 1989) have been considered.

Evaluations of two different feedback controller configurations for hip and trunk in the coronal plane have been undertaken at the Cleveland VAMC Motion Study Laboratory. In one study (Abbas and Chizeck, 1991), a feedback controller of coronal plane hip angle was implemented. The two-stage controller consisted of a modified PID stage in cascade with a nonlinear single-input, multiple-output costimulation map. The controller's performance was evaluated by comparing the response of the feedback-controlled system to that of the open-loop system. In an evaluation based on temporal response characteristics, the feedback-controlled system exhibited a 43% reduction in rms error, a 54% reduction in steady-state error, and a 25% reduction in the rms error calculated with respect to steady state. However, a set of subjective ratings by clinicians indicated that these control-system design criteria alone may not be appropriate indicators of the desired performance characteristics (Abbas and Chizeck, 1989). In a second study, the control of both hip and trunk angles using two parallel independent controllers was investigated (Abbas, 1989). The results suggested that coordination between the hip and trunk controllers is needed for adequate maintenance of posture in the presence of disturbances. They also suggest that future mathematical models and computer simulations used to develop and test such controllers should not lump the hips, head, and trunk into a single component.

Recent work in our laboratory has demonstrated the ability to control individual joints in paraplegic patients using feedback control. It also demonstrates the need to carefully coordinate the control of each joint, so as to achieve functionally appropriate response of the overall system. In work directed toward the characterization of disturbance responses of paraplegic subject during FNS standing (Moynahan, 1990), evidence was found for the need to provide time-sequence coordination of feedback control actions. Feedback control of electrical stimulation to the muscles of the lower extremity, based upon knee-angle measurements was used to maintain stance despite disturbances. The disturbance response of a paraplegic subject using open-loop stimulation of the hamstrings, gluteus maximus, and erector spinae, and feedback-controlled stimulation of the quadriceps to maintain stance, was evaluated. The PW/SP controller described above, modulating both stimulus period and pulse width in response to changes in knee position, was used (at both knees) during these trials. The controller algorithm was tuned to provide a burst-like response to changes in joint position. It provided knee recovery to extension after repeated flexion disturbances were applied to the knees. The time course of several biomechanical responses was analyzed for each flexion disturbance and a repeatable pattern of events was found to exist. Tilt of the upper body and changes in force exerted by the subject on the support device showed early responses which could not be attributed to voluntary reaction times. The subject's perception of his supporting effort was related to the actual amount of effort exerted during the disturbance trials. These standing evaluations have generated new insight regarding the relationships between the goals of individual controllers and more general, clinical goals.

Current research on the use of lower level controllers during the supporting phases of gait is focusing on the need for predictive capabilities in these joint controllers to account for the delays of stimulation and computation. For example, our current open-loop portable walking system achieves knee trajectories in paraplegic patients such as the one shown in Figure 14–8, as opposed to the more normal trace shown

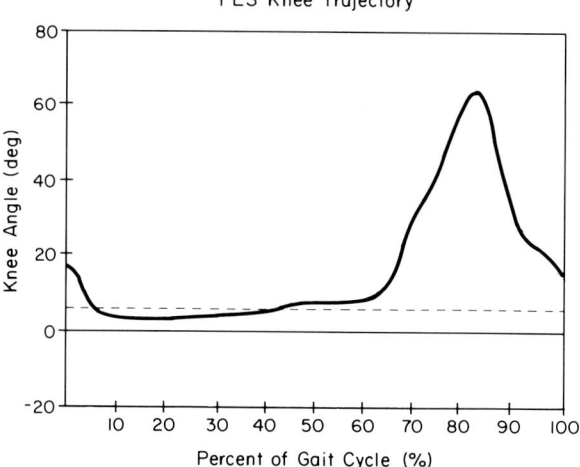

Figure 14–8 Typical knee-angle trajectory achieved by a complete paraplegic patient using 48 channels of open-loop stimulation, delivered through percutaneous intramuscular electrodes. Compared with a typical knee-angle trajectory of an unimpaired individual, it is seen that the first flexion occurrence is missing, and the second is significantly delayed. This lack of flexion during the stance phase of gait contributes to the unusual appearance of the gait and may lead to hyperextension of the knee. (Adapted from Willemin, 1991, with permission.)

in Figure 14–9. The lack of flexion during the support phase results in unnecessary vertical motion of the center of mass of the patient during locomotion. Preliminary results (Willemin and Chizeck, 1989) indicate that a more natural knee trajectory can be attained, which may resolve this excess energy expenditure.

Nonlinear Muscle Models and Nonlinear Control Using Feedback Linearization

In this section and the next, two approaches to nonlinear control will be described. These methods can potentially exploit the nonlinear properties of muscles, geo-

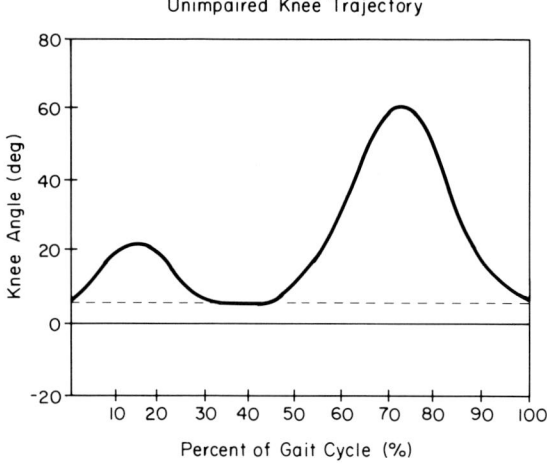

Figure 14–9 Knee-angle trajectory of an unimpaired individual, through the gait cycle. (Adapted from Willemin, 1991, with permission.)

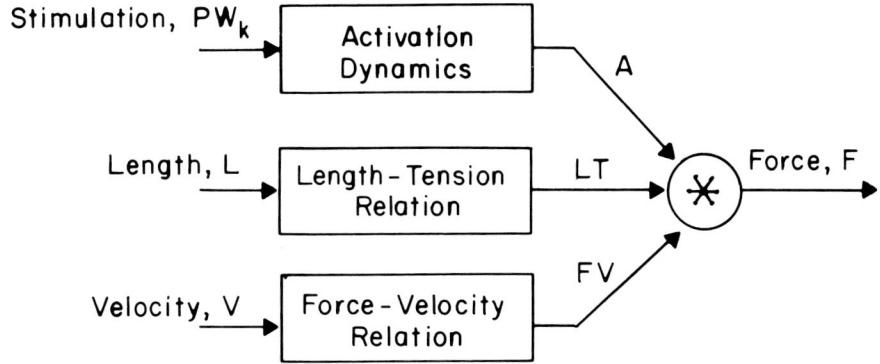

Figure 14–10 Block diagram of the three-factor muscle model. Force is the product of three factors: activation dynamics, the length-tension relationship, and the force-velocity relationship. Note that both stimulation and muscle length (and hence velocity) are inputs. (Adapted from El-Bialy, 1990, with permission.)

metrical couplings, and biomechanical couplings. To date, neither has been tested in an actual motor neural prosthesis, however. Consider the three-factor muscle model, represented schematically in Figure 14–10. Muscle output force is generated by the product of muscle activation dynamics, a length-tension factor, and a force-velocity factor (Crago et al., 1990). Discrete time versions of this three-factor nonlinear muscle model have been fit to animal data (Geng, 1989; Shue, 1990). This model can be used to design nonlinear controllers of muscle. One approach to doing this is reported in Veltink et al. (1989, 1992), where this model's parameters were experimentally identified (off-line), and then "inverted" as a feed-forward controller design. This was combined with a PID controller.

An alternate approach is to design a controller that explicitly accounts for and exploits the nonlinear input-output properties of electrically stimulated muscle, as well as the nonlinear effects of biomechanical coupling in multiple-DOF limb movements. This is an alternative to the use of controller designs that assume that muscle can be well modeled as a linear system. Methods for the control of nonlinear systems are currently an intense topic of theoretical research.

One approach, most often referred to as exact linearization or feedback linearization involves the design of nonlinear feedback and forward loop dynamic compensators based upon a known nonlinear input-output or input-state model of the system to be controlled. These compensators are, in general, time varying and can involve multiple inputs and outputs. The basic idea is that these coordinate transformations convert the inherently nonlinear system into a linear one (eg., Isidori, 1989):

Through the use of nonlinear state or output feedback and forward loop elements based upon the model of a nonlinear dynamic system, this system can be represented mathematically (in terms of a different, artificial input signal) as an "equivalent" linear system. The forward and feedback loop elements essentially map the system into a mathematically different coordinate setting where it is linear.

This is illustrated in Figures 14–11 and 14–12. Figure 14–11 shows a nonlinear dynamic system with input vector u, state vector x, and output y. A linearized version

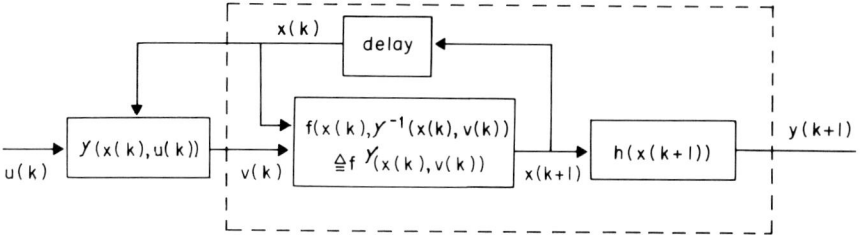

Figure 14–11 The nonlinear system (described by f, h, and the delay with state x and output y). The γ mapping here converts input u to v; its inverse (applied to x and v, inside of f) undoes this. This diagram represents that same situation as if the γ box were deleted, and f operated as f[x(k), (u(k)]. (Adapted from El-Bialy, 1990, with permission.)

is shown in Figure 14–12. Here, γ and T^{-1} are the linearizing coordinate transformations. The vector z is the state variable in the new coordinate setting. Matrices A, B, and vector c are the linearized model, and v is the input vector signal in the linearizing coordinate space.

A controller for this equivalent linear system can then be designed (mathematically) using standard methods. Together, the "linearizing" transformations and the controller of the equivalent linear system comprise the desired controller.

These methods have been developed in the literature for both general continuous-time and discrete-time linear systems. It is assumed that system parameters are known exactly in these derivations. In El-Bialy (1990), the discrete-time theory is extended and specialized, to handle a class of dynamic systems that includes the three-factor muscle input-output model. The resulting controllers can also account for and exploit the nonlinear biomechanical couplings that result from multiple-DOF, multiple-joint, multiple-muscle geometries, if models of these phenomena are available. The application involved determination of the equivalent system (and the necessary transformation mappings) and then the application of two feedback controller designs: one based on traditional digital PID control of linear systems and one based upon the linear quadratic control methods of "modern" control theory. These controllers were evaluated in computer simulation, for a hypothetical double-muscle, single-joint system, under various conditions of measurement noise and parameter variations. The feedback linearized quadratic controller exhibited the best noise tolerance.

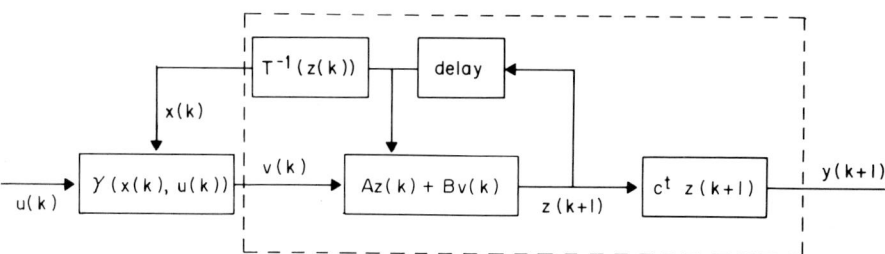

Figure 14–12 The nonlinear system of Figure 14–11 (defined by f, h, and the delay) has now been feedback linearized. The system from input signal v to output y is linear. The state variable of this linear system is indicated by z(k). T is a nonlinear mapping that converts the original state space X into a new state space Z [and its inverse converts z(k) into x(k)]. γ converts the actual input u(k) into the linearized system input v(k); note that γ is parameterized by x(k). Here A, B, and c^t are suitably dimensioned matrices or vectors. (Adapted from El-Bialy, 1990, with permission.)

Combination of real-time identification of nonlinear models of electrically-stimulated muscle with either of the nonlinear control methods described above yields an adaptive nonlinear controller. For example, the three-factor discrete-time model of electrically stimulated muscle can be identified (in real time) from input-output data using a sequential nonlinear least-squares algorithm (Shue, 1990). This identification can be combined with the methods described in Chia et al. (1991) to simultaneously identify recruitment nonlinearities in real time. The nonlinear model can be then be incorporated into an indirect adaptive controller.

The applicability of feedback linearization methods for motor neural prostheses is not yet clear. On-line identification of model parameters and the use of robust controllers around the linearized system may dominate the undesirable effects associated with inversion errors resulting from incorrect models. However, the determination of these nonlinear maps is generally computationally difficult. With currently available technology, the required level of computational and the available time between stimulation cycles makes this type of nonlinear control inappropriate for on-board, real-time use in a motor neural prosthesis.

Nonlinear Control Using Artificial Neural Nets

In this section, a method is described for the control of a class of nonlinear dynamic systems using feedback linearization, when the nonlinear models are not well known. In this approach to nonlinear adaptive control, the coordinate transformation maps are essentially "learned" using an artificial neural network (ANN). The design of this controller involves two ANNs and a two-step training process. The basic idea of this method (Loparo and Teixeira, 1990; Teixeira et al., 1991b) is to choose the overall compensator structure so that one artificial neural network (ANN_1) is forced to learn the inverse dynamics of the nonlinear system to be controlled (Figure 14–13A). This is done in advance of real-time operation by training and back-propagation, using data obtained from the system or its computer simulation. Then a second ANN is trained to learn the feedback control laws that make the system under control behave like a desired system (Figure 14–13B). Training is complete once the output of ANN_2 which is the input to the nonlinear system, converges to the output of ANN_1 (which is the input that is applied to the nonlinear system to obtain the same output as the desired system). Note that if the desired system is linear, then a "feedback linearizing control law" has been obtained.

After training, the system and the compensating ANN_2 together provide the approximate desired system performance (Figure 14–13C). This combination could be combined with one of the lower level linear system controllers described earlier (e.g., the PID or the adaptive controllers). In Teixeira et al. (1991a), this method is applied to the control of electrically stimulated muscle. Data obtained from experiments with an intact animal muscle (Shue, 1990) is used to construct a computer simulation.

In principle, the weights of both ANNs can be adaptively adjusted as well. Between each update of the ANN weights (which might occur periodically, each time a certain number of times steps pass), the two ANNs would be adjusted, via back-propagation.

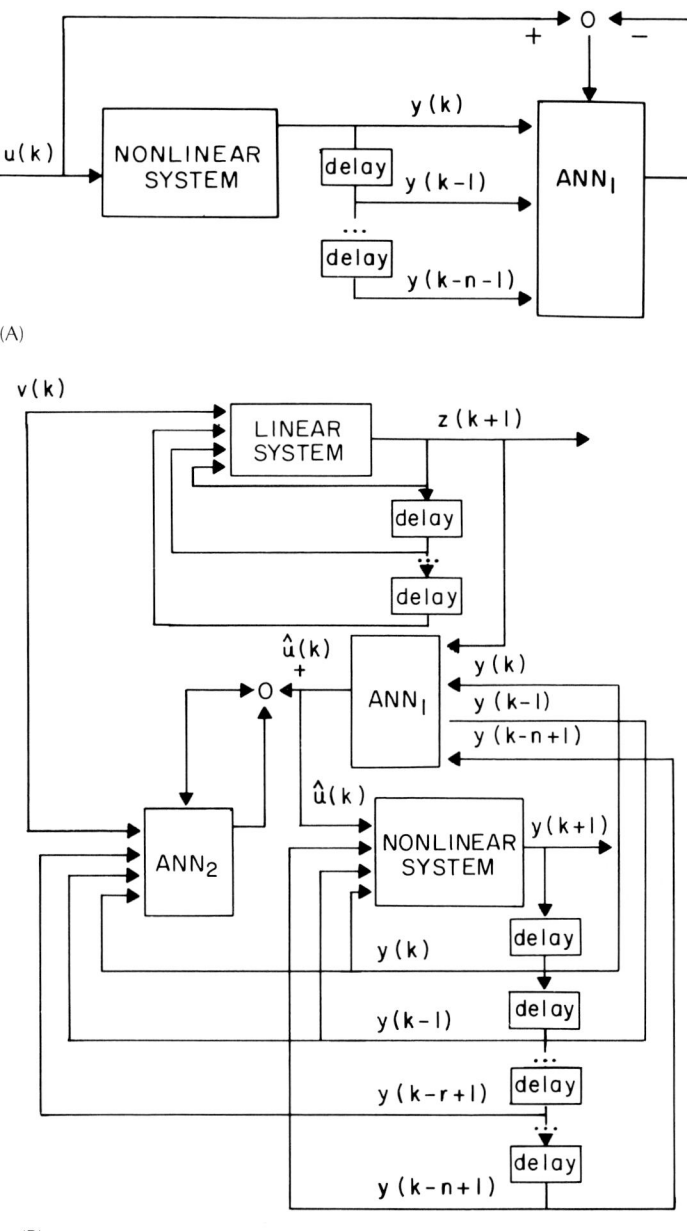

Figure 14–13 The use of artificial neural nets to obtain nonlinear control and feedback linearization. (A) The nonlinear system (or its computer simulation) is used in this configuration to train the artificial neural net ANN_1 to learn its inverse dynamics. Back propagation is used to fit the weights of the net, so that its output sequence (in response to the output sequence $\{y(k)\}$ of the nonlinear system), matches the input sequence, $\{u(k)\}$, to the nonlinear system. (B) Next, the tuned inverse dynamics net ANN_1 is used, in this configuration, to train the controller neural net, ANN_2, to make the output of the nonlinear system follow the output that a desired, linear system might produce. (C) When this has been accomplished, the trained controller net ANN_2 is used to operate the nonlinear system. If the desired system is linear [as in (B)], then ANN_2 has, in fact, learned the linearizing coordinate transformation for the nonlinear system. (Adapted from Teixeira et al., 1991b, with permission.)

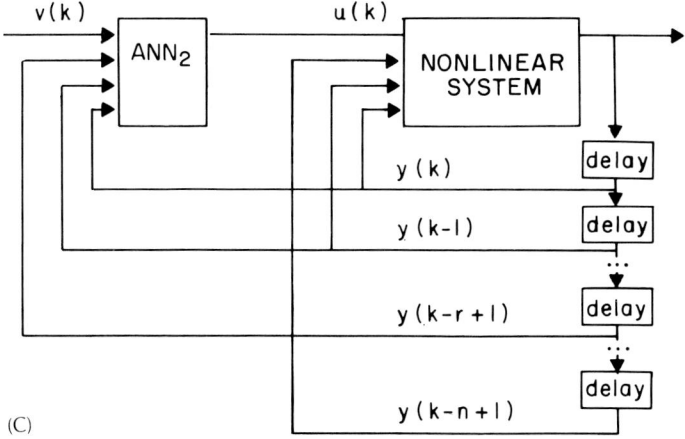

(C)

Figure 14–13 (Continued).

UPPER LEVEL CONTROLLERS

As described in the first section, control of FNS involves two levels of activity. One is servomechanism-like control of individual joints or groups of joints so that they track desired angle trajectories. The second level of control involves coordination tasks and the adjustment of future task segments based on past performance. Both aspects of control are applicable for FNS systems with and without orthoses.

One approach to the control of electrical stimulation, that is essentially all "upper level control," is to switch between stored stimulation patterns (time courses of stimulation parameters for each electrode), based upon a determination of which phase of the activity the patient is in. Locomotion has been obtained in this way by FNS research groups; different approaches include the use of flexion-withdrawal reflexes (Bajd et al., 1983, 1985; Kralj and Grobelnik, 1973); systems with preprogrammed computer-controlled stimulation patterns (Kralj et al., 1980, 1983; Vance et al., 1983); EMG-triggered stimulators (Graupe et al., 1983, 1984); stimulation triggered by sole-mounted footswitches (Kobetic and Marsolais, 1985); and by other sensors (Andrews et al., 1987; Petrofsky and Phillips, 1983, 1985a,b; Chizeck et al., 1985).

A number of specific stimulation control issues and problems have been identified, from analysis of the performance of paraplegic subjects using up to 48 channels of open-loop intramuscular stimulation (Marsolais and Kobetic, 1987). These include excessive physiological effort requirements and an inability (of complete paraplegic individuals) to effectively maneuver with crutches. Transitions between quasi-static and dynamic situations, such as at the start and end of FNS crutch walking, during crutch-assisted stair climbing and descent, during crutch-assisted sidestepping and backstepping, and during crutch-assisted rising from or settling into a chair are not sufficiently smooth and reliable in paraplegic patients. In addition, there is insufficient control of dynamics during crutch walking. Functional neuromuscular stimulation crutch walking is not sufficiently smooth, predictable, and efficient in paraplegic subjects. Stability is less than adequate.

Because of the inherent time delays in muscle stimulation, as well as the time delays of controller computation, for many tasks the use of feedback information to modify the upper level of control will involve changing what will happen "next time" that the task segment is performed. This is because the task segment under way may no longer be modifiable. This is particularly true for FNS gait.

In our current work (Willemin, 1991), predictive feedback control of knee (and ankle) angles of the supporting leg, from heel strike until toe-off, is being incorporated into the open-loop stimulation patterns for walking. We anticipate that improved controller design (upper and lower level) will result in improvements in the energy efficiency of FNS locomotion in three ways. Energy savings will be obtained through reduction in unnecessary motion during locomotion. In addition, if enhanced coordinated control of the hip, trunk, knees, and ankles yields improved balance during FNS locomotion (especially with crutches), then a reduction in upper body effort (primarily from arm support) should reduce the physiological effort required. A third reduction of energy expenditure, as measured relative to distance is achieved if the subject walks faster. Improved control of joint motion during FNS locomotion should facilitate the achievement of greater walking velocities.

The development of automatic methods to modify preprogrammed portions of the electrical stimulation of gait for the next step, based upon measurements of the current and past steps, can be accomplished in (at least) two ways. One approach is through the use of a rule-based expert system (driven by detection of gait events). A second method is the construction of an artificial neural network controller which modulates the activity of functionally synergistic groups of muscles, so as to generate coordinated patterned movements.

For the rule-based approach, the goal is to automatically adjust and synchronize stimulation patterns based upon sensor-based discrete event detection (e.g., thresholds in angles, accelerations, foot pressure), based upon a set of logical rules. Preliminary efforts in rule classification for a paraplegic gait are described in Simon et al. (1987). These rules are the result of prior experimentation, both with the real system and with computer simulations of models of it. Such rules may be learned iteratively, by experimental trial and modification. Alternatively, so-called "inference engine" software can be applied to extract rules from large numbers of samples of sets of sensor data records and their corresponding (expert-derived) time-sequence determinations of events. Recent computer hardware advances (in particular, fuzzy logic chips) make the use of this type of controller more feasible for onboard systems.

In the artificial neural net approach, the idea is to develop an artificial neural network controller for a neural prothesis. For FNS gait, conceptually this might be done in three stages: the development of an artificial neural net pattern generator; the incorporation of sensor (feedback) information into this pattern generator, and the addition of an on-line adaptation feature to the pattern generator. Initial investigations of this idea are currently being investigated by Abbas (1992). The architecture of the artificial pattern generator is a simplification of that in Grillner et al. (1988). Although these ideas are very speculative, similar techniques have been used successfully for the much simpler system of an "artificial cockroach" (Chiel and Beer, 1989; Beer et al., 1990).

To tune an artificial neural net (through back-propagation techniques) to become a pattern generator that produces a nominal sequence of stimulation parameters for paraplegic FNS gait requires a large number of training examples (stimulation pattern sequences and resulting motions). Practicality considerations require that this be done using a computer simulation of the system that is a good predictor of experimentally obtained paraplegic FNS gait. The nomimal pattern of stimulation parameters produced by the artificial neural net should generate locomotion, in a noiseless fixed-parameter model computer simulation, that is qualitatively similar to experimental results (in paraplegic patients).

A second stage of this development will be to provide the artificial neural network with the ability to make adjustments to the nominal stimulation pattern for the current cycle based on feedback information. These modifications are directed at providing robustness in the presence of external forces or varying initial conditions. This feedback will affect the functioning of the network for the current cycle only; it will not affect the nomimal trajectory for future cycles. Two types of feedback might be incorporated into the network: that which is used for timing, and that which is used for scaling. Feedback for timing adjustments will be provided to the neural net to trigger the initiation or termination of the various phases of gait. Feedback for scaling will be provided to the synergist neurons for modulating the activation levels of the synergist group of muscles.

The third stage of this effort will be to provide the network with the ability to modify its internal parameters based on feedback information such that the nominal trajectory for future cycles will be modified. This learning facility should be directed at fine tuning the network parameters and making adjustments for varying system parameters. Adaptation facilities for both the timing of the activation of synergies and for adjustment of the scaling of the activation of the synergies might be included.

CONCLUDING REMARKS

The control of motor neural prostheses challenges the limits of adaptive and nonlinear control theory, incorporating the latest information gleaned from the diverse fields of science, and is implemented using the latest in available technology. Although motor neural prostheses must be designed using primitive technology when compared to the original equipment that they repair, the "existence proof" of human motor function make this a most exciting field of applied science and engineering.

> No, a thousand times no; there does not exist a category of science that can be called applied science. There is science and the applications of science, bound together as the fruit to the tree which bears it. [Louis Pasteur, 1871]

REFERENCES

Abbas, J.J. (1989). *Feedback Control of Coronal Plane Hip and Trunk Angles in Paraplegic Subjects Using Functional Neuromuscular Stimulation.* M.S. Thesis. Case Western Reserve University, Cleveland, OH.

Abbas, J.J., and Chizeck, H.J. (1987). Feedback control of the hip and trunk in paraplegic subjects using functional neuromuscular stimulation. *Proc. 9th IEEE/EMBS Conf.*

Abbas, J.J., and Chizeck H.J. (1989). FNS control system tuning and clinical ratings of performance. *Proc. 11th Ann. IEEE Eng. in Med. and Biol. Conf.*, 1494–1495.

Abbas, J.J., and Chizeck, H.J. (1991). Feedback control of coronal plane hip angle in paraplegic subjects using functional neuromuscular stimulation. *IEEE Trans. Biomed. Eng.*, in press.

Abbas, J.J. (1992). Ph.D. Thesis. Case Western Reserve University, Cleveland, OH.

Allin, J., and Inbar, G.F. (1986). FNS control schemes for the upper limb. *IEEE Trans. Biomed. Eng.*, **33**, 818–828.

Andrews, B.J., and Bajd. T. (1984). Hybrid orthoses for paraplegics. *Proc. of the 8th Internat. Symp. on ECHE (suppl.)*, **55**. Dubrovnik.

Andrews, B.J., Baxendale, R.M., Barnett, R., and Phillips, G. (1987). A hybrid orthosis for paraplegics incorporating feedback control. *Proc. 8th ECHE*, Dubrovnik.

Astrom, K.J., and Wittenmark, B. (1989). *Adaptive Control*. Reading, MA: Addison-Wesley.

Bajd, T., Kralj, A., Turk, R., Benko, H., and Sega, J. (1983). The use of a four channel electrical stimulator as an ambulatory aid for paraplegic patients. *Phys. Ther.*, **63**, 1116.

Bajd, T., Andrews, B.J., Kralj, A., and Katakis, J. (1985). Restoration of walking in patients with incomplete spinal cord injuries by use of surface electrical stimulation—preliminary results. *Prosthet. Orthot. Int.*, **9**, 109–111.

Beer, R.D., Chiel, H.J., and Sterling, L.S. (1990). A biological perspective on automonous agent design. *Robotics and Automonous Systems*, **6**, 169.

Bernotas, L.A., Crago, P.E., and Chizeck, H.J. (1986). A discrete-time model of electrically stimulated muscle. *IEEE Trans. Biomed. Eng.*, **33**, 829–838.

Bernotas, L.A., Crago, P.E., and Chizeck, H.J. (1987). Adaptive control of electrically stimulated muscle. *IEEE Trans. Biomed. Eng.*, **34**, 140–147.

Brindley, S., Polkey, C.E., and Rushton, D.N. (1979). Electrical splinting of the knee in paraplegia. *Paraplegia*, **16**, 248.

Caldwell, C.W., and Reswick, J.B. (1975). A percutaneous wire electrode for chronic research use. *IEEE Trans. Biomed. Eng.*, **22**, 429–432.

Chang, C.W. (1984). *Stiffness Regulation via Feedback Control*. M.S. Thesis. Case Western Reserve University, Cleveland, OH.

Chia, T.L., Chow, P.C., and Chizeck, H.J. (1991). Recursive parameter identification of constrained systems: An application to electrically stimulated muscle. *IEEE Trans. Biomed. Eng.*, in press

Chiel, H.J., and Beer, R.D. (1989). A lesion study of a heterogeneous artificial neural network for hexapod locomotion. *Proc. IJCNN I*, 407–413.

Chizeck, H.J., Lalonde, R., Chang, C.W., Rosenthal, J.A., and Marsolais, E.B. (1985). Performance of a closed-loop controller for electrically-stimulated standing in paralyzed patients. *Proc. 8th Rehab. Eng. Soc. N. Am. Conf.*, 231–233.

Chizeck, H.J., Crago, P.E., and Kofman, L.S. (1988a). Robust closed-loop control of isometric muscle force using pulse width modulation. *IEEE Trans. Biomed. Eng.*, **35**, 510–517.

Chizeck, H.J., Kobetic, R., Marsolais, E.B., Abbas, J.J., Donner, I., and Simon, E. (1988b). Control of functional neuromuscular stimulation systems for standing and locomotion of paraplegics. *Proc. of IEEE*, **76**, 1155–1165.

Chizeck, H.J., Streeter-Palmieri, L., and Crago, P.E. (1989). Feedback control of electrical stimulation of muscle using simultaneous pulse width and frequency modulation. *Proc. IEEE Eng. Med. Biol. Soc. Conf.* 1155–1164.

Clarke, D.W. (1984). Self-tuning control of nonminimum-phase systems. *Automatica*, **20**, 501–517.

Crago, P.E., Peckham, P.H., and Thorpe, G.B. (1980). Modulation of muscle force by recruitment during intramuscular stimulation. *IEEE Trans. Biomed. Eng.*, **27**, 679–684.

Crago, P.E., Chizeck, H.J., Neuman, N., and Hambrecht, F.T. (1986). Sensors for use with functional neuromuscular stimulation. *IEEE Trans. Biomed. Eng.*, **33**, 256–268.

Crago, P.E., Lemay, M., and Liu, L. (1990). External control of limb movements involving environmental interactions. In: J.M. Winters and S.L. Woo, eds., *Multiple Muscle Systems: Biomechanics and Movement Organization*, New York: Springer-Verlag.

Crago, P.E., Nakai, R.J., and Chizeck, H.J. (1991). Feedback regulation of hand grasp opening and contact force during stimulation of paralyzed muscle. *IEEE Trans. Biomed. Eng.*, **38**, 17–28.

Cybulski, G.R., and Jaeger, R.J. (1986). Standing performance of persons with paraplegia. *Arch. Phys. Med. Rehabil.*, **67**, 103–108.

Dong, Y., and Chizeck, H.J. (1990a). A horizon-recursive form for predictors and their computation. *Proc. 29th IEEE Conf. Decision and Control.*

Dong, Y., and Chizeck, H.J. (1990b). A time-horizon recursive algorithm for predictive controllers. *Systems Engineering Department Technical Report.* Case Western Reserve University, Cleveland, OH.

Dong, Y., and Chizeck, H.J. (1991a). A unified approach to the analysis and design of predictive control. *Proc. 1991 Am. Control Conf.*, 1744–1745.

Dong, Y., and Chizeck, H.J. (1991b). A unified approach to predictive control. *Systems Engineering Department Technical Report.* Case Western Reserve University, Cleveland, OH.

Donner, I. (1986). *Electrical Stabilization of the Hip in the Lateral Plane via a Feedback Controller.* M.S. Thesis. Case Western Reserve University, Cleveland, OH.

Durfee, W.K., and Hausdorff, J.M. (1990). Regulating knee joint position by combining electrical stimulation with a controllable friction brake. *Ann. Biomed. Eng.*, **18**, 575–596.

El-Bialy, A. (1990). *Control of Multiplicative Discrete-Time Systems.* Ph.D. Thesis. Case Western Reserve University, Cleveland, OH.

Geng, K. (1989). *Parameter Identification of Nonlinear Discrete-Time Models of Electrically Stimulated Muscle.* M.S. Thesis. Case Western Reserve University, Cleveland, OH.

Gorman, P.H., and Mortimer, J.T. (1983). The effect of stimulus parameters on the recruitment characteristics of direct nerve stimulation. *IEEE Trans. Biomed. Eng.*, **30**, 407–414.

Grandjean, P., and Mortimer, J.T. (1986). Recruitment properties of monopolar and dipolar epimysial electrodes. *Ann. Biomed. Eng.*, **14**, 53–66.

Graupe, D., Kohn, K., Kralj, A., and Basseas, S. (1983). Patient controlled electrical stimulation via EMG signature discrimination for providing certain paraplegics with primitive walking function. *J. Biomed. Eng.*, **5**, 270–276.

Graupe, D., Kohn, K., Basseas, S., and Naccarato, E. (1984). Controlling electrical stimulation of paraplegics via EMG-based posture-mapping. *Proc. 6th IEEE Eng. Med. Biol. Soc. Conf.*, 4–8.

Grillner, S., Buchanan, J.T., and Lansner, A. (1988). Simulation of the segmental burst generating network for locomotion in lamprey. *Neurosci. Lett.*, **89**, 31–35.

Handa, Y., Handa, T., and Nakatsuchi, Y. (1985). A voice-controlled functional electrical stimulation system for the paralyzed hand. *Jpn. J. Med. Elec. Biol. Eng.*, **23**, 292–298.

Holle, J., Thoma, H., Frey, M., Gruber, H., Kern, H., and Schwanda, G. (1984). Walking with an implantable stimulation system for paraplegics. *Proc. 2nd Conf. Rehabil. Eng.*, 551.

Isidori, A. (1989). *Nonlinear Control Systems.* New York: Springer-Verlag.

Jaeger, R.T. (1986). Design and simulation of closed-loop electrical stimulation orthoses for restoration of quiet standing in paraplegics. *J. Biomech.*, **19**, 825–835.

Khang, G., and Zajac, F.E. (1989a). Paraplegic standing controlled by functional neuromuscular stimulation: Part I—computer model and control system design. *IEEE Trans. Biomed. Eng.*, **36**, 873–884.

Khang, G., and Zajac, F.E. (1989b). Paraplegic standing controlled by functional neuromuscular stimulation: Part II—computer stimulation studies. *IEEE Trans. Biomed. Eng.*, **36**, 885–894.

Kobetic, R., and Marsolais, E.B. (1985). Automated electrically induced paraplegic gait. *Proc. 38th ACEMB*, 293.

Kralj, A., and Grobelnik, S. (1973). Functional electrical stimulation—a new hope for paraplegic patients. *Bull. Prosth. Res.*, 10–20.

Kralj, A., Bajd, T., and Turk, R. (1980). Electrical stimulation providing functional use of paraplegic patient muscles. *Med. Prol. Technol.*, **7**, 3.

Kralj, A., Bajd, T., Turk, R., Krajnik, J., and Benko, H. (1983). Gait restoration in paraplegic patients: A feasibility demonstration using multichannel surface electrode FES. *J. Rehabil. Res. Dev.*, **20**, 3.

Lan, N., Crago, P.E., and Chizeck, H.J. (1990). A pertubation control strategy for FNS motor prostheses. *Proc. 12th IEEE Eng. Med. Biol. Conf.*, 2327–2328.

Lan, N., Crago, P.E., and Chizeck, H.J. (1991a). Control of end-point forces of a multi-joint limb by functional neuromuscular stimulation. *IEEE Trans. Biomed. Eng.*, **38**, 953–965.

Lan, N., Crago, P.E., and Chizeck, H.J. (1991b). Feedback control methods for task regulation by electrical stimulation of muscles. *IEEE Trans. Biomed. Eng.*, **38**.

Lemay, M.A. (1991). *Automated Tuning of a Closed Loop Hand Grasp Neuroprosthesis*. M.S. Thesis. Case Western Reserve University, Cleveland, OH.

Liu, L. (1990). *Tuning of Active Stiffness Regulation for Robust Control of FNS Hand Grasp*. M.S. Thesis. Case Western Reserve University, Cleveland, OH.

Loparo, K., and Teixeira, E. (1990). A new approach for adaptive control of a nonlinear system using neural networks. *IEEE Intl. Conf. Systems, Man and Cybernetics*.

Marsolais, E.B., Ko, W., and Masiello, A. (1985). Finger switch for a portable microprocessor system to restore walking in paraplegics. *Proc. 8th Annual RESNA Conf.*, 376–378.

Marsolais, E.B., and Kobetic, R. (1983). Functional walking in paralyzed patients by means of electrical stimulation. *Clin. Orthop.*, 175.

Marsolais, E.B., and Kobetic, R. (1986). Implantation techniques and experience with percutaneous intramuscular electrodes in the lower extremities. *J. Rehabil. Res. Dev.*, **23**, 1–8.

Marsolais, E.B., and Kobetic R. (1987). Functional electrical stimulation for walking in paraplegia. *J. Bone Joint Surg.*, **69**, 728–733.

McNeal, D.R., Waters, R., and Reswick, J. (1977). Experience with implanted electrodes. *Neurosurgery*, **1**, 228–229.

Mortimer, J.T., Bayer, D.M., Lord, R.H., and Swanker, J.W. (1974). Shoulder position transduction for proportional two axis control of orthotic/prosthetic systems. In: *The Control of Upper Extremity Prostheses and Orthoses*. C.C. Thomas.

Moynahan, M. (1990). *Characterization of Paraplegic Disturbance Response During FNS Standing*. M.S. Thesis. Case Western Reserve University, Cleveland, OH.

Naples, G.G. (1987). *An Implantable Spiral Cuff Electrode for Electrical Stimulation of Peripheral Nerve*. M.S. Thesis. Case Western Reserve University, Cleveland, OH.

Pasteur, L. (1871). La Science en France. *La Revue Scientifique*, 73–77.

Pletomaa, A., and Koivo, H.N. (1983). Tuning of a multivariable discrete time PI controller for unknown systems. *Int. J. Control*, **38**, 735–745.

Peterson, D.K., and Chizeck, H.J. (1987). Linear quadratic control of a loaded agonist-antagonist muscle pair. *IEEE Trans. Biomed. Eng.*, **34**, 135–140.

Petrofsky, J.S., and Phillips, C.A. (1983). Computer controlled walking in the paralyzed individual. *J. Neurol. Orthop. Surg.*, **4**, 153–164.

Petrofsky, J.S., Phillips, C.A., Larson, P., and Douglas, R. (1985a). Computer synthesized walking: An application of orthosis and functional electrical stimulation (FES). *J. Neurol. Orthop. Med. Surg.*, **6**, 219–230.

Petrofsky, J.S., Phillips, C.A., Douglas, R., and Larson, P. (1985b). Integration of orthosis with computer-controlled movement. *IEEE Trans. Biomed. Eng.*, 32.

Rosenthal, J.A. (1984). *Control Electrically-Stimulated Standing for Paraplegics.* M.S. Thesis. Case Western Reserve University, Cleveland, OH.

Schwirtlich, L., and Popovic, D. (1984). Hybrid orthoses for deficient locomotion. *Proc. of the 8th Int. Symp. ECHE.* Dubrovnik.

Shue, G. (1990). *Multiplicative Model of Stimulated Muscle for FNS Control.* M.S. Thesis. Case Western Reserve University, Cleveland, OH.

Simon, E., Kobetic, R., Chizeck, H.J., Marsolais, E.B. (1987). Control of FNS gait based on the detection of discrete events. *Proc. 9th Ann. IEEE Eng. Med. Biol. Conf.*, 1575–1576.

Smith, B., Peckham, P.H., Keith, M.W., and Roscoe, D.D. (1987). An externally powered multichanneled, implantable stimulator for versatile control of paralyzed muscle. *IEEE Trans. Biomed. Eng.*, **34**, 499–508.

Stanic, U., and Trnkoczy, A. (1974). Closed-loop positioning of hemiplegic patient's joint by means of functional electrical stimulation. *IEEE Trans. Biomed. Eng.*, **21**, 365–370.

Szeto, A.Y.J., and Riso, R.R. (1987). Sensory feedback using electrical stimulation. In: R.V. Smity and J.H. Leslie, eds. *Rehabilitation Engineering.* Boca Raton, FL: CRC Press.

Teixeira, E., Jayaraman, G., Shue, G., Crago, P.E., Loparo, K., and Chizeck, H.J. (1991a). Feedback control of nonlinear multiplicative systems using neural nets: An application to electrically stimulated muscle. *IEEE Intl. Conf. Syst. Eng.*, in press.

Teixeira, E., Loparo, K., and Gomide, F. (1991b) Feedback linearization using neural networks. *Systems Engineering Department Technical Report.* Case Western Reserve University, Cleveland, OH.

Thoma, H., Frey, M., Holle, J., Kern, H., Reiner, E., Schwanda, G., and Stor, H. (1983). Paraplegics should learn to walk with their fingers. *Proc. IEEE Eng. Med. Biol. Soc. Conf.*, 579–582.

Timmons, W.D., Chizeck, H.J., and Katona, P.G. (1991). Adaptive control is enhanced by background estimation. *IEEE Trans. Biomed. Eng.*, **38**,

Tomovic, R., Vukobratovic, M., and Vodovnik, L. (1972). Hybrid actuator for orthotic systems: Hybrid assistive systems. *Proc. 4th ECHE.* Dubrovnik.

Vance, F., Kobetic, R., Marsolais, E.B. and Chizeck, H.J. (1983). Portable microprocessor-controlled stimulation for activation of paralyzed muscles. In M. Hamza, ed., *Mini and Microcomputers and Their Applications*, ACTA Press.

Veltink, P.H., El-Bialy, A., Chizeck, H.J., and Crago, P.E. (1989). Nonlinear control of an artificially stimulated muscle-skelton-load system. *Proc. 11th IEEE Eng. Med. Biol. Conf.*, 969–970.

Veltink, P.H., Chizeck, H.J., Crago, P.E., and El-Bialy, A. (1992). Nonlinear joint angle control for artificially stimulated muscle. *IEEE Trans. Biomed. Eng.*, **39**, in press.

Voss, G.I., Katona, P.G., and Chizeck, H.J. (1987). Adaptive multivariable drug delivery: Control of arterial pressure and cardiac output in anesthetized dogs. *IEEE Trans. Biomed. Eng.*, **34**, 617–623.

Wilemon, W.K., Mooney, V., McNeal, D, and Reswick, J. (1970). Surgically implanted peripheral neuroelectric stimulation. *Rancho Los Amigos Hospital Internal Report.* Downey, CA.

Willemin, D., and Chizeck, H.J. (1989). Feedback control of the knee during the stance phase of paraplegics FES gait using a stiffness regulator. *Proc. 12th Rehab. Eng. Soc. N. Am. Conf.*, 399–400.

Willemin, D. (1991). M.S. Thesis. Case Western Reserve University, Cleveland, OH.

15
The Transfer of Technology From the Laboratory to the Real World

GERALD E. LOEB AND JOSEPH H. SCHULMAN

Research projects on neural prostheses are usually preoccupied with obtaining functioning laboratory prototypes, often to the exclusion of considering many other factors that are critical to the success or failure of commercial products. Functional neuromuscular stimulation has yet to produce such products, but many important lessons can be learned from the fields of cardiac pacemakers and cochlear prostheses. We have collected many examples of personal, political, fiscal and administrative shortcomings that have had at least as much influence on the course of product development as the technical feasibility of the original invention. Specific strategies are suggested for coping with critical tasks of project management that are often foreign to bench scientists and engineers, including securing and developing intellectual property rights, maintaining extended interdisciplinary collaborations, targeting commercially viable clinical applications, and selecting and approaching industrial partners.

After a quarter-century of technical promise, reasonable financial support, and growing complexity, researchers in the field of functional neuromuscular stimulation (FNS) are facing increasing pressure to produce clinical and commercial successes. Two other sophisticated applications of neural control have approached such a threshold and gone in opposite directions: cochlear prostheses are now being implanted worldwide at an increasing pace (Loeb, 1990), while overt attempts to build visual prostheses went out of fashion almost 20 years ago (Loeb, 1987), only recently to reemerge in the light of new technology (Bak et al., 1990).

The foregoing chapters of this book are concerned primarily with the scientific and technological problems that must be overcome to achieve success in the laboratory. However, experience suggests that even when such problems have been solved, there is no guarantee that this will lead to success in the clinic and in the marketplace. This chapter examines the factors that affect this latter process as seen from the perspective of the academic researcher. Unfortunately, the process of technology transfer tends to be described infrequently and nonspecifically, particularly if there has been failure. Thus, we must beg the forgiveness of both our readers and our colleagues for presenting a largely unreferenced collection of personal experiences, industry gossip, and broad generalizations, at least some of which may contain minor factual errors. The general lessons that we hope to convey transcend the details of the examples, but the lessons are hard to appreciate without many concrete examples, which we have tried to present concisely. We particularly thank many of our colleagues for sharing their recollected experiences.

LESSONS FROM COCHLEAR PROSTHETICS

Cochlear prostheses are frequently cited as the leading example of a successful, sophisticated, implantable interface with the nervous system. However, there have been over 25 different designs in as many years and only one is currently being marketed in North America (see review by Loeb, 1990). Thus, this field is also the leading example of hi-tech failure. It is particularly ironic that the one successful product to date, the Nucleus-22 from Cochlear Corp., was developed in Australia, starting about 6 to 8 years after three separate groups in California pioneered the first clinical implants in deaf patients. All four efforts were initiated by clinical otolaryngologists, but the projects soon developed very different personalities.

Stanford University: Emphasis on Engineering Technology

Founded by Blair Simmons, this group operated principally out of the microelectronics laboratory under the direction of Robert White. Most of the NIH-funded research consisted of graduate student projects to develop integrated-circuit techniques to build electrode arrays and digitally controlled, multichannel stimulators. An eight-channel cochlear stimulator was developed using several sophisticated, custom integrated-circuit chips (Soma, 1980), at least one of which required nonstandard processes that made the chip set unattractive to industry. Neurophysiological and psychophysical input to the design was weak, few clinical implants were done, and results were unimpressive. A simplified single-channel device was spun off to a venture-funded start-up company that was badly managed and went bankrupt. The project eventually faded away.

UCSF: Emphasis on Basic Science

Founded by Robin Michelson, this group operated principally out of a neurophysiological laboratory directed by Michael Merzenich. They conducted critical studies of the biophysics of electrode design (Merzenich and White, 1977), but were hampered in constructing multichannel prostheses based on these designs by a lack of engineering expertise and facilities. A small number of patients were implanted with a prototype device that produced very promising results (Schindler and Kessler, 1987), but an attempt to transfer the system to Storz Instrument Company (a manufacturer of surgical instruments) failed because the company was unable or unwilling to correct inherited design problems and limitations in packaging and electronic design. The whole system has since been completely reengineered by Minimed Technologies, incorporating additional speech-processor strategies developed independently at Research Triangle Institute (Wilson et al., 1988). It is due to begin investigational device trials in early 1991, 20 years after the first implant at UCSF.

House: Emphasis on Clinical Practice

Founded by William House in Los Angeles, this group remained under the control of clinicians dedicated to achieving widespread acceptance of a very simple single-channel device. Dozens of satellite groups were trained and thousands of patients were implanted. The device was sold to and manufactured by the 3M Corporation almost without change for several years (Fretz and Fravel, 1985). In attempting to correct a minor design flaw, a serious mistake led to a high failure rate and a product recall. This, plus the growing appreciation of the superior performance of the multichannel Nucleus system, led to 3M's withdrawal from the entire field [and the orphaning of a promising single-channel device developed in Austria by Burian et al. (1986), whose rights 3M had acquired]. However, it is arguable that without the vigorous proselytizing of the House group, the field of cochlear prosthetics might not exist today.

Nucleus: Emphasis of Product Development

Founded by Graeme Clark at the University of Melbourne, this effort was rapidly brought under the wing of a large pacemaker company through the financial support of the Australian government. Several key strategic decisions led to a multichannel design that was technically sophisticated, but which made some scientific compromises to minimize development time (Franz et al., 1987). It was ready for clinical trials in 4 years and was market-approved by the Food and Drug Administration (FDA) 3 years after that, in 1985. The Nucleus-22, with some evolutionary design changes, now dominates the world market.

CATEGORIES OF FAILURE AND SOME EXAMPLES

Every stage of the process of product development offers opportunities to fail, and failure at any stage dooms the product. Thus, it is not surprising that so few hi-tech ventures succeed (10% is considered good). This is why venture capital is often raised by funds that spread the risk over many projects. Unfortunately, most researchers do not have the opportunity to participate personally in more than one or two such projects during the course of their careers. Thus, it behooves us to try to anticipate potential problems and to make our commitments even more selectively.

Technical

As in most electronic devices, the most likely components to fail in medical devices tend to be connectors and leads. In the early days of the pacemaker industry, it was common to borrow connector technology from more conventional applications, where there was extensive experience. Unfortunately, the environment provided by the human body (warm salt water in constant motion) generates failure modes that are new and overcome only with novel materials and mechanical configurations. In one case, a coaxial connector that had been used successfully in one pacemaker failed in another because its different pulse waveform accelerated corrosion around the pins.

Often, fixing one problem creates new problems. Mercury batteries worked well in epoxy-encapsulated packemakers because the small amount of hydrogen gas that they evolve could diffuse out through the epoxy. Problems with inward water permeation through epoxy led to hermetically sealed cans; these solved the corrosion problem but experienced rupture of the hermetic seals due to hydrogen gas build-up. One manufacturer added a "getter" material to chemically bind the hydrogen, but the reaction produced water vapor inside the can, nullifying the attempt to prevent water-damage by using an hermetic package.

Manufacture

The process of transferring fabrication procedures from the prototyping laboratory to the production line requires special attention to the capabilities of production workers and the need to maintain quality in the absence of high levels of motivation and expertise. What is often overlooked is that this process is a continuing challenge rather than a one-time exercise. Because of personnel turnover and the cumulative effects of apparently innocuous procedural changes, manufacturers often discover that they have "forgotten" how to perform successfully some step that has never caused any problems. Failures may then arise in final testing, perhaps even in the field, that can be very difficult to trace to processes that were believed to be secure and thus were not being adequately quality-controlled. Sterilization is a process that is notorious for failing in production despite its apparent simplicity.

Sometimes, changes in procedure can produce the appearance of a problem that doesn't really exist. In one case, a new janitorial service used an alkali wax stripper on the floors in a nonlaboratory space; the fumes spread through the air conditioning duct and caused a sensitive chemical test to indicate falsely that hermetic seals were leaking.

Fiscal

It is a truism that no hi-tech project is ever brought in on schedule and within budget. In the complex world of medical devices, the potential for budget overruns during product and market development is virtually open-ended. Whether the project is pursued or abandoned in the face of each new setback should depend simply on the difference between the estimated gain of success (weighted by the probability of success) and the expenses that would have to be written off as a loss or extended as a gamble. Unfortunately, this straightforward calculation is often subverted by arbitrary limits imposed by the size and fiscal health of the company and the limited imagination of management. Serious players need "deep pockets" and the willingness to dig into them deeply without losing their nerve. Small companies can usually work faster and more efficiently on research and development, but they may get to the bottom of their pockets sooner, especially if they are engaged in other risky ventures. For example, the LAURA multichannel cochlear prosthesis developed at the University of Antwerp was transferred to Forelec, a relatively small manufacturer of electrical equipment. With the assistance of the Belgian government, Forelec proceeded with two hi-tech projects at the same time: LAURA and remote controllers for domestic use. LAURA was actually proceeding fairly well, but the market for domestic controllers developed slower than anticipated and the company went bankrupt. LAURA is now being pursued by Antwerp Bionic Systems, a small venture capital company.

Marketing

If you build a better mousetrap, the world can indeed beat a path to your door to buy it. If you build a better neural prosthesis, market accessibility is less certain. This is because the customer who realizes the benefit (patient) is different from the customer who recommends the purchase (physician) and the customer who pays the bill (medical insurer). This results in three different assessments of cost/benefit ratio, each of which must appear favorable to the relevant party. In the case of neural prostheses, the government agency that must often pay the bills is usually not the agency that will realize the savings produced by rehabilitating the patient. Conversely, in the case of cardiac pacemakers, there was substantial resistance among physicians to simple, cheap implants, at least in part because their fees were tied to device cost and complexity.

Political

The regulatory environment for medical devices remains generally favorable, at least compared to pharmaceuticals. However, specific issues can become politicized without warning. In the 1970s, there was one alleged but undocumented incident in which a microwave oven interfered with a cardiac pacemaker. Unfortunately, this coincided with well-publicized concern about over-the-horizon radar, which produced massive pulsating radiation that could inhibit a demand pacemaker. The Air Force tested and rated all pacemakers for sensitivity to such intense emissions. Despite the fact that commercial ovens were well shielded and emitted no radiation that posed a risk to pacemakers, manufacturers were forced to incorporate a number of expensive modifications to their designs. In one case, a titanium shell fitted as an RF shield over a then-conventional and quite reliable epoxy pacemaker resulted in a large number of sterile abscesses in patients. It was rumored that about 20,000 pacemakers had to be surgically replaced.

Bureaucratic

The limiting factor in pacemaker life is battery life. In the 1960s, the available mercury batteries would last less than 2 years, requiring multiple reoperations in the typical patient (ironically, they lasted 7 years when tested in the laboratory, a discrepancy that was ultimately traced to the deleterious effects of constant motion). Thus, there was great interest in the nuclear pacemaker, which utilized a tiny amount of radioactive material to power itself almost indefinitely. However, the rules governing the transport and disposal of this material were so cumbersome that this technically successful device failed as a product.

At one point, the mercury battery problem was solved by a major American manufacturer of household appliances, whose batteries would last for 15 years. However, bad press resulting from a small recall of appliances apparently caused the corporate bureaucracy to drop their cardiac pacemaker line. Eventually the battery-life problem was solved with the advent of lithium cells.

TOWARD HEALTHIER ATTITUDES AND STRATEGIES

Threshold of Clinical Utility

Cochlear prosthetics succeeded as a field because it turned out that a primitive device could produce worthwhile benefit for a substantial number of patients. However, in the field of FNS, a similarly simple and effective device for correcting footdrop in stroke patients was commercially unsuccessful simply because the relatively small benefits did not exceed the aggregate "costs" to the patient [including surgery, fitting, maintenance, and repair (Waters et al., 1985)] and because some benefit could be obtained from an inexpensive, albeit awkward, mechanical brace. At the opposite end of the spectrum, achieving complete, integrated sensorimotor functions such as walking using FNS alone would clearly be an enormous benefit, but current attempts should be considered strictly academic research projects, far ahead of general feasibility given the current state of the art.

It seems likely that the first commercially successful systems for walking will be hybrid devices involving both FNS and braces, which will be both more expensive than braces and less attractive cosmetically than fully implanted systems. Thus, these hybrids will have to produce a high degree of function from the outset. This, in turn, suggests that the first commercially successful FNS applications will be in less ambitious areas such as assists for partially functional limbs. Such devices will require more tailoring to the special conditions in each individual patient, which has led us to focus on a modular family of implantable devices (Loeb et al., 1990). This in turn will create the need for a more sophisticated clinical environment than is required for cochlear prostheses, where "one size fits all."

Figure 15-1 illustrates the problem of finding clinical applications that are amenable to current technology. Over time, the curve on the left advances and overtakes more and more of the curve on the right, which in turn shifts rightward as projects reach completion. For a highly constrained subset of all clinical applications of technology (e.g., FNS), and at a given point in time, it may be that no projects lie

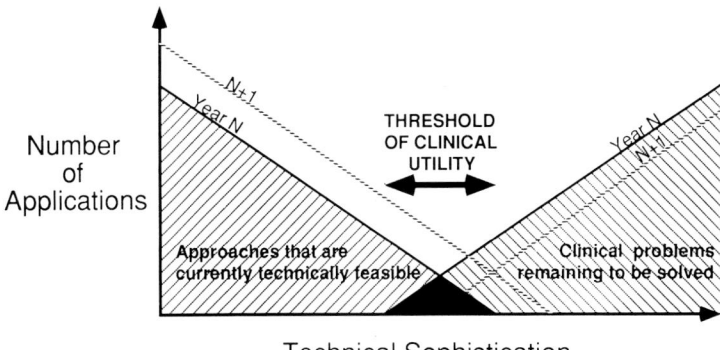

Figure 15-1 At any given time (year N), there are more simple projects that can be accomplished with the currently available technologies than there are complex projects (shaded curve on left). Conversely, clinical problems that remain to be addressed tend to require more sophisticated technology (shaded curve on the right). With time, both curves move toward the right. The overlapping region in the middle (black) is where one may find applications that have crossed the threshold of clinical utility: they are worth doing and they can be done. Unfortunately, for a given field of endeavor at a given time, there is no guarantee that any projects actually lie in this zone.

in the overlap zone. While it may be useful to continue to pursue demonstration projects in the zone to the right or to accelerate the motion of the technology curve on the left, it should be remembered that neither of these efforts is, by itself, clinically or commercial viable.

Planning an Orderly Transition from Laboratory

Although the details vary for different countries, institutions, and clinical areas, the general considerations, processes, and players are now fairly standardized in the medical device field:

1. Development and animal testing of prototype devices, usually performed with at least some peer-reviewed research funding and subject to preapproved procedures for intramural oversight.
2. Initial use of the device with human patient volunteers. In some jurisdictions, this again involves only local review by a human research committee, but obviously the stakes are higher in terms of both potential liability and the beginnings of a database of clinical experience that will eventually form the basis for an application for premarket approval from a regulatory agency. The thoroughness and understandability of your informed consent procedures are critical, including a complete analysis of the alternatives available to the patient, estimated probabilities of obtaining both positive and negative clinical outcomes, and procedures and responsibilities for handling unforeseen complications.
3. In the United States, even the initial clinical testing of a medical device comes under the rules for investigational device exemption (IDE) of the FDA. This procedure has been designed to speed and simplify compliance. For an institution-based investigator, it is largely a notification to the FDA that such research

and internal review procedures are underway; unless the FDA takes specific action (usually a request for further information), you may proceed after 30 days. If you already have an industrial partner, applying for the IDE under their auspices will facilitate eventual market approval; the rules are the same but the material demonstrating safety and the procedures for evaluating efficacy will probably be reviewed more thoroughly. If the partner is supporting the research in cash or in kind, this is essential. Note that the scale and duration of the IDE phase is usually difficult to predict. The FDA would generally prefer it to be overstated rather than understated so that you will not appear to be returning prematurely for premarket approval (PMA). During the IDE period, your industrial partner can charge a reasonable price reflecting the costs of manufacture (but not profit) of the devices being tested, but all such testing must occur under the auspices and procedures approved in the IDE.

4. Most countries have some formal procedure for designating that a device may be generally sold to and used by licensed practitioners and/or patients according to prescribing rules (e.g., PMA in the U.S. FDA). Such approval is usually tied to the availability of paying customers either formally (through inclusion in the lists of approved therapeutics in national health services) or informally (through willingness of private or public third-party insurers to reimburse costs). Generally, the requirement for this approval is a demonstration of both safety (relative to the risks of the untreated condition) and efficacy (measurable benefit to the patient). Note that efficacy in centrally administered health care systems usually includes cost effectiveness vis-à-vis competing therapies, whereas in free-market systems (e.g., U.S. FDA) only *some* net benefit must be demonstrated relative to risk, not cost.

5. Once a device has gained market approval, the institutions and investigators participating in its development effectively lose all legal control over the further technical development and clinical practices related to the device (except as may have been prenegotiated in licensing agreements). Your relief at giving birth may be tempered by the realization that it's an unpredictable world out there. Your ability to continue to influence this world will now depend on the evolving strategies of your industrial partner, your personal scientific and medical stature, and your willingness and ability to integrate the realities of the marketplace into your scientific thinking.

Putting the Profit Motive in its Proper Place

Many truly unpleasant misunderstandings among researchers, administrators, and entrepreneurs arise from misconceptions about the process of converting ideas into profits. Most of the time, we accept the notion that researchers seek only intellectual recognition for their creativity (i.e., fame), while entrepreneurs seek monetary reward for financial risk-taking (i.e., fortune). However, at the cutting edge of technology, it is sometimes the case that creative ideas provide an inside track to profitability, for which entrepreneurs are willing to pay. The problem is that even with an inside track, the race is long, risky, and expensive (see Figure 15–2). In highly technical and heavily regulated areas such as implantable medical devices, the investment required to produce the prototype is usually less than 5% of the investment

Typical cost factors associated with hi-tech medical devices:

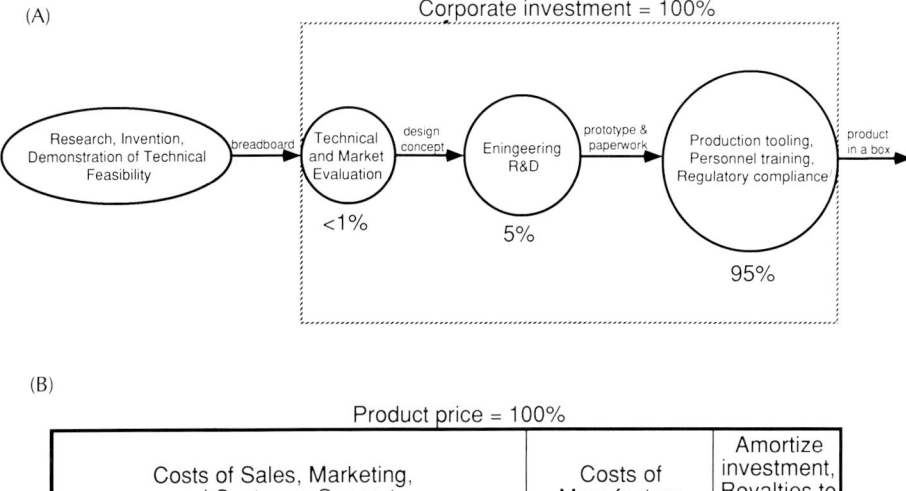

Figure 15–2 (A) Once there has been a "breadboard" level demonstration of feasibility (usually funded by government agencies), industry faces three successive categories of investment with progressively greater costs (expressed as percentage of total investment). (B) Once there is a product, the sales price is the sum of three categories of "cost."

required to get the product into a cardboard box at the end of a production line. After that, the cost of production is further dwarfed by the cost of advertising, marketing, clinical training, and regulatory complicance. Thus, the prudent entrepreneur can afford to pay only a small fraction of the highly uncertain profits to the inventor, and almost none of this is likely to be "up-front" money that might be useful to further the immediate research effort.

There are just enough success stories around to whet the unnatural appetite for fortune in researchers, particularly when goaded by aggressive but often naive university administrators. However, we would hazard the guess that most of these success stories are related more to good fortune than clever tactics. There are also tragedies of missed opportunities. However, most of these are egregious failures to identify and secure obvious inventions (see next section), rather than victimization by sharp practices.

Experience suggests to us one approach that might maximize the ability of researchers to participate usefully in the process of commercialization while minimizing the personal angst, intellectual distraction, and professional jealousy that often accompanies the process. In most institutions, researchers now have the obligation to identify potential inventions to their administrations. While the individual inventor and the institution often share equally in any profits, it must be remembered that the inventor's primary professional interest is "fame" while the institution's main interest is "fortune." Thus, it is appropriate for the inventor to aggressively seek a commercial developer for his invention, but he should rely on his institution to negotiate the terms. If the terms turn out to be overly generous to the manufacturer, the researcher is still fairly well served by having his ideas leverage the huge investment needed to convert an invention into a successful product. Meanwhile, he can get on with further invention and improvements whose significance may be better recognized in the next round. If the institution shows no interest, it should be possible to obtain a release so that intellectual property rights can be secured and marketed independently; however, this course is fraught with problems for a commercially unsophisticated scientist with a thoroughly nonobjective affection for his own ideas.

The Rules of Intellectual Property

Scientists, accustomed to the way that other scientists think about ideas, discoveries, and inventions, often find the law of patents and copyrights to be particularly confusing and even offensive. This is largely because the logic behind these rules flows primarily from legal and commercial considerations, where it matters more that there is internal consistency than technical sense. This in turn means that even the most knowledgeable scientist or engineer must rely heavily on the expertise of outsiders who are often technically ignorant and may not even be expert in patent law nor highly motivated (a frequent problem in the legal offices of universities). Finally, in the area of complex medical devices, the patentable aspects of an invention may not emerge until considerable development and testing has been pursued, which may itself require the resources of an industrial partner.

Fortunately, there are rules and circumstances that work in the inventor's favor. Current policy in most granting agencies is to permit grantee institutions to own and to sell patent rights developed through government-funded research (precisely to insure that private enterprise can be motivated to make the huge additional investment required to develop products and markets). The "1-year clock" (in the United States and some other jurisdictions) permits an inventor to file patent applications up to 1 year after public disclosure (e.g., press conference, publication in journals, clinical use in patients), although usually all foreign patent rights are lost. Thus it may be possible to interest an industrial partner in pursuing the patent rights, thereby drawing on considerably more expertise and motivation than can usually be obtained at home. However, be prepared for some very difficult questions. Successful industrialists and venture-capitalists got that way by worrying about the bottom line in a way that is much more rigorous than the section of your grant application that you entitled "clinical relevance."

Be sure to exchange disclosure agreements which protect information beyond that reported publicly, including both the information that you provide to the company and that which they provide to you (which may actually be more valuable, at least to them). One need not be particularly paranoid about this; no serious businessman is going to jeopardize a million-dollar investment in a product by trying to short-change the rightful inventors. However, these exchanges often do include enjoinders of 1 to 2 years, during which time you may not be free to pursue other industrial opportunities even if the first contact does not pan out. Thus, disclosure agreements should not be entered into lightly, particularly in highly competitive fields. (Fortunately or unfortunately, FNS shows no signs yet of being commercially highly competitive).

If a commercialization deal is struck, it is important to include nonperformance clauses. If possible, there should be definite milestones regarding production and marketing which, if not met, would allow the invention to be transferred to an organization that may be better prepared to develop the product. These milestones will be much more conservative than the optimistic hype that often accompanies these deals and their attendant publicity. Their role is not to harrass a well-meaning effort because of unforeseen difficulties but rather to protect against catastrophes such as bankruptcy, major management shifts, and deliberate sandbagging of technology that might compete with an existing product line.

Finally, one must eschew the temptation to punt on all of these hassles by deliberately placing inventions in the public domain by refusing to pursue patent and copyright protection. This path may seem altruistic, but it is the "kiss of death" for most potential products. No company is going to pour millions of dollars into developing a product, a market, and a favorable regulatory environment if another company can then come along and usurp it with a cheap copy. An aggressive approach to securing intellectual property rights is essential, and it should not be confused with personal greed. As discussed above, your role and goal as a scientist or engineer is well served by making sure that someone secures these rights and develops the product whether or not you or your institution gets rich.

Understanding Corporate Structure

You would probably be amused if a prospective graduate student tried to get a position in your laboratory by taking your secretary to lunch, but you may be guilty of similar organizational naiveté in approaching industry. Unfortunately, corporate organization is less stereotyped than university department structures, so some individual research is required.

First, recognize that there are three parts to every company: (1) the part that makes products; (2) the part that sells products; and (3) the part that manages the money. These parts are controlled by different people, often with very different personalities and attitudes. The decision-making power in a company may reside in any one of these parts. As companies mature, power tends to shift naturally from production to marketing to fiscal management.

The researcher is most likely to develop initial contacts with product-oriented personnel, who may have little decision-making power in a large company. These contacts are very valuable, because it is often very difficult to attract the attention of senior management through outside "cold" approaches. On the other hand, it is important to determine discretely how and where to proceed. Remember that the kindred spirits whom you find in the research and development department may be just as uncomfortable with senior management as you are going to be, but you have no choice. You may have to push through several layers of middle management before you find someone who can make decisions. Occasionally, the opportunity arises to make your pitch under unusually friendly circumstances—for example, the owner's son is a paraplegic. Beware. You may not enjoy the hard-nosed process of

Device Development

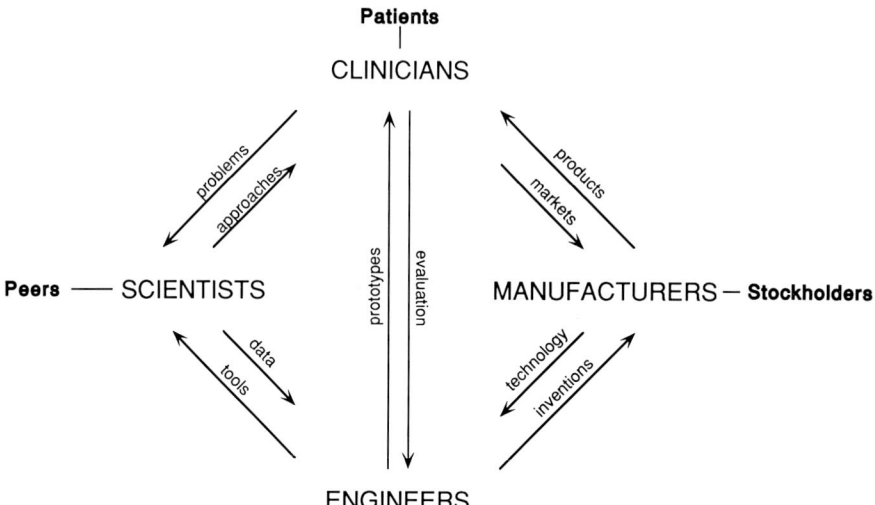

Figure 15-3 Medical device development requires the active contribution of four types of players: scientists, clinicians, manufacturers, and engineers. The first three players are free to participate in the development only to the extent that their activities are responsive to the demands of outsiders: peers, patients, and stockholders, respectively. All of the players need to be involved in reciprocal relationships to assure their continuing enthusiastic and productive participation in the project.

strategic planning, but you desperately need it and it's hard to find people who do it well.

Closing All of the Loops

Figure 15-3 presents the major players who must be involved in the development of any successful hi-tech medical device and summarizes the interactions that motivate their continuing contribution to the effort. It is important to note that, except for the engineers, each of these players (basic scientists, clinicians, and manufacturers) are beholden to outsiders who have no direct interest in an invention, at least until it becomes a product. These outside influences may be seen as disincentives to continue on the project unless the interactions indicated between the players are perceived as important and fruitful. The situation is quite different than in the usual industrial research and development project, where it is typically possible to hire and thus control all of the key technical input and to create demand in the end market directly rather than through intermediaries. This, in turn, demands project management skills that are more akin to diplomacy and psychology than to traditional laboratory or business management. The four different cochlear prosthesis projects described above reflect the four different poles in Figure 15-3. The weaknesses of these projects can each be related directly to the difficulty of nurturing those parts of the loops that involve players who are not part of the management team. Unfortunately, the administrative headaches are directly related to the number of different types of players that you try to represent on this management team.

CONCLUSION

Neural prosthetic projects such as those being pursued for FNS represent some of the most complex systems ever attempted by man, both in terms of their required range of science and technology and in terms of their interactions with social institutions. As the critical pieces of science and technology have been amassed over the past 25 years, the limiting factors have shifted from specific questions and problems to the ability to manage the emergent complexity of these systems. A researcher who wishes to work on such systems must plan on being a part of large, heterogeneous teams that must include scientists, engineers, clinicians, and manufacturers. Those who would direct such projects must ask if they have the teams and the leadership skills to see their ideas all the way to successfully marketed products.

REFERENCES

Bak, M., Girvin, J.P., Hambrecht, F.T., Kufta, C.V., Loeb, G.E., and Schmidt, E.M. (1990). Visual sensations produced by intracortical microstimulation of the human occipital cortex. *Med. Biol. Eng. Comput.*, **28**, 257–259.

Burian, K., Hochmair-Desoyer, I.J., and Eisenwort, B. (1986). The Vienna cochlear implant program. *Otolaryngol. Clin. North Am.*, **19**, 313–328.

Fretz, R.J., and Fravel, R.P. (1985). Design and function: A physical and electrical description of the 3M-House cochlear implant system. *Ear Hear. (Suppl.)*, **3**(6), 205–235.

Franz, B.K., Dowell, R.C., Clark, G.M., Seligman, P.M., and Patrick, J.F. (1987). Recent developments with the Nucleus 22-electrode cochlear implant: A new two formant speech coding strategy and its performance in background noise. *Am. J. Otolaryngol.*, **8**, 516–518.

Loeb, G.E. (1987). Whatever happened to the visual prosthesis? In: J.D. Andrade et al., eds., *Artificial Organs*, New York: VCH Publishers, Inc. pp. 457–466.

Loeb, G.E. (1990). Cochlear Prosthetics. *Annu. Rev. Neurosci.*, **13**, 357–371.

Loeb, G.E., Zamin, C.J., Schulman, J.H., and Troyk, P.R. (1990). An injectable microstimulator for functional electrical stimulation. *Proc. North Sea Conf. Biomed. Eng.* Antwerp, and *Med. Biol. Eng. Comput.*, in press.

Merzenich, M.M., and White, M.W. (1977) Cochlear implant. The interface problem. In: F.T. Hambrecht and J.B. Reswick, eds., *Functional Electrical Stimulation: Applications in Neural Prostheses*, pp. 321–340. New York: Marcel Dekker.

Schindler, R.A., and Kessler, D.K. (1987). The UCSF/Storz cochlear implant: Patient performance. *Am. J. Otolaryngol.*, **9**, 247–255.

Soma, M. (1980). Design and fabrication of an implantable multichannel neural stimulator. *Technical Report #G908-1*, Integrated Circuits Lab, Department of Electrical Engineering, Stanford, CA: Stanford University.

Waters, R.L., McNeal, D.R., Faloon, W., and Clifford, B. (1985). Functional electrical stimulation of peroneal nerve for hemiplegia. *J. Bone Joint Surg.*, **67A**, 792–793.

Wilson, B.S., Schindler, R.A., Finley, C.C., Kessler, D.K., Lawson, D.T., and Wolford, R.D. (1988). Present status and future enhancements of the UCSF cochlear prosthesis. In: P. Banfai, ed., *Cochlear Implant: Current Situation*, pp. 279–282. Erkeleng, FRG: Rudolf Bermann GmkbH.

Index

Actuator 17, 37, 52, 65–66, 137, 239–245, 267–270
Amputation 154
Artificial neural network (ANN) 319–323
Atrophy, disuse 11, 168, 176

Brace (*see* Orthosis)

Calcium 35, 44–45, 49–50
Clonus 291
Compliance (*see* Stiffness)
Contracture 214, 216–217, 233–236, 244
Control
  adaptive 286–290, 310–312, 319–321
  closed-loop (*see* Feedback)
  feedback 12, 18, 88–90, 99–100, 107–108, 117–122, 129–130, 133–136, 140–142, 235, 245–247, 258–264, 281–294, 298–323
  feed-forward 89, 112, 118, 129–130, 133–145, 168, 243–245, 256–259, 263, 273, 286, 304–305, 313, 315–317
  heirarchical 246, 271
  length 281–285
  myoelectric 10, 169, 175–176
  non-numerical 235, 245
  open-loop (*see* Feed-forward)
  shoulder 11, 175–6
  servo 140, 281–284
  switch 175–176, 214, 237, 243, 255
  voluntary 11, 148, 154–160
crutches 9, 255, 321

Dynamic scaling 138–139, 143–145
Dynamic similarity 191–193
Dynamics, intersegmental 259–261, 265–267
  inverse 257, 260, 263, 313
  muscle 259

Electricity, animal 4
Electrode, cuff 67, 68, 89, 103–104, 106–115, 238, 302
  epimysial 10, 68, 170–171, 175, 238, 302, 305
  implanted 9–10, 68, 89, 170, 173–174, 179–181, 234–235
  longevity 104–106
  micro 104–108
  percutaneous 9–10, 89, 162, 168–172, 175, 179–181, 207, 234, 238, 301

Electrode (*Continued*)
  platinum-iridium 10, 104, 170
  skin 6–11, 162, 181, 207–208, 211, 216, 220, 234–238, 301
  stainless steel 10, 103, 169
Electrometer, 3–4
Electromyogram (EMG) 10, 39, 103, 107, 110–113, 149–158, 172, 237, 286–290
Electroneurogram (ENG) 103, 108–122
Energy 23, 25, 28, 46–50, 195–197, 199–200, 208, 216, 220–227, 322
Equilibrium point hypothesis 141, 281, 284–285

Force-length relation (*see* Length-tension relation)
Force-velocity relation 20, 23, 29, 33–38, 42, 49, 64, 69–72, 75–82
Froude number 192–200

Gait (*see* Locomotion)
Golgi tendon organ 283–285
Grasp (*see* Prehension)

Heart rate 224
Heat (*see* Energy)
Hemiplegia, 8, 99, 118, 121–122, 153, 162, 165, 179, 238, 314
Hybrid 121, 137–140, 208, 233, 239–244, 255–256, 272–274
  assistive system (HAS) 233, 239–244

Inhibition 290–291
Interpulse interval (*see* Rate coding)

Joint stabilization 172–173

Length-tension relation, muscle 29, 35–37, 43, 69–72, 76–82, 172
  sensor 90–92
Locomotion 8–9, 58–59, 65, 99–100, 118, 121, 192–200, 202–230, 236–247, 270–273, 286

model 192–200
stiff-leg 205–206
Magnetism, 5
Model identification (*see also* Gait model; Muscle model, Nerve model) 58–84, 129–143, 302–314
  autoregressive moving average (ARMA) 310
  Hammerstein 41, 63, 70
  Wiener 41, 63
Motor (*see* Actuator)
Motor neuron, alpha 8–9, 282–284, 286, 292–293
  gamma 140, 282–284, 291–293
Muscle, 5–11, 17–52, 58–84, 132, 143–145, 162–183, 202–230, 233–247, 252–274, 282–294, 307–314
  activation 29, 33–37, 39–50, 67, 167–169, 268, 306–314
  fatigue 10–11, 67, 70, 88–89, 99, 112–115, 118–120, 168, 176, 211, 233–234, 244, 258, 269, 286
  model
    cross-bridge 17, 21–31, 43, 49, 51–52, 61
    distribution moment 17, 21–24, 29, 43–52
    Hill-type (*see* Viscoelastic)
    Huxley-type (*see* Cross-bridge)
    viscoelastic 17, 20–23, 31–38, 43, 49–52, 61, 64, 69, 71–77, 81, 267–271, 317
  sarcomere 23, 41–43
  spindle 133, 281–284

Nerve, adaptation 100–102
  denervation 172–174, 178–179, 240–243
  model 10–11
  recording 103–132, 285
  sensory 99–132, 285, 281–294

Orthosis 9, 162, 172, 176, 178, 182, 191, 199–200, 202–230, 236, 239–247, 255, 286, 300–302
  floor-reaction 255, 286
  hip-guidance (HGO 204, 222–226, 272
  knee-ankle-foot (KAFO) 203, 254, 272
  long-leg (LLB) 203, 221–225
  reciprocal gait (RGO) 202–204, 207–229, 239, 255–256, 273
Osteoporosis 233–236

Index

Optimization, dynamic 263–264
  static 262–263

Pacemaker 5, 332–334
Paralysis, cerebral 165, 236
Paraplegia (*see also* Spinal cord injury) 9, 99, 118–122, 151–152, 202–230, 314–316, 321
Prehension, 9, 59, 65, 89–90, 100–102, 118–119, 162–183, 306–310
  lateral 9, 163–168, 172, 175–177
  palmar 9, 163–168, 172, 175–177
  precision 100–102, 118
  synthesis 167–169, 171–174
Prosthesis, 3–12, 17, 52, 58–59, 65–67, 71, 81, 162–183, 202–230, 298–323, 329–341
  assessment 176–182, 221–224
  cochlear 329–331, 334
  cost 227–228, 332–333
  history 3–12
  visual 329
Pulse width (*see* Recruitment)

Quadriplegia (*see also* Spinal cord injury) 9, 59, 89–90, 118, 122, 152, 162–183, 306–310

Rate coding, 35, 39, 46, 48, 67–69, 168, 312
Recruitment (*see also* Muscle, activation) 35, 67, 69–80, 89, 112, 168, 171, 174, 229, 306–313
Reflex 18, 58, 151, 235, 255, 281–294, 303
  artificial 286–287
  cutaneous 294
  gain 285–289
Running (*see* Locomotion)

Sclerosis, multiple 152, 236
Sensor, 8–12, 68, 88–97, 137, 183, 285, 298–307, 313–314
  capacitative 88, 95
  conductive 88–89, 91
  force 68, 88–97, 104, 109–111, 285, 301, 314
  Hall-effect 176

natural (*see* Nerve, sensory)
  optical 88, 96
  piezoelectric 88, 96
  position 97, 104, 121, 285, 301, 314
  shoe 8, 121
  silicon 88, 91–92, 94
  strain gage 94–95
  tactile 88, 90–93, 97
Simulation 252, 264, 303
Slip detection 102, 114–117
Spasticity 11, 152, 167, 182, 214, 233, 236, 244, 290–291
Spinal cord, injury 9, 59, 89–90, 99–100, 118–122, 151–152, 162–183, 202–230, 233–247, 252–274, 285–286
  (*see also* Paraplegia, Quadriplegia)
  reorganization 154
  testing 152–154
Splint (*see* Orthosis)
Stance 9, 99–100, 118, 121, 206, 218–219, 236–237, 243–245, 266, 269–270, 286–289, 314
Stiffness 18–20, 23, 25–28, 30–38, 42–44, 46, 49, 142–145, 259, 281, 284–285, 306–309, 314
  regulation 281, 284–285, 306–308, 314
Stimulation, brain 148–160
  functional electrical (FES) 9, 88–90, 99–100, 107–122, 130, 145, 162–183, 202–230, 233–247, 252–274, 281, 286, 291, 294, 298–323
  functional neuromuscular (FNS; *see* Functional electrical)
  sensory 174–176
Stimulator (*see also* Stimulation, Functional electric)
  electric 148
  faradaic 5–7
  implantable 9–10, 12, 170–174, 178, 239, 302
  magnetic 148–149
Stroke (*see* hemiplegia)

Technology transfer 179–182, 329–341
Tendon transfer 168, 172–73, 182
Tenodesis 9, 173
Transducer (*see* Sensor)
Tremor 40

Walker 9, 212, 217–218, 237, 245, 255
Walking (*see* Locomotion)